The Lung Transplantation Handbook

SECOND EDITION

by Karen A. Couture

Former Title:
Things You Should Know
About Lung Transplantation:
Before, During and After

Order this book online at www.trafford.com
or email orders@trafford.com

Most Trafford titles are also available at major online book retailers.

Print information available on the last page.

ISBN: 978-1-5521-2504-5 (sc)

Trafford rev. 10/19/2018

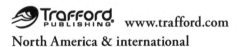 www.trafford.com

North America & international
toll-free: 1 888 232 4444 (USA & Canada)
fax: 812 355 4082

*To my family and
donor family. . . Without
your help, I would not be
alive today and the creation
of this book would not
have been possible.*

> *"Obstacles are those frightful things you see when you take your eyes off your goal."*
> *– Henry Ford*

Acknowledgments:

No book is ever written without the input of many people. Therefore, there are many I need to thank for their help with this book. As a transplant recipient who has lived through transplantation and not someone with a medical background, I am especially grateful to the many transplant professionals who gave so generously of their time, experience and perspective: Maher Baz, M.D.; Wendy Swafford, R.N., B.S.N.; Le McGinn, R.N., B.S.N., Laura Thomas, R.P.R.T.; Daniel Martin, Ph.D., P.T., F.A.C.S.M.; and Ian Jamieson, M.B.A., all of Shands Hospital at the University of Florida. Also, Pegi Shaner, R.N., B.S.N., St. Louis Children's Hospital; Jeffery D. Punch, M.D., University of Michigan Medical Center; Jason McDowell, R.N., B.S.N., University of Florida Organ Procurement Organization; Lynn Cravero, R.N., C.P.T.C., and Candace L. Wilson, R.N., B.S.N., C.P.T.C., University of Miami Organ Procurement Organization. I am lucky that there are so many in the transplant field that really care about the work they do.

As always, I am eternally grateful to members of UNOS for responding to my many requests for information: Denise Tripp and Samia Buckingham, UNOS Research Department; Joel D. Newman, M.S., Bob Spieldenner, A.P.R.; Angela William, B.S. and Kimberly M. Whitehead, M.P.H., Professional Services; William G. Lawrence, J.D., Division of Patient Affairs; and the staff of UNOS' News Bureau. Keep up the good work guys!

A special thank you goes out to the medical staff who helped review the section on medications: Geoffrey M. Cook, Novartis Pharmaceuticals Corp.; Paul Blahunka, Pharm.D., Fujisawa Healthcare Inc.; Charlotte Berlin, SangStat Medical Corp.; Franco Quagliata, M.D., Faro Pharmaceuticals Inc.; Mark Faust, R.P.H., Apothecon; Tammy Law, Pharm.D. candidate, Alza Pharmaceuticals Corp.; J. Jaffess, Pharm.D., Ortho-McNeil Pharmaceuticals; Constance A. McKenzie, Pharm.D., Glaxo Wellcome Inc.; Marissa Buttaro, R.Ph., M.P.H., and Kelli Walker, R.Ph., Wyeth-Ayerst Pharmaceuticals; Linda J. Dawson, B.S., Pharm.D., Glaxo Wellcome; Michael B. Barrett, Monarch Pharmaceuticals Inc.; Patricia Wilkinson, Pharm.D., M.S., Janssen Pharmaceutica; Helene Panzer, PhD., Pfizer Inc.; Ellen M. Martin, Xoma; Patricia C. Layton, R.N., B.S.N., and Ruchi Rastogi, Pharm.D., Ortho Biotech; Jessica Scharf, Pharm.D., and Karen Cohen, Pharm.D., Bristol-Myers Squibb Co.; Ellen Antal, Pharm.D., and Jane S. Jones, Pharmacia & Upjohn; and the staff at Roche Pharmaceuticals.

Also, I am indebted to Marilyn D. O'Brien, American Lung Transplant Association of Florida Inc.; Dick Hauboldt, Milliman and Robertson Inc.; Kathryn Bloom, Biogen Inc.; Amy Hunter, Porter Novelli; Lisa Coscia, R.N., B.S.N., C.C.T.C., National Transplant Pregnancy Registry; E. Steve Woodle, M.D., F.A.C.S., and Tom Beebe, R.N., B.S.N., the Israel Penn Transplant Tumor Registry; Cheryl Campbell, R.N., and Sharen Thompson, L.C.S.W. for generously contributing some of their time to this book.

A very special note of thanks to Paul Scott Abbott for reviewing the entire manuscript and providing his invaluable support and experience. And finally, a big thanks to all those who shared their personal experience with lung transplantation. My appreciation goes out to all of you, but especially to Andrea Aulbert, Gene Downey, Cathy Foreman, Richard Heering, Karen Hoelzel, Janet Kolish and Darelene Reitz who are now breathing free at last.

Author's Note:

When I had my lung transplant in 1996, there was no ONE source to turn to for practical information about lung transplantation. The information was out there all right, but it wasn't all in the same place and not always easy to access. Back in 1997, when I wrote the first edition of this book, called *Things You Should Know About Lung Transplantation,* my idea was to try to fill that gap and provide patients with everything they needed to know to plan for, and ultimately get, a lung transplant and live a long life afterward.

Transplantation can be a very scary thing, but once you have the power that comes with knowledge you will feel better-equipped to handle it. In this era of managed care, overworked hospital staff, shrinking health insurance coverage and physicians who are too busy, too arrogant or just too baffled, it is imperative that patients take charge of their own health care. There's too much at stake. Seek out as much information as possible, from everywhere you can; after all, it is your life.

In this edition, you will find that the basic format of the book hasn't changed much, only that things are dealt with in greater detail. I have also included a glossary and some blank worksheets for you to use in the back of the book. But, the most important difference between this edition and the last is that I have included short stories written by people who have gone through or who are going through transplantation, called "The Voice of Experience." It is my belief that some of the best information about lung transplantation can be gotten from patients because they will tell it like it is.

When reading this book, I have several words of caution for readers. Even though I am very knowledgeable about lung transplantation, I don't have a medical background. However, all attempts have been made to ensure the information in this book is medically accurate. In addition, you may find things referred to that you aren't familiar with, but every transplant experience is different and every transplant center is different. Plus, advances in transplantation, organ allocation and transplant medications continue at a rapid pace. This book is only a snapshot of this ever-changing process. Therefore, it should be regarded as just a supplement to your most important resource – YOUR transplant team.

By the time this book is published I will have celebrated the fifth anniversary of my lung transplant! I am amazed that I have survived this long and am doing this well. I attribute much of my success to being actively involved in my treatment. When I first learnt about lung transplantation, I remember reading that I had a 40% to 50% chance of surviving five years. Well, it's five years now and I don't appear to be going anywhere anytime soon. I have been very fortunate to see and do many things since my transplant. My hopes now are for many more years of the same for me AND for you!

– Karen A. Couture
bilateral-lung transplant recipient

Contents:

PART TWO: During Transplantation

1 Before Transplantation

HISTORICAL PERSPECTIVE:

"May your wait be short and your new lungs perfect!"
– Beth Kern

Transplantation, as defined by *Taber's Medical Dictionary*, is the "grafting of living tissue from its normal position to another site or the transplantation of an organ or tissue from one person to another." The physical replacement of failing organs and tissues has been a dream of physicians since the days of the ancient Greeks. Saints Cosmas and Damian, twin physicians, removed a man's infected leg and replaced it with the healthy leg of a man who had just died. During the 18th century, surgeons experimented with animal transplants, but it wasn't until the early 1900s that transplantation became a serious pursuit.

Over the years, many attempts were made at transplantation without success. At that time, little was understood about the immune system and those early transplants eventually failed due to rejection. However, in 1954, Dr. Joseph Murray, of Peter Bent Brigham Hospital in Boston, performed the first successful transplant of a kidney from a healthy man into the body of his identical twin, who was dying. The recipient lived for eight years.

In the early 1960s, scientists began employing powerful immunosuppressant drugs (azathioprine and prednisone) to prevent rejection. Now it was possible to transplant a kidney from one relative to another. Successful heart and liver transplants were next to come. However, it wasn't until the development of cyclosporine in early 1980s that transplantation became widely performed.

During the 1980s and '90s, transplantation has evolved from a rare, experimental procedure into a common occurrence. The success of organ transplantation would not have come about without improvements in surgical techniques and the development of methods to suppress the recipient's immune system. These advances have made transplantation the preferred method of treatment for end-stage organ failure of the kidneys, heart, liver, lungs and pancreas.

In the past 30 years, transplantation has experienced outstanding growth. Today, approximately 21,000 solid organ transplants are performed each year. Kidney transplantation accounts for more than half of all transplant procedures, followed by liver, heart, kidney-pancreas, lung, pancreas, multi-organ, heart-lung and intestine transplantation. The patient survival rates for all organs have increased significantly since the early days. Currently, the one-year patient survival rates are as follows: living-

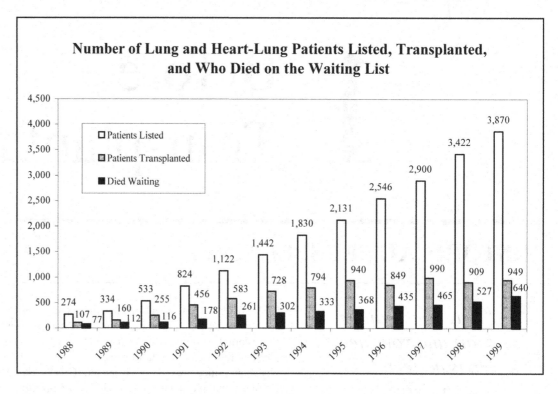

Number of Lung and Heart-Lung Patients Listed, Transplanted, and Who Died on the Waiting List

Legend: Patients Listed, Patients Transplanted, Died Waiting

1988: 274, 107, 77
1989: 334, 160, 12
1990: 533, 255, 116
1991: 824, 456, 178
1992: 1,122, 583, 261
1993: 1,442, 728, 302
1994: 1,830, 794, 333
1995: 2,131, 940, 368
1996: 2,546, 849, 435
1997: 2,900, 990, 465
1998: 3,422, 909, 527
1999: 3,870, 949, 640

Chart 1. The number of lung and heart-lung patients on the waiting list, transplanted, and who died while on the waiting list. (Data based on UNOS' OPTN/Scientific Registry as of April 15, July 15 and Dec. 31, 2000.)

related kidney, 97.7%; pancreas, 95.2%; cadaveric kidney, 94.1%; liver, 88.7%; heart, 85.5%; lung, 77.5%; and heart-lung, 63%.

The History of Lung Transplantation:

In 1963, the very first human lung transplant was performed by Dr. James Hardy, at the University of Mississippi, for an isolated cancer of the lung. The patient lived for 18 days, then died of kidney failure. Between 1963 and 1980 there were more than 40 attempts at lung transplantation around the world, but only two recipients lived longer than one month. This disappointing start contributed to a halt in lung transplantation until cyclosporine was introduced, which renewed interest in the procedure.

In 1981, Dr. Bruce Reitz, of Stanford University Hospital, performed the first successful heart-lung transplant for pulmonary vascular disease by inserting the heart and lung as one. At the time, lung transplantation occurred only in the setting of heart-lung transplantation, until 1983, when Dr. Joel Cooper performed the first successful single-lung transplant, at Toronto General Hospital. The patient lived for seven years, but later died from complications of immunosuppression.

This breakthrough was quickly followed by the very first double-lung transplant at Toronto General Hospital. This procedure involved transplanting two lungs as a group (or en bloc) into patients with bronchiectasis, cystic fibrosis and emphysema. This surgery offered the first glimmer of hope for cystic fibrosis patients who suffer from infections in both lungs. However, the en bloc double-lung transplant had a high death rate due to problems with the surgical connection. In 1989, the procedure was changed to the bilateral sequential lung transplant, whereby each lung is removed and attached separately, and that is the procedure used today.

In the past 15 years, lung transplantation has evolved from an experimental procedure to an effective therapy for end-stage lung disease. Many factors have contributed to its success, including refined surgical techniques; more effective methods to diagnose and treat rejection and infection; and enhanced postoperative rehabilitation programs.

As lung transplantation became more successful, the need for organs increased as more and more patients were listed for the procedure. However, the supply of organs has not kept up with this demand. In a desperate attempt to save more lives, living-lobar lung donors are being employed as a last resort. Dr. Vaughn A. Starnes, of Stanford University Medical Center, did the first successful, living-lobar lung donor transplant on a cystic fibrosis patient in 1990. Living-lobar lung donor transplants account for only 15 to 25 of the lung transplant surgeries performed in the U.S. each year. There has been approximately 150 living-lobar lung donor transplants performed in this country so far.

The success of lung transplantation in adults has led to the use of lung transplantation in children. However, experience in children – especially preadolescent children – remains limited. Approximately 50 to 60 pediatric (<17 years old) lung transplants are performed in the U. S. each year, and less than 50 have been performed on children less than one year old.

Today, many patients who would otherwise have died from end-stage lung disease are benefiting from transplantation. In 1999, 949 patients in the United States received lung and heart-lung transplants, which accounts for approximately 4% of all organ transplants performed. There have been more than 13,500 lung-related transplants done worldwide, over 8,000 of them in the United States alone. However, the number performed each year appears to have reached a plateau since 1995.

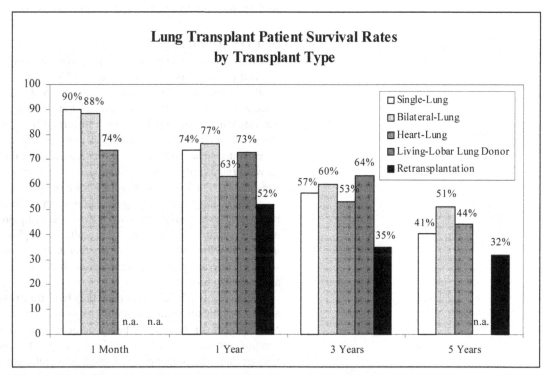

Chart 2. *Patient survival rates by transplant type for all transplants performed from 1988 to 1998. (Data based on UNOS' OPTN/Scientific Registry as of June 1 and Sept. 7, 1999; n. a. denotes not available.)*

Functional Outcomes:

Following lung transplantation, both lung function and exercise capacity are dramatically improved, and often results are seen immediately following transplantation. In addition, supplemental oxygen is usually no longer required once patients are discharged from the hospital. According to the 17th Annual Data Report of the International Society of Heart and Lung Transplantation, 56% of lung transplant recipients had no activity limitations one year after transplantation. Exercise capacity improves enough to allow the majority of patients to resume an active lifestyle.

As a general rule, patients receiving bilateral-lung transplantation approach normal pulmonary function, while patients receiving single-lung transplant gain less than normal function. For example, following single-lung transplantation for chronic obstructive pulmonary disease, the forced expiratory volume in one second (FEV_1) increased to approximately 50% to 60% of predicted. However, some patients may gain more pulmonary function. Patients who receive bilateral lobes taken from healthy living donors have been shown to approach near-normal function. In a study of 37 patients, preoperative FEV_1 increased from 19% to 73% after surgery.

Pulmonary function, including forced expiratory volume in one second (FEV_1), forced vital capacity (FVC), maximal voluntary ventilation (MVV), diffusing capacity and arterial pO_2 are all significantly improved after lung transplantation. How soon and how much improvement a patient receives depends on your original lung disease, how sick you were before the transplant, whether you received a single or bilateral-lung replacement and if you had any complications during or after surgery. Peak lung function levels reached varies from patient to patient, but in general a patient may reach peak, then level off anywhere from six months to a year following surgery, providing you had an uncomplicated course.

Survival Rates:

As transplant centers gain more experience with lung transplantation, survival rates are bound to improve. The United Network for Organ Sharing (UNOS) tabulates survival rates that include ALL transplants performed since the inception of the procedure. Therefore, a certain amount of learning curve is included in these numbers. It is important to remember that survival rates are based on PAST experience and patients being transplanted today will surpass those figures. Even though the one-year survival rate is only 77.5% nationally, most transplant centers are reporting one-year survivability well over 77% for transplants performed in 1999.

Despite these results, a significant number of grafts (organs) fail, either because of severe early graft failure, airway healing problems, infection or, most likely, chronic rejection. As a result, retransplantation becomes necessary. While ethicists debate whether patients should be eligible for a second transplant given the organ donor shortage, more and more centers are doing the procedure.

These centers believe that once they have transplanted a patient, they are responsible for them and should perform additional transplants as long as the patient can be restored to a good quality of life. Retransplantation accounts for only 2% to 3% of all lung transplants. Ambulatory, nonventilator dependent patients undergoing retransplantation who are more than two years after their first transplant had a one-year survival rate of 64%, vs. 33% for nonambulatory, ventilated patients.

THE ORGAN DONOR SHORTAGE:

"I am not sure where people get the idea that you have to be extra brave if you want to live. I always thought that the idea of dying was a little more scary."
– Larry E. Cloud

S uccessful lung transplantation depends largely on the availability of organs. However, the scarcity of organs is one of the major obstacles. Even though donation rates are slowly increasing, the number of patients being listed is growing even faster.

In 1999, new registrations outpaced lung transplants by a ratio of 4:1. According to UNOS, a new name is added to the waiting list every 14 minutes and 17 patients die each day while on the waiting list. Further complicating this shortage, only 10% to 20% of potential donors end up having suitable lungs for donation. This means that out of the 20,794 organs recovered in 1998, only 1,385 lungs were recovered for transplantation. The remaining lungs had to be discarded or were donated for research purposes.

However grim these figures may seem, during 1998, the number of organs recovered from donors increased 4%. This was the largest one-year increase since 1994 and can be attributed to an increased use of older donors and living donors.

Organ procurement programs and transplant clinicians are working hard to find ways to increase the number of available organs in order to decrease the number of lives lost while waiting for a transplant. However, traditional approaches to reduce the organ donor shortage will lessen, but not eliminate, this shortage.

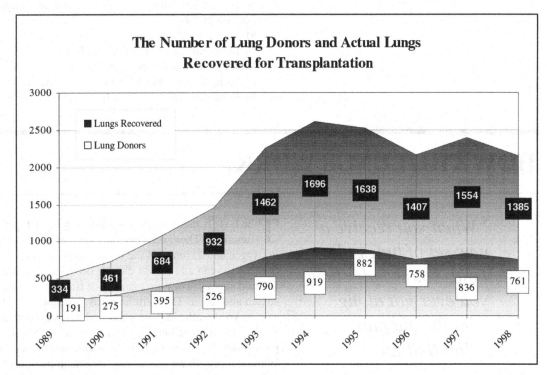

Chart 3. *The number of lung donors and the number of actual lungs recovered for transplantation from 1988 to 1998. (Data based on UNOS' OPTN/Scientific Registry as of Sept. 21, 1998 and Sept. 7, 1999.)*

Expanding the Donor Pool:

Several innovative strategies for increasing the number of donated organs have emerged over the last couple of years. Federal legislation now requires that all Medicare- and Medicaid-participating hospitals notify the local organ procurement organization of all individuals whose death is imminent or who have died. Failure to do so will result in the loss of Medicare and Medicaid reimbursement. The State of Pennsylvania, whose legislation was used as a model, experienced a 59% increase in the rate of donation. Other strategies to overcome the limited number of donor lungs include:

1) Maximizing the Use of Available Organs:
   a) Expanding the indications for single-lung transplants, while restricting the use of bilateral-lung and heart-lung transplantation only when absolutely necessary;
   b) Exploring the use of marginal donors selected from patients with less-than-perfect chest x-ray results or with evidence of chest trauma. Accepting donors older than 55 years old, or with a smoking history greater than 20 pack years (number of years multiplied by the number of packs smoked per day) or accepting those with less than optimal blood gas volumes, or longer cold ischemic times;
   c) Utilizing the technique of split-lung transplantation, where a single lung is divided into two portions, each being transplanted into the left and right side of a single recipient, for patients needing a double.
2) Exploring the use of medical or surgical alternatives for conditions currently managed with lung transplantation:
   a) Lung volume reduction surgery for emphysema;
   b) Using prostacyclin infusions for primary pulmonary hypertension.
3) A more critical review of the use of donated lungs for indications with poor prognosis:
   a) Retransplantation;
   b) Lung transplantation in the elderly.
4) Seeking alternative sources for organs:
   a) Using living-related lung donors in specific circumstances;
   b) Exploring the use of non-heart beating donors.

HOW THE LUNGS WORK:

"When you receive a new set of lungs like I did, you wonder how you ever got along with the old pair."
– Jim Bellizzi

The body is made up of billions of cells, which perform various functions. These cells can only survive in an environment that: 1) takes in oxygen and 2) removes the waste product carbon dioxide. The exchange between oxygen and carbon dioxide occurs in your lungs. Normal lungs are soft and spongy. They are made up of elastic tissue that allows them to stretch and recoil. The right lung has three lobes and the left has two.

As you breathe in, your chest and lungs expand, and air is drawn in. As you breathe out, the lungs go back to their smaller size, and the air is pushed out. The diaphragm is the main muscle used in regular breathing. When it moves down (contracts), we breath in, and when it moves up (relaxes), we breathe out. Extra muscles in the chest and neck are used when breathing becomes difficult.

Life Goes On! Living with O2.

I was just shy of 30 in 1988 when I discovered that the bad cold I thought I had acquired was actually a rare lung disease, eosinophilic granuloma. I was placed on four liters of oxygen, 24 hours a day, and a lobectomy was scheduled in hopes that it would improve my breathing. The lobectomy didn't improve my breathing, although it did provide a diagnosis and a bleak prognosis – two to eight years to live without a lung transplant.

I decided to postpone the inevitable lung transplant as long as possible. I returned to work and started pulmonary rehabilitation at the same time. I worked four hours in the morning and went to rehab from 12:30 until 4:30 everyday for a month. I was lucky. I worked for seven years on oxygen. I never considered the oxygen a burden, but a lifesaver and thought of it the same as I would of needing my glasses.

In 1992, I had our daughter, Sarah, while on oxygen and never needed to turn up the oxygen for labor thanks to pursed-lip breathing. My husband, Richard Merritt, was always supportive and by my side. I listed for a transplant in September of 1994. I quit my job in March of 1995 when my need for oxygen exceeded the six-liter limit of the portable when not at rest.

I never stopped living my life. If I had died during transplant surgery, it would not have been tragic. I was transplanted March 25, 1996 and I am happy, healthy, productive and grateful to God and my donor family for giving me these last three years of new life.

– Kathryn Flynn, bilateral-lung transplant recipient,
March 25, 1996

Evaluating whether your lungs are working properly is determined by a number of methods, but the most common one is by pulmonary function tests and arterial blood gas analysis. In addition, pulse oximetry and exercise testing can prove useful tools as well.

Understanding Your Pulmonary Function Test:

Pulmonary function testing (PFT) refers to a diagnostic test or series of tests that provide an objective method for assessing the functional status or changes in a patient with known or suspected lung disease. When properly performed and interpreted, they help diagnose the cause of a symptom (such as shortness of breath), the extent of a disease (how far advanced the condition is) and help determine the effectiveness of therapy.

Usually when a new patient is evaluated, a complete array of tests are performed. After the initial visit, smaller tests may be given to monitor a patient's status. Repeated testing helps to determine any improvement or deterioration. In addition, a patient can track the rate their pulmonary function is declining by plotting the results on a line graph. This can be a useful tool in predicting when you should get listed for a lung transplant.

PFTs can be very difficult to perform for a patient with impaired lung function; if done correctly, they require maximum, consistent efforts on the part of the patient. Standards have been established by the American Thoracic Society for what constitutes a normal or "predicted" score. These figures are based on the height, age, sex and race of healthy subjects. Your score is presented in actual values as well as a percentage of the predicted value. There are three main categories of testing and they are as follows:

SPIROMETRY is defined as the measurement of breathing and is the most basic test performed. It involves the assessment of airflow during maximal forced expiration, i.e. the patient breathes out as hard and as fast as possible. These tests reflect the condition of the airways.

Three good trials are required for an accurate test. If the spirometry is abnormal, a bronchodilator is given and the test repeated. Any improvement after the inhalation of the medication suggests the patient may benefit from the use of drugs. From these tests, several measurements can be determined. These include:

Forced Vital Capacity (FVC) represents the amount of air that can be forcefully blown out of the lungs after a maximal inhalation. During the FVC maneuver, the small airways can close prematurely, thereby trapping air in the lungs. If the disease is restrictive, e.g. pulmonary fibrosis or sarcoidosis, the FVC will be reduced. If the disease is obstructive, e.g. emphysema, asthma or cystic fibrosis, the FVC could be within normal limits, but most likely will be reduced. This maneuver is also called a "Flow-Volume Loop," which is graphically displayed comparing volume and flow rate.

Forced Expiratory Volume in the 1st Second (FEV_1) is the amount of air that can be forcefully blown out during the first second of expiration

Patterns of Pulmonary Function Impairment

	Obstructive Lung Diseases, such as Asthma and Chronic Bronchitis	Obstructive Lung Diseases, such as Emphysema and A1AD	Restrictive Lung Diseases, such as Pulmonary Fibrosis	Mixed lung Disease, such as Cystic Fibrosis, BOOP or Bronchiectasis
FVC	Normal or ↓	Normal or ↓	↓	↓
FEV_1	Normal or ↓	Normal or ↓	↓	↓
FEV_1/FVC	↓	↓	Normal or ↑	Normal or ↑
FEF_{25-75}	↓	↓	↓	↓
FRC	↑	↑	↓	↑
RV	↑	↑	↓	↑
TLC	Normal or ↑	Normal or ↑	↓	↑
DLCO	Normal	↓	↓	↓
bronchodilator response	Yes	Seldom	No	Seldom

Table 1. When analyzing PFTs, abnormalities are usually categorized into one of two patterns (or a combination of the two); an obstructive pattern, characterized mainly by obstruction to airflow, vs. a restrictive pattern, with evidence of decreased lung volumes but no airflow obstruction.

after a maximum inspiration. This will usually be reduced in restrictive disease and is almost always severely reduced in obstructive disease.

FEV$_1$/FVC represents the ratio of the amount of air forced out in the first second to the total amount forced out. This is a good measure of the level of obstruction to airflow. In the normal lung, 80% of the total volume is blown out in the 1st second. If the disease is restrictive, e.g. sarcoidosis or interstitial fibrosis, the FEV$_1$/FVC is normal, or even greater than normal, whereas the FEV$_1$/FVC is decreased in obstructive disease.

Forced Expiratory Flow Rate between 25% and 75% of Vital Capacity (FEF $_{25-75}$) is the rate of airflow during the middle half of expiration (between 25% and 75% of the volume expired during the forced vital capacity). This is a measurement of airflow in the small to medium-sized airways. The FEF $_{25-75}$ is a more sensitive indicator of early airway obstruction than the FEV$_1$. The FEF $_{25-75}$ is reduced in both restrictive and obstructive disease. This test is also known as the maximal mid-expiratory flow rate (MMFR or MMEFR). This measurement is decreased in restrictive and obstructive lung disease.

LUNG VOLUMES represent the measurement of how much air is in the lungs during normal breathing. This measurement is a good indicator of the elasticity of the lungs. During this test, the patient breathes a mixture of gases for at least two minutes or sits in a glass chamber and performs a series of panting maneuvers. The following measurements are made:

Function Residual Capacity (FRC): is the volume of gas in the lungs when at resting state or at the end of a normal breath. Changes in the elastic properties of the chest result in changes to the FRC. Loss of elastic recoil in emphysema increases FRC, whereas the increased stiffness of sarcoidosis or interstitial fibrosis results in decreased FRC. The FRC is made up of two components; the Residual Volume; and the Expiratory Reserve Volume. (FRC = RV + ERV)

Residual Volume (RV) is the volume of air remaining in the lungs after maximal expiration. This is also called "dead space" or the nonworking volume of air in the lungs. In normal lungs, this would be the air that remains in the airways after a maximal expiration. In restrictive disease the residual volume is reduced, while in obstructive disease the residual volume is increased. (RV = FRC – ERV)

Expiratory Reserve Volume (ERV) is the amount of air that can be blown out after a normal exhalation. (ERV = FRC – RV)

Total Lung Capacity (TLC) is the volume of air within the lungs after a patient inhales as much as possible. This includes the working (vital capacity) and nonworking (dead space or RV) part of the lungs. The TLC is composed of two volumes; the vital capacity and residual volume (TLC = VC + RV).

Vital Capacity (VC) is the volume of air that can be expired slowly and completely after a maximal inhalation. (VC = TLC – RV)

Difficult Decisions

The decision whether or not to get listed for a transplant has been a decision in the making for quite awhile, but only recently has taken on a life of its own. I was diagnosed in January 1994 with early-stage pulmonary fibrosis. With treatment, my condition was stabilized and I actually felt that everything was under control. Then I got viral pneumonia and spent 26 days in the hospital, and things have never been the same since.

When first confronted with the possibility of a transplant, my immediate response was NO WAY. I don't like pain, and I don't like sickness or hospitalization. I was also aware that lungs didn't have as much long-term success as the other organs do.

In a discussion with my psychiatrist, he simply said to me, "The decision has already been made." I went home mulling that over and discovered that he was right. The decision was already made. I would go forward with the transplant if I could get listed.

I have been married to the same wonderful man for 34 years and my illness has been as hard on him as it has been on me. Given my prognosis, we have been emotionally separating ourselves from one another. But once the decision to go ahead was made, I could feel a veil lift. We are now closer than ever and we are actually laughing again – something that we haven't done in quite awhile.

I don't have many places to choose from if I plan to live at home. I considered San Diego, which is about 1,000 miles away, but felt that I didn't want to be separated from my husband. All my support is here and there is a lot to be said about living at home – familiar surroundings, familiar bed, support people and family.

Of course, I am nervous and maybe even scared. I still have to choose a center and go through the evaluation. But the most important part has been done. The decision to go ahead and seek transplant. With God's help, the rest will fall into place.

– Cathy Foreman, single-lung transplant recipient,
May 6, 2000

DIFFUSION CAPACITY is the final component of a complete PFT. This test measures how fast carbon monoxide moves from the smallest areas of the lungs, called alveoli, to the smallest division of the vascular system, called capillaries. In this test the patient exhales fully, then breaths in a mixture of gas, which includes a very small amount of carbon monoxide. When the patient exhales after about 10 seconds of breath-holding, the expired breath is collected in an airtight bag and analyzed. From this measurement, gas exchange efficiency is made.

The results of the diffusion capacity test correlates with the body's ability to extract oxygen from the lungs. A decreased capacity in obstructive disease is consistent with the clinical diagnosis of emphysema as opposed to other obstructive diseases, e.g. asthma or chronic bronchitis. A decreased diffusing capacity in the presence of otherwise normal pulmonary function test results may be a sign of early pulmonary fibrosis, pulmonary vascular disease or a physiologic vascular shunt. The main measurement for diffusion capacity is the DLCO or Diffusing Lung Capacity of Carbon Monoxide.

Understanding Your Arterial Blood Gas Analysis:

Despite the extensive information that pulmonary function tests provide, they don't show the net effect of lung disease on gas exchange. This information can be easily assessed by tests performed on arterial blood. To obtain a blood sample for arterial blood gas analysis (ABG), a needle is usually placed in the radial artery in the wrist. This procedure can be somewhat painful, but if it is performed by someone who does them regularly, than it can be done swiftly. Three main measurements are obtained: arterial pH, pa_{O2} and pa_{CO2}.

ARTERIAL pH measures the blood's acid-base equilibrium. This balance is controlled by several factors, primarily metabolism and oxygenation of the blood. Normal values run between 7.35 to 7.45. Values less than 7.35 are considered to be acidic, while those greater than 7.45 are more alkaline. A blood pH <7.35 or >7.45 is abnormal and is a sign of an acute, rather than chronic state, regardless of the oxygen and carbon dioxide levels.

ARTERIAL pa_{O2} measures the actual pressure of oxygen in the blood. A normal value is between 80 and 100 mm Hg (depending on age), but oxygen saturation is not seriously affected until it falls below 60 mm Hg. A low pa_{O2} can damage other organ systems and oxygen therapy is usually given.

ARTERIAL pa_{CO2} measures the body's ability to remove CO (carbon dioxide). A normal pa_{CO2} is between 35 and 45 mm Hg. An elevated pa_{CO2} is a sign of respiratory failure and may be associated with problems in blood oxygenation.

Understanding Your Pulse Oximetry:

A pulse oximeter is a photoelectric apparatus for determining the percent of red-blood cells in the body that are saturated with oxygen. A small probe, in the form of a clip, that has both a transmitting and receiving side, is placed on the finger. The receiving side measures the light that passes through the nail bed. This test is not as accurate as the values obtained from an ABG, but can give a general measurement. A normal Sa_{O2} is 95% to 100%. Oxygen therapy is generally required when the Sa_{O2} is less than 86%.

Exercise Testing:

The study of patients during exercise provides valuable information about their exercise limitations. Adding measurements of arterial blood gases during exercise provides an additional dimension and shows whether gas exchange problems contribute to the impairment.

During this test, the patient exercises on a treadmill or stationary bicycle while breathing through a mouthpiece or mask. Many measurements are made, but essentially how much oxygen the lungs and heart can supply to the leg muscles at anaerobic threshold (or the point when you body can no longer supply O_2 to the muscles) and peak exercise are the most significant. This is valuable in differentiating disability based on respiratory vs. cardiac vs. sedentary causes. This testing is a useful measurement when the patient is beginning a rehabilitation program.

DO YOU NEED A LUNG TRANSPLANT?

"No one, not even your doctors can tell you what the course of your un-transplanted disease will be; they carry stethoscopes not crystal balls."
– Stan Robbins

The decision to receive a transplanted organ is a major one and should not be made without a great deal of thought for several reasons. First, transplantation is a major surgical procedure which involves some degree of risk. Second, transplantation requires a sincere and definite commitment by you to the maintenance of a rigid post-transplant regimen, which needs to be followed for the rest of your life. Many patients find that following the strict diet, medication, exercise and clinic visit schedule requires big changes in lifestyle. And, third, the medications you take after transplant can have serious side effects, which may cause other medical problems.

The doctor, patient and family should ask themselves the following basic questions to determine whether a transplant is necessary:

1) Have all other therapies (e.g., physical rehabilitation, medications or lung volume reduction surgery) been tried or excluded?
2) Is the patient likely to die without the transplant? Generally, does the patient have a life expectancy that is less than one without a transplant?
3) Is the person in good health other than the lung or heart-lung disease?
4) Can the patient adhere to the lifestyle changes – including complex drug treatments and frequent examinations – required after transplant?

What Are the Surgical Options?

There are many types of lung disease which cause end-stage pulmonary disease. The type of transplant chosen depends on the patient's lung disease, heart function, age and current condition. At present, there are four surgical options for lung transplantation:

1) Replacement of one lung (single-lung transplantation)
2) Replacement of both lungs (bilateral-lung transplantation)
3) Replacement of both the heart and lungs (heart-lung transplantation)
4) Living-lobar lung donor transplantation (where the patient receives a portion/or lobe of a lung from two living persons).

Patients presenting with failure of more than one organ have, on occasion, been considered for multi-organ transplantation. Some liver and lung, and kidney and lung transplants have been performed. Experience in this area is limited and only well-established centers with transplant programs in each of the organs involved should consider such a procedure.

Patients considered for retransplantation are patients with acute graft failure, airway complications or chronic rejection (Obliterative Bronchiolitis Syndrome). Five types of retransplantation are available:

1) Redo single-lung transplantation on the same side
2) Redo single-lung transplantation on the opposite side
3) Single-lung redo after bilateral or heart-lung transplantation
4) Redo bilateral-lung transplantation
5) Bilateral-lung retransplantation after a first single-lung transplantation.

Common Indications for Single-Lung Transplantation:

Single-lung transplantation is a simpler and shorter operation with a lower postoperative complication rate than bilateral-lung transplantation. Thus, it may be the procedure of choice for those patients who are older or are considered high-risk. Also, in view of the organ donor shortage, single-lung transplantation allows the transplantation of two patients instead of only one. However, in single-lung transplantation, concerns about hyperinflation of the native lung with resulting compression of the donor lung are valid. In cases where the donor lung is too small, or if bullous disease is present, a bilateral-lung transplant may be indicated.

EMPHYSEMA/COPD begins with the destruction of air sacs (alveoli) in the lungs, which is where oxygen from the air is exchanged for carbon dioxide in the blood. Damage to the air sacs is irreversible and results in permanent holes in the tissue of the lower lungs. The air sacs are destroyed, this results in hyperinflation, and the lungs are unable to transfer oxygen to the bloodstream, causing shortness of breath. The overly inflated lungs cause obstruction of airflow leaving the lungs. Another term for emphysema is COPD or chronic obstructive pulmonary disease.

Single-lung transplantation is the procedure of choice for emphysema patients; most recipients do not have pleural adhesions, so taking out the native lung is easy. Pulmonary function for emphysema patients is restored to acceptable levels, with most patients achieving a forced expiratory volume in one second (FEV_1) in the 50%-of-predicted range. Although there is evidence that long-term survival is slightly better in bilateral

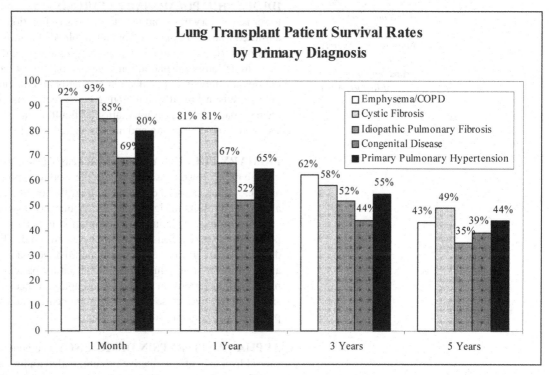

Chart 4. *Lung transplant patient survival rates by primary diagnosis. (Data based on UNOS' OPTN/Scientific Registry data as of Sept. 7, 1999.)*

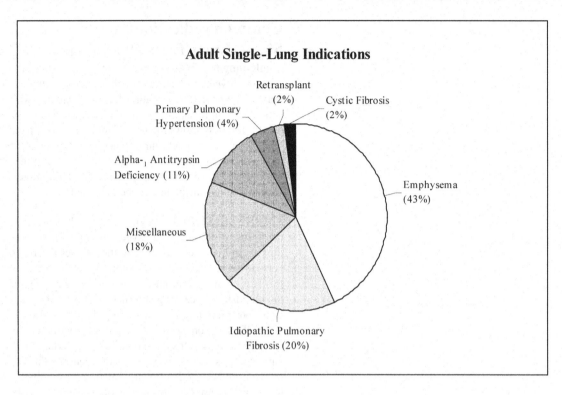

Adult Single-Lung Indications

Retransplant (2%)

Cystic Fibrosis (2%)

Primary Pulmonary Hypertension (4%)

Alpha-$_1$ Antitrypsin Deficiency (11%)

Miscellaneous (18%)

Emphysema (43%)

Idiopathic Pulmonary Fibrosis (20%)

Chart 5. Adult single-lung indications for transplants performed from 1982 to 1999. (Data based on the Registry of the International Society for Heart & Lung Transplantation 17th Annual Report, April 2000.)

recipients than in single-lung recipients, the shortage of organs continues to dictate the use of single-lung transplantation whenever possible.

IDIOPATHIC PULMONARY FIBROSIS is a group of diseases of the lower respiratory tract that lead to the loss of functional alveolar units, and a limited transfer of oxygen from air to blood. There is widespread inflammation and accumulation of scar tissue within the lung tissue.

Single-lung transplantation is a good option for patients with pulmonary fibrosis since infection is usually absent. However, this procedure is technically challenging given recipients often have shrunken pleural spaces, making implantation difficult. As a result, these transplants are more time-consuming and are associated with longer ischemic times.

PRIMARY PULMONARY HYPERTENSION is a rare obliterative disease of unknown cause, involving the medium and small pulmonary arteries, which causes a decrease in the diffusion of oxygen across the alveoli, and results in right-sided ventricular heart failure.

Performing single-lung transplantation in patients with primary pulmonary hypertension is somewhat controversial. These patients are difficult to care for in the early postoperative period and difficulties can arise. However, single-lung transplantation for patients with primary pulmonary hypertension can be a good option, especially if the patient is of small stature, lives close to the transplant center and cannot afford the potentially longer wait for a pair of lungs.

ALPHA-$_1$ ANTITRYPSIN DEFICIENCY is a genetic disease that is caused by a lack of a protective protein, called alpha-$_1$ antitrypsin (A1AT). A1AT protects the lungs from a natural enzyme (neutrophil elastase) that helps fight bacteria. This enzyme, which is normally helpful, will attack the

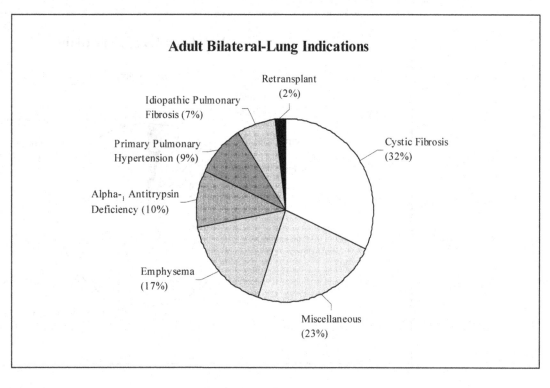

Adult Bilateral-Lung Indications

Retransplant (2%)

Idiopathic Pulmonary Fibrosis (7%)

Primary Pulmonary Hypertension (9%)

Alpha-$_1$ Antitrypsin Deficiency (10%)

Emphysema (17%)

Miscellaneous (23%)

Cystic Fibrosis (32%)

Chart 6. Adult bilateral-lung indications for transplants performed from 1982 to 1999. (Data based on the Registry of the International Society for Heart & Lung Transplantation 17th Annual Report, April 2000.)

walls of alveoli causing destruction. The lungs lose their elasticity, causing patients great difficulty in exhaling.

BRONCHIOLITIS OBLITERANS is the inflammation of the bronchioles usually due to a viral infection. The peripheral airways are primarily affected, and the arterial pO_2 will be low due to a mismatching of air movement (ventilation) and blood flow (perfusion).

LYMPHANGIOLEIOMYOMATOSIS (LAM) is a rare disease characterized by an unusual type of muscle cell that invades the lung, the airways, blood and lymph vessels. Over time, these muscle cells grow into the walls of the airways, causing them to become obstructed. Later, the muscle cells block the flow of air, blood and lymph to and from the lungs, preventing the lungs from providing oxygen to the rest of the body.

SARCOIDOSIS is a disease of unknown origin, although it is generally thought to be an autoimmune disease. Very small growths, called granulomas, are associated with it; they can occur in the lungs, lymph nodes, eyes, skin and spleen. These growths may clear up on their own or cause permanent damage. The resulting pulmonary dysfunction may be obstruction, restriction, impairment of diffusion (exchange of oxygen and carbon dioxide in the blood) or any combination of the three.

Common Indications for Bilateral-Lung Transplantation:

Bilateral-lung transplantation is mandatory for those patients with chronic pulmonary infection, and for those patients where there is significant risk that the native lung would adversely affect the newly transplanted lung.

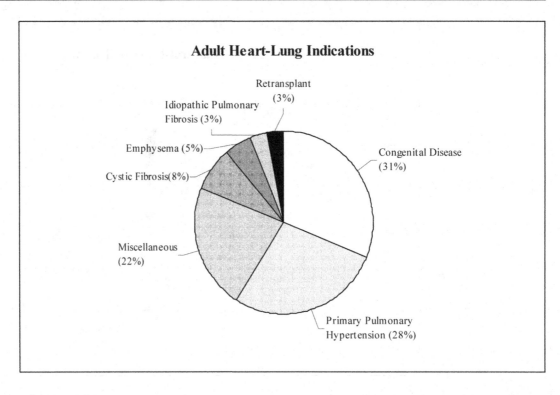

Adult Heart-Lung Indications

Retransplant (3%)

Idiopathic Pulmonary Fibrosis (3%)

Emphysema (5%)

Cystic Fibrosis (8%)

Miscellaneous (22%)

Congenital Disease (31%)

Primary Pulmonary Hypertension (28%)

Chart 7. Adult heart-lung indications for transplants performed from 1982 to 1999. (Data based on the Registry of the International Society for Heart & Lung Transplantation 17th Annual Report, April 2000.)

Depending on organ availability, some centers will perform a bilateral-lung transplant in younger patients. Despite a more lengthy operation, pulmonary function is better restored following bilateral transplantation, and, in the event of chronic rejection, a bilateral has a better reserve.

CYSTIC FIBROSIS (CF) is the most common inherited disease in the Caucasian population. CF causes the body to produce an abnormally thick, sticky mucus. This abnormal mucus clogs the lungs and can lead to fatal infections. The thick mucus also obstructs the pancreas, preventing enzymes from reaching the intestines to digest food.

Bilateral-lung transplantation is the only transplant procedure of choice for patients with cystic fibrosis. However, the surgery can be technically challenging because of the underlying infection and pleural adhesions.

BRONCHIECTASIS is a chronic disease that damages the muscle and elastic tissue within the airways of the lungs. Permanent dilation of the airways results from the damaged bronchial wall. Dilation can be a uniform enlargement or it may be irregular, which results in the formation of pouches. These pouches are susceptible to infection since bacteria can thrive in warm, dark and moist areas.

Common Indications for Heart-Lung Transplantation:

Heart-lung transplantation is for those patients with severe lung disease and, in addition, with heart disease, due to any of the conditions listed previously. Since heart-lung donors are in such short supply, repairing simple cardiac defects simultaneously with lung transplantation has reduced the number of heart-lung transplants being performed.

EISENMENGER'S SYNDROME is a congenital heart defect consisting of ventricular septal defect or arterial septal defect, pulmonary hypertension with pulmonary artery enlargement, and increased size of the right ventricle. It is also called acquired pulmonary hypertension.

Common Indications for Living-Lobar Lung Donor Transplantation:

Living-lobar lung donor transplantation is most often performed in children, adolescents and small adults with cystic fibrosis. This technique has also been performed in other diagnoses, including primary pulmonary hypertension, idiopathic pulmonary fibrosis and obliterative bronchiolitis. The advantage living-lobar lung donor transplantation has over cadaveric transplantation is the opportunity for the surgery to take place within a controlled time frame. Patients who will not survive the wait for a cadaver organ, and are at high risk of being deemed inoperable with time, benefit the most from living-lobar lung donor transplantation.

However, living-lobar lung donor transplantation is only used as a last resort since it requires two appropriate living donors. Therefore, putting three people, instead of one, in the position of having to undergo major surgery. In addition, this approach is not applicable to infants and young children since an adult lower lobe is too large for the chest of a young child.

Common Indications for Pediatric Lung Transplantation:

There are more diseases that lead to end-stage pulmonary and/or vascular disease in children than in adults. In the infant age group (<1 year), congenital abnormalities and primary pulmonary hypertension are two most common diagnoses. In the one- to 10-year-old age group, cystic fibrosis is the most common, followed by primary pulmonary hypertension, retransplantation, idiopathic pulmonary fibrosis and congenital anomalies. In the 11- to 17-year-old age group, cystic fibrosis is the most common indication.

Common Indications for Lung Retransplantation:

Patients considered for retransplantation have marked deterioration in respiratory capacity and functional decline. The most common indication for retransplantation is chronic rejection, otherwise known as Obliterative Bronchiolitis Syndrome (OB). Less common indications are acute graft failure, airway complications, severe acute rejection, among others.

LOOKING FOR A TRANSPLANT CENTER:

"Somewhere in my life I found out that my judgment is no better than my information. I cannot make good, sound judgments without some type of information to base them on."
– Larry E. Cloud

When looking for a transplant center, you should realize that many excellent centers exist. (A complete list of all active lung transplant programs can be found on page 240.) Gather all the information that you can. Ask for the names of some patients who have been transplanted there and ask for their opinion.

Also, it is important not to focus TOO much on statistics. You should realize that a center that does only five transplants a year, while it may be an excellent place, can be devastated by bad luck statistically. Each patient lost can cut their survival rate down drastically. Also, a lower survival statistic might indicate that a particular center does more high-risk transplants. In addition, survival rates include all types of transplant patients, including the young and the old, the sickest and the healthiest, with all types of diseases, and those with and without complications. Therefore, these numbers need to be taken with a grain of salt.

UNOS has launched the Transplant Patient DataSource, which is a website containing a wealth of information for patients. Visitors can find center-specific data, searchable by region or state, for each organ, as well as detailed information on transplant programs and OPOs (Organ Procurement Organizations). Transplant Patient DataSource is designed to provide the latest statistics on survival rates, information about the size of waiting lists and waiting time, and the current supply of donated organs nationally, by state, and by transplant center. It is part of UNOS' Transplant Living and can be found at http://www.patients.unos.org/tpd. Patients without Internet access can call in requests for information to a UNOS network administrator at 888-TX-INFO-1 (888-894-6361).

In addition to survival figures, a patient should consider the availability of family, friends or others to help before, during and after the transplant. When it comes to employment, caregivers and patients are protected by the Family Medical Leave Act (FMLA). Generally speaking, if you or your family are eligible, your company is required to provide 12 weeks per year during which a job is protected and available upon return from a sick leave. To find out more about the FMLA, call 800-959-FMLA (800-959-3652).

Another important factor when looking for a lung transplant center is the cost of living, in addition to convenience in terms of routine checkups, and possible emergency care. Don't forget to consider the time and costs associated with travel and lodging if you choose a center far from home.

If waiting time is critical, you may want to look at newly opened centers because their lists will be quite short compared to centers that have been open for awhile. Also look at the performance of the organ procurement organization serving that particular transplant center to determine how successful they are in providing needed organs. Generally speaking, the more OPOs per state, the better.

UNOS has published the "1997 Report of the OPTN: Waiting List, Activity and Donor Procurement," however, its information is somewhat dated. The report is an historic accounting of waiting times across the country for patients registered for transplant between 1994 and 1996. This report presents comprehensive data for examining geographic waiting times according to some of the primary factors that influence waiting times, e.g., blood type, location, age group and race. *(To see the median waiting times from this report, turn to page 261.)*

Sample Questions a Patient Might Ask:

1) How many lung transplant have you performed? How many single-, bilateral- and heart-lung transplants have you performed? (Studies have found that volume is a significant indicator of quality.)
2) What type of transplant is recommended for my diagnosis?
3) How many transplants have you done on my particular disease?
4) Approximately how many lung transplants do you perform each year?
5) What is your patient survival rate?
6) How many surgeons do you have to perform this kind of operation?
7) How long of a wait do you think I will have?
8) How many patients are waiting on the local waiting list?
9) How many other patients share my blood type on the local list?

THE VOICE OF EXPERIENCE

When the Stakes are High

After living with idiopathic pulmonary fibrosis for about 13 years, my pulmonologist told me it was time to get listed at a transplant center. I was told four years earlier my only chance for survival was ultimately a transplant, but I hoped to put it off as long as possible. He recommended Loyola University in Maywood, IL., a Chicago suburb. However, my position was I wanted this procedure performed by the best in the world since my life was at stake. I asked my pulmonologist, whom I trusted completely, what he thought of Barnes Hospital in St. Louis, and he said that would also be a good choice.

I then proceeded to obtain approval from my insurance company, expecting all kinds of problems. After a couple of weeks, I called them and was told they hadn't received my doctor's request or any of my medical records. I then called the supervisor in charge of referrals at my pulmonologist's office, to whom I said, in a nice voice, that I didn't want to die waiting for a transplant just because someone sat on the paper work. She replied that she would fax it that afternoon. The next day I got a call from my insurance company, and was told I had been approved. WOW, that was fast!

I proceeded to call Barnes and was fortunate to get an appointment within a couple of weeks. I would go through three days of testing and shortly thereafter I was listed. At the same time, a friend of the family made inquires on my behalf to transplant physicians in Switzerland, and they suggested I reconsider Loyola. Their abilities and statistics were just as good as Barnes, but Loyola would be close to home. But, more importantly, my wife and I would be able to continue working until I was transplanted. If we left our jobs for an extended period of time, we could have lost our medical coverage, as well as our income.

I contacted Loyola and, with a few additional tests, was accepted. I was able to transfer my accrued waiting time and received my transplant in 11 months. I have been blessed with such good fortune throughout my experience I wish it could be that way for everyone. Transplant is not easy, but the pleasure I receive in simple things makes it one of my life's greatest experiences.

– Damian Neuberger, bilateral-lung transplant recipient,
Oct. 19, 1997

10) How many of your patients have died while waiting?
11) Do I need to move closer to the transplant hospital after I am put on the waiting list? If so, do you provide housing before the transplant and how much will is cost?
12) If I do not have to live closer to the transplant center, how will I get there when I get the call?
13) How much does my transplant cost? How much will I have to pay?
14) How long is the average hospital stay?
15) Do you provide housing after the transplant operation? If so, how much will it cost?
16) Do you have a support group? If not, is there one in this area?

(Turn to page 265, and copy the worksheet provided to help you evaluate the differences among various transplant centers.)

THE EVALUATION:

"Your medical record is really what counts, as well as your attitude and outlook on life. They are looking for people who WANT to live."
– Nancy Yoakum

Before you can be accepted for a lung or heart-lung transplant, a careful evaluation is necessary. This process usually starts with a referral to the transplant program from your physician or pulmonologist. The transplant center will ask your doctor to send a copy of your medical records, along with your most recent chest x-ray and pulmonary function test. For heart-lung patients, they may also want a copy of your most recent echocardiogram (ECHO), electrocardiogram (EKG) and heart catherterization. Once they receive that information, and they think you might benefit from a transplant, you will be scheduled for an initial visit.

Initial Visit:

During your initial visit, you and your family members will meet with the transplant physician to learn more about the procedure, including the pros and cons of transplantation. This visit is designed not only for the transplant team to gather information about you, but for you to learn more about their program and what it means to live with a transplanted organ.

In addition to reviewing your medical history and performing a comprehensive physical exam, you may have a chest x-ray, pulmonary function test and an arterial blood gas. If, after discussing this with your family, you decide to pursue transplantation, you will go onto the next step in the process, which is a formal evaluation.

Formal Evaluation:

The formal evaluation can be done either as an inpatient or as an outpatient. As an inpatient, the evaluation usually consists of three to five days of tests; as an outpatient, it takes approximately three weeks. The purpose of this evaluation is to collect data to help determine if you are a good candidate, establish a baseline and identify those patients for whom transplantation would pose too great a risk.

In addition to the following tests, you can expect to meet some of the other members of the transplant team who will educate you and your family about what is involved in the process. The person who will work most closely with you before, during and after your hospitalization is the transplant coordinator. The coordinator will see you through the evaluation process and, most likely, will be the person who contacts you when a donor organ becomes available.

During the time of your formal evaluation, you will undergo many tests. Additional tests may be required depending on your transplant center. The most common ones are:

CHEST CT SCAN is a computerized x-ray scan of the chest, which gives a more detailed picture of the lung and lining of the chest wall (pleura). This test is used to rule out any cancers, to see the extent of lung disease and determine which lung is in worse condition. For those considering single-lung transplantation, this study may help decide which side would be better served by the surgery.

ELECTROCARDIOGRAM (EKG) records your heart rhythm and shows how fast your heart is beating, as well as any abnormal beats. It can also show if there are any signs of old heart attacks. Electrodes are placed on the chest, arms and legs and a recording is made.

CARDIOVASCULAR STUDIES are taken to assess the size and function of your heart, and to rule out coronary artery disease. These studies may include the following:

Echocardiography (ECHO) uses sound waves to look at the heart's muscle, valves and the presence of any abnormal heart function. As the patient lies on a table, a technician moves a hand-held device (transducer) over the chest, which takes pictures and records the function of the heart.

Left-Heart Catheterization. If you are being evaluated for single- or bilateral-lung transplantation and are more than 40 years of age, or have any history of heart problems, you may need this study to ensure heart function and blood supply to the heart muscle are adequate. This procedure is performed in a "Cath Lab," and involves inserting a catheter into an artery at the groin and advancing it into the heart.

Pressure in the heart chambers is measured, and dye is injected through this catheter to take pictures of your heart and coronary arteries. The prep time and procedure takes about an hour and a half and is done while you are awake, but you will get medications to help you relax. Afterward, you will need to lie flat for at least six hours to prevent bleeding at the point where the catheter was inserted.

Right-Heart Catheterization measures the specific pressure in your lungs and the right side of your heart. By inserting a catheter into a large vein, usually in the groin, and advancing it into the heart, pressures in the chambers of your heart are measured and recorded. This procedure is usually done along with a left-heart catherterization, and is performed in a "Cath Lab." This procedure can take 15 minutes to a half-hour. You will be administered medications to help you relax. You will need to lie flat for two to four hours afterward to prevent bleeding at the point where the catheter was inserted.

VQ LUNG SCAN shows how much air movement (ventilation) and blood flow (perfusion) goes to each lung. This is used to rule out pulmonary embolism, and to see which lung gets the best blood flow and ventilation. This information helps in deciding which lung to transplant in the case of single-lung transplantation, and which lung to do first, in the case of bilateral-lung transplantation. A radioactive medication is injected through a small intravenous catheter, then pictures are taken by a scanner.

LABORATORY WORK includes a number of blood samples taken to determine your blood type (or ABO grouping), tissue type, kidney and liver function, what viruses you have been exposed to and to look for the presence of infection.

PANEL REACTIVE ANTIBODY (PRA) is also performed to see how many antibodies are in your blood (or sensitivity). These antibodies can be made in response to blood transfusions, pregnancy or previous transplants. A high percentage rate indicates a high level of antibodies and a greater chance of rejection.

SPUTUM CULTURE for cystic fibrosis and bronchiectasis patients, to look for the presence of infection, and determine which antibiotics would be most effective at the time of transplant.

SINUS X-RAYS to rule out sinus disease.

SINUS CT SCAN for all cystic fibrosis patients with sinus disease.

ABDOMINAL ULTRASOUND to rule out the presence of gallstones, kidney stones or masses in the liver or kidney.

SIX-MINUTE WALK TEST consists of walking for six minutes (with oxygen, if needed) at your own pace, with no incline. This test is done to see what happens to your oxygen saturation with exercise, and to measure your endurance by the distance you can cover in six minutes.

SKIN TESTING to check for exposure to tuberculosis, valley fever, etc.

24 HOUR URINE COLLECTION to test kidney function.

STOOL TEST to check for hidden blood in the stool. Additional studies of the gastrointestinal tract may be required if blood is detected.

GYNECOLOGY CONSULT AND PAP SMEAR for female patients, to rule out malignancies. Also, a mammogram is sometimes required for women more than 35 years old.

DIGITAL RECTAL PROSTATE EXAM AND PSA (Prostate-Specific Antigen) for male patients with a family history of prostate cancer, to rule out malignancies.

ROUTINE DENTAL AND EYE EXAMINATIONS, respectively, are necessary to identify any potential sources of infection in the mouth, and provide a baseline vision test and to evaluate for glaucoma.

Covering Your Bases

At the age of 10, I was diagnosed with cystic fibrosis. I led a relatively normal life until my late 20s and early 30s, when I began a steady decline in my pulmonary function. It was during this time that my pulmonologist introduced the idea of transplantation. She explained the importance of being proactive in this situation. Once placed on the list, I would begin accruing time, which was crucial in the process. She also explained if my health stabilized and it was determined that the transplant could wait, I would be placed on in-active status without losing any accrued time. This made it an easy decision for me to pursue transplantation. I felt it was a win-win situation, and I would have my bases covered either way.

I was evaluated three months before my 31st birthday and it was determined that my lung functions were too high to be placed on the list. Around the time of my evaluation, it was discovered that I had become resistant to all antibiotics. In order to combat this problem, I was immediately taken off all these drugs. This brought about a substantial drop in my FEV$_1$ and FVC. Shortly after that, I received a call from my pulmonologist. My transplant center had reviewed my latest test results, and I was now eligible to be put on the waiting list. However, in order for the transplant to take place, I would have to become sensitive to antibiotics again. This meant limiting the use of antibiotics only when it was absolutely necessary. I landed in the hospital for a 15-day stay. It was a challenge to remain off antibiotics and still maintain my health.

I knew deciding to pursue transplantation would be a big step for me and would bring a whole new set of challenges. But, I have always looked upon transplantation as a positive solution to my situation. It was presented to me in a very straightforward but very optimistic way. That was the mind frame I had going into it and right up until I was put to sleep in the OR, and I have maintained that outlook to this day. My waiting period, which lasted for 20 months, was definitely worth it. I had a very successful double-lung transplant in April 1999!

– Randy E. Sims, bilateral-lung transplant recipient,
April 9, 1999

DIETARY CONSULT, is especially important for patients whose weight is significantly greater than or less than ideal body weight. Your nutritional status is extremely important in maintaining your health during the waiting period, lowering the risk of the surgery and speeding your recovery.

CLINICAL SOCIAL WORKER CONSULT, in which you and your family members will meet with the transplant social worker to review psychosocial issues and concerns, to further discuss the transplant process, and to answer any questions you might have.

FINANCIAL CONSULT with a financial adviser to assist you in determining how the surgery and long-term medications will be paid for. Most insurance companies and medical assistance programs cover lung transplantation. *(For more information about financing transplantation, turn to pages 43 and 211.)*

PSYCHIATRIC OR PSYCHOLOGICAL CONSULT to assess your present and past psychological function, including assessment for depression and anxiety, which are relatively common in people with serious illnesses. Transplant centers differ in what they ask and how they apply information from this consultation. A history of major depression, for example, makes for a higher risk of postoperative depression, and puts the staff on alert for symptoms so that it can be treated aggressively. The psychiatric consult is also used to determine your ability to adhere to medical regimen. Poor compliance in the past is correlated with poor compliance in the future. In addition, they want to know the quality of your social supports and relationships; having at least one high quality support person is associated with better outcomes, both medically and psychologically.

The psychiatric consult is also used to find out what your coping style is like. Patients who have an avoidance coping style, more or less pretending that nothing is wrong, often do worse psychologically than people who use a more approach-oriented style, meeting things head on and doing what is necessary.

During the psychological consult, your intellectual and psychological functioning will be evaluated. Although some centers are hesitant to list people with significant impairment, in general, most centers will not turn down someone strictly on the basis of a psychological exam. More typically, the information is used to determine how best to help each person through the difficulties encountered during transplantation.

CHILD LIFE SERVICES, with a child life specialist meeting you and your child to introduce you to their services. Using a variety of play therapy techniques, the child life specialist works with your child to explain and brighten the often traumatic hospitalization experience.

Living-Lobar Lung Donor Transplantation Evaluation:

Candidates for a living-lobar lung donor transplant are evaluated the same way as other lung transplant candidates, although tissue typing and cross-matching are performed. Tissue typing, also called histocompatibility testing, is a test that identifies the HLA (or human leukocyte antigens) for both donor and recipient to see if they match. Each person has several different types of antigens located on the surface of their white-blood cells. HLA antigens are the ones that come under attack by the recipient's immune system after transplantation. Cross-matching is where the blood of the recipient is combined with the donor's to see if there is any reaction.

The donor selection for a living-lobar transplant is done very cautiously since the donor may have a small, but measurable, decline in lung function as a result of donating a part of their lung. The donor postoperative FEV_1 decreases approximately 18%. However, this drop does not result in any noticeable impairment to the donors.

The potential donor must have the same blood type, be between 18 and 55 years old and be free of medical problems. The donor also must be without pressure to donate, and his or her motives must be altruistic. In addition to a careful physical evaluation (which includes a medical history, physical exam, lab studies, pulmonary function tests, EKG, ECHO, chest x-ray, chest CT, VQ Lung Scan, among others), the potential donor will also undergo an extensive psychological evaluation.

Pediatric Transplantation Evaluation:

Like adults, a nonambulatory condition prior to transplantation is likely to have a long-term impact on survival after lung transplantation. Therefore, most pediatric transplant centers prefer to transplant children who are not on mechanical ventilatory support.

In addition, infants and children often have congenital heart defects and/or a more rapid decline than most adult patients with primary pulmonary hypertension necessitating early referral. Guidelines for listing infants and children, although similar to those for adults, need to be approached on a case-by-case basis. However, since children are heavily dependent on their parents and caretakers, the requirements for competence, commitment and resources on the part of the parents needs to be addressed before transplant takes place.

Retransplantation Evaluation:

Repeat lung transplantation is performed in only a small percentage of patients, and, if performed at all, patients should meet strict criteria. These surgeries are considered high-risk since candidates for retransplantation are often suffering from rejection and immunosuppression and are often debilitated by opportunistic infections. Nonambulatory, ventilated patients should not be considered for retransplantation with the same priority as other candidates. In addition, any patient who lost his or her transplant due to deliberate noncompliance would not be a good candidate for retransplantation.

Inclusion Criteria:

Traditionally, each center uses its own criteria for listing patients on the transplant waiting list. However, UNOS has approved guidelines for the selection of lung and heart-lung transplant patients. It is important to note that these are guidelines only and not every patient will fit them exactly. For example, some centers have transplanted patients more than 65 years old, so don't think you'd be automatically disqualified because of your age. However, lung transplantation is rarely an option for critically ill patients.

To be considered a candidate for lung transplantation, you should have end-stage pulmonary and or/vascular disease with:

1) A projected life expectancy less than one you would have with a lung transplant. These calculations should take into account the waiting time necessary for an organ to become available; and
2) A New York Heart Association (NYHA) Class III or IV functional level with rehabilitation potential; which means patients who are comfortable at rest, but have symptoms with less than ordinary effort or patients who have symptoms at rest.

IDIOPATHIC PULMONARY FIBROSIS (IPF): Patients with IPF may be listed for lung transplantation when they have not responded to high dose corticosteroids and their forced vital capacity (FVC) is less than 65% of predicted.

CYSTIC FIBROSIS (CF): Patients with CF may be listed when their forced expiratory volume in the first second of expiration (FEV_1) is less than 30% of predicted or when a patient is experiencing a rapid functional

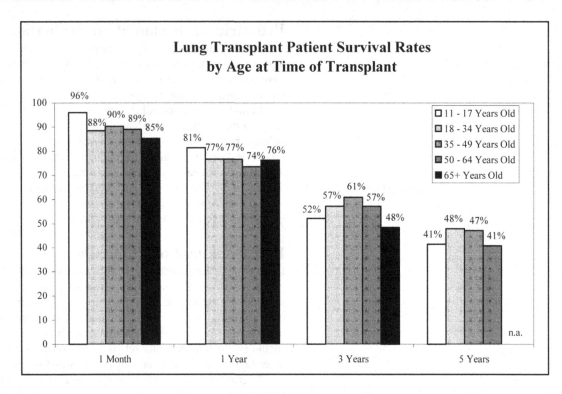

Lung Transplant Patient Survival Rates by Age at Time of Transplant

Chart 8. Lung transplant patient survival by age at time of transplant. (Data based on UNOS' OPTN/ Scientific Registry data as of Sept. 7, 1999; n. a. denotes not available.)

decline despite optimal therapy. Such a patient may still function at a better than NYHA Class III level. Children, especially girls, may need to be listed earlier in the course of their disease since they appear to decline more rapidly than other patients with CF do.

PRIMARY PULMONARY HYPERTENSION (PPH): There are various parameters that correlate with survival in patients with PPH, such as the right arterial pressure, pulmonary artery pressure and cardiac index. Nevertheless, therapy with vasodilators, such as prostacyclin (Flolan), may alter the natural history of this disease. All patients who are potential candidates should be listed and followed carefully while on IV prostacyclin to determine the appropriate timing for transplantation.

EISENMENGER'S SYNDROME: Patients with Eisenmenger's syndrome, or pulmonary hypertension secondary to congenital heart disease, usually follow a course of gradual functional deterioration over many decades. Nevertheless, no published data exists regarding the natural history of these different cardiac defects. Therefore, these patients should be listed for lung transplantation when they experience progression of symptoms despite therapy and are unsatisfied with their quality of life.

EMPHYSEMA: Patients with emphysema may be listed for lung transplantation when their post-bronchodilator FEV_1 is less than 25% of predicted or when cor pulmonale (increase in size of the heart or failure of the right ventricle) is present.

Relative Contraindications:
The following are a list of general medical conditions that are felt to have a negative impact on the long-term outcome of lung transplantation. Medical

or psychosocial treatment to address these issues should be instituted when appropriate in patients who do not currently, but may ultimately, meet the criteria for lung transplantation. However, in most cases, referral should not be delayed while patients are undergoing corrective treatment.

WEIGHT OUTSIDE OF ACCEPTABLE RANGE: Nutritional issues are an important predictor of surgical outcomes. Patients with body weight less than 70% or greater than 130% of ideal require either weight gain or weight loss to become eligible for transplant.

SURGICAL PLEURODESIS: Prior thoracic procedures are not contraindications with the exception of surgical pleurodesis. It can become a problem because of the danger of hemorrhage during the removal of the native lungs while anticoagulated on cardiopulmonary bypass.

PHYSIOLOGIC AGE: Although no reliable data exists regarding age as a criterion for a lung transplantation, the generally accepted maximal limits for age for consideration of lung transplantation are as follows:
- Less than 65 years old for single-lung transplantation
- Less than 60 years old for bilateral-lung transplantation
- Less than 55 years old for heart-lung transplantation.

PREDNISONE USE: The use of corticosteroids pre-transplant has been liberalized from previous recommendations. Although a pre-transplant prednisone dose of less than 20 mg per day is preferable, there are no upper limit steroid doses that would be a contraindication to transplantation.

PSYCHOSOCIAL INSTABILITY (or Incapacitating Mental Illness): Psychosocial problems, that have a likelihood of negatively impacting outcome and cannot be controlled or resolved with therapy, e.g., poorly controlled major psychological disturbance or disorder, are relative contraindications to transplantation. A documented history of noncompliance with medical treatment is a relative contraindication.

In addition to a strong psyche, the care from and support of a significant support structure is essential to a successful transplant.

SUBSTANCE ABUSE: Candidates for lung transplantation must be free of substance addictions, e.g., alcohol, tobacco or narcotics, for at least six months. However, if a patient can prove complete abstinence for a period of six months, then this may not be an obstacle to transplantation.

MECHANICAL VENTILATION: The requirement for invasive ventilation results in more significant disease and a longer recovery period post-transplant. Patients receiving noninvasive ventilatory support, e.g., CPAP, BiPAP, are eligible for lung transplantation.

INTRINSIC RENAL DISEASE: This is a relative contraindication because of the toxic nature of cyclosporine and Prograf to the kidneys.

SIGNIFICANT PERIPHERAL VASCULAR DISEASE: This is a relative contraindication because of the potential of blood clots to form during the early post-transplant period. It may also represent a significant impairment to physical rehabilitation later post-transplant.

IMPAIRED LEFT HEART FUNCTION: Because lung transplantation puts a significant stress on the heart, and heart failure is the third most common cause of death after lung transplantation, impaired left-heart function is a relative contraindication for lung transplantation unless a heart-lung transplant is being considered.

SEVERE CHEST WALL DEFORMITY: A significant chest wall deformity is a relative contraindication because it can impair the breathing capacity of the lungs and can impair physical rehabilitation post-transplant.

SYMPTOMATIC OSTEOPOROSIS: This is a relative problem to transplantation because it can impair physical rehabilitation post-transplant.

SPUTUM WITH PAN-RESISTANT BACTERIA: The presence of bacteria that is resistant to all classes of antibiotics is a relative contraindication because of the risk of infection post-transplant. The presence of atypical mycobacteria in the sputum or history of adequately treated infection with mycobacterium tuberculosis are not contraindications.

HEPATITIS B or C INFECTION: Infection with hepatitis B virus (HBV) or with hepatitis C virus (HCV) is relative contraindications because of the probability of accelerated liver disease in the setting of systemic immunosuppression post-transplant.

Medical conditions which haven't resulted in organ damage and are well-controlled are generally acceptable in candidates for lung transplantation. These may include hypertension, noninsulin and insulin dependant diabetes and ulcer.

Absolute Contraindications:

BONE MARROW FAILURE: Bone marrow failure is an absolute contraindication because of the likelihood of complications related to bleeding, infection and transfusion requirements.

CIRRHOSIS OF THE LIVER: Significant cirrhosis of the liver is an absolute contraindication because of a propensity for clotting, dysfunction of the brain and/or accelerated liver failure post-transplant.

MALIGNANCY PRECLUDING LONG-TERM SURVIVAL: Any recent malignancy likely to preclude long-term survival is a contraindication to transplantation.

Other life-limiting conditions such as HIV, multiple sclerosis, amyotrophic lateral sclerosis (also known as Lou Gehrig's disease) represent absolute contraindications to lung transplantation.

Medical Review Board:

After your evaluation is complete, the transplant team, along with some other medical professionals, meets as a medical review board. The results of your tests are presented and discussed. At this time a determination will be made in regard to your candidacy for transplantation. Your transplant coordinator will contact you to discuss the results of your evaluation.

THE WAITING PERIOD:

"There were many times when Mom was ready to throw in the towel. To those of you waiting for transplants, NEVER give up, it does actually happen!
– Amy Clark

O nce it has been determined that you are a good candidate for transplantation, you are then placed on the national waiting list with UNOS in hopes of finding a suitable donor for you. You are then given a beeper so the transplant center can get in touch with you should a donor organ become available.

Waiting for a suitable organ to become available may take anywhere from several days to many months or years. This time has been described by many patients and their families as the most difficult part of the transplant process. Fear, anxiety and uncertainty are normal reactions. Since this can be a frustrating and demanding time, it is often helpful for you and your family members to attend a support group. Contact your transplant social worker about the availability of support groups in your area. *(For more information on support groups, see page 215.)*

The Waiting List:

In the early '80s, before there was a centralized computer network for organ sharing, patients in need of a transplant had difficulty in obtaining organs and some resorted to media exposure to seek assistance. It wasn't until 1984 that Congress passed the National Organ Transplant Act (NOTA), which established a legal framework for allocating organs in the United States and prohibited the sale of human organs. NOTA created the Organ Procurement and Transplantation Network (OPTN) to ensure a fair, safe and effective system for donation, procurement, allocation and transplantation. In 1986, the OPTN awarded the federal contract to establish and operate the OPTN to the United Network for Organ Sharing (UNOS).

Originally, UNOS began its operations in 1977 as a national service provided by the SouthEastern Organ Procurement Foundation with more than 90 transplant centers across the country. In 1984, it was incorporated as a separate company, and, in 1986, it received the contract to create and operate the organ allocation system we know today.

UNOS, located in Richmond, Va., maintains a centralized computer network linking all the organ procurement organizations and transplant centers in the country. This computer network is accessible 24 hours a day, seven days a week. By working with medical professionals, patients and donor families around the country, UNOS facilitates some 20,000 matches annually between donors and recipients, and has helped match some 185,000 organs since its inception. While most people have heard of the waiting list, few understand how organs are allocated among the 70 active lung transplant centers in this country.

When a patient's name is added to the list, his or her medical profile is entered and stored in the UNOS computer. Patients are listed according to blood type and size. The system is blind to the recipient's age, race, nationality, religion and ability to pay. For kidney, bone marrow and some heart transplants, a tissue match is made, which takes eight to 12 hours. But for lungs and heart-lungs, tissue matching isn't practical due to the need to retransplant the organs as soon as possible. Lungs and hearts are only viable without a blood supply for four to six hours, which eliminates tissue

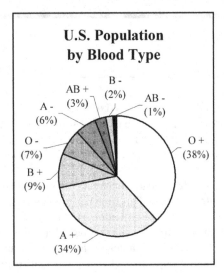

**U.S. Population
by Blood Type**

AB +
(3%)

B -
(2%)

A -
(6%)

AB -
(1%)

O -
(7%)

O +
(38%)

B +
(9%)

A +
(34%)

*Chart 9. U.S. population by blood type.
(Data provided by the American
Association of Blood Banks.)*

typing and the range organs can be shared around the country.

When a donor becomes available, the local Organ Procurement Organization (OPO) runs its waiting list according to size, blood type, waiting time accrued and distance between donor and recipient. It then generates a list of patients that most closely match the donor's characteristics. Transplant candidates get points for the right blood match and size, how long they've waited and distance from the donor hospital.

After receiving a printout of the waiting list, the procurement coordinator at the OPO contacts the transplant surgeon to see if he or she wants to and is able to accept the organ. Sometimes, the top patient will not get the organ for one of several reasons. He or she must be accessible, healthy enough to undergo major surgery and be willing to be transplanted immediately.

Position on the List:

There are a number of factors that go into your position on the transplant list. You could be No. one on your local list by waiting time, having waited longer than everyone else has. However, if you're blood type B and a type A organ becomes available, you'll be automatically passed over; the organ would go to the first person with the matching or compatible blood type. The same is true for organ size. Even if you're at the "top of the list" you may not get the next organ because you may not live geographically close to where the organ is recovered. However, organs are most often transplanted into one of the first 10 candidates identified on the match run. If you are interested in knowing your position on the list, ask your transplant coordinator. UNOS will not give out this information to patients.

Medical Urgency:

UNOS does not figure medical urgency or status into its allocation of lungs as it does for other organs, such as livers and hearts. The policy is "first-come, first-served." As the patient's condition worsens, he or she is more likely to be rejected as being too sick for transplantation. Optimally, lungs are transplanted during what is called, a "window of opportunity;" which means a period of time when you are sick enough to warrant the operation, but not so sick that you might not survive it.

Fortunately for patients listed with idiopathic pulmonary fibrosis, UNOS has made adjustments to its rule. Once they are placed on the waiting list, they immediately get an additional three months credit added to their waiting time. This is due to the fact that these patients often deteriorate quite rapidly and have the highest mortality rate while waiting for a suitable donor. In addition, patients with chronic obstructive lung disease have a higher rate of survival on the transplant waiting lists than do patients with pulmonary fibrosis, cystic fibrosis or pulmonary hypertension. UNOS' policy states:

3.7.6 Status of Patients Awaiting Lung Transplantation. All patients awaiting isolated lung transplantation are considered to be the same urgency status for the purposes of thoracic organ allocation.

3.7.9.2 Waiting Time Accrual for Lung Candidates with Idiopathic Pulmonary Fibrosis (IPF). A lung transplant candidate diagnosed with IPF shall be assigned 90 days of additional waiting time upon the candidate's registration on the UNOS Patient Waiting List.

How Long is the Waiting Period?

The length of time you wait depends on your blood type, height and weight and lung disease. According to UNOS, in 1998, the national median waiting time for a lung transplant was 703 days, or approximately two years. In 1997, the median waiting time for a heart-lung transplant the wait was 795 days, or approximately 26 months. Waiting times are generally shorter for patients waiting for a single-lung transplant compared to those waiting for bilateral-lung or heart-lung transplants.

In addition to the medical criteria, the present system of organ allocation relies heavily on geographic distribution and the availability of donor organs in your area because of the short ischemic times for lungs and hearts. The United States is divided into 59 local organ procurement areas that service various transplant programs.

When a donor organ becomes available, its medical criteria is entered into the UNOS computer, and the host OPO checks the local waiting list. If no match is available through the local list, the search is expanded within a 500-mile radius of the donor hospital. If still no match, the search is expanded again to within a 1,000-mile radius of the donor hospital. Because there are so many patients waiting in any given area, a donor/recipient match is often made before it is necessary to go to the regional or national level. UNOS' policy for lung and heart-lung allocation is as follows:

3.7.2 Geographic Sequence of Thoracic Organ Allocation. Thoracic organs are to be allocated locally first, then within the following zones in the sequence described in Policy 3.7.10. Three zones will be delineated by concentric circles of 500 and 1,000 nautical mile radii with the donor

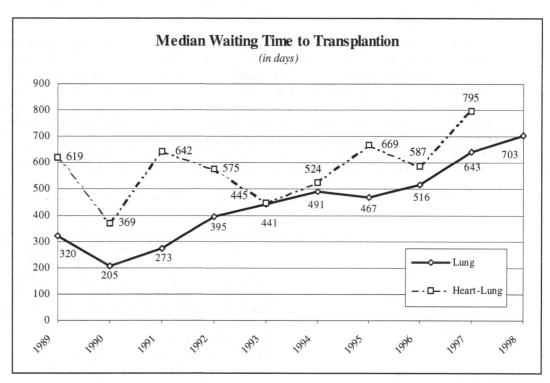

Chart 10. *Median waiting time to transplantation in days. (Data based on UNOS' OPTN/Scientific Registry data as of Sept. 8, 1998, Sept. 7, 1999 and Aug. 26, 2000.)*

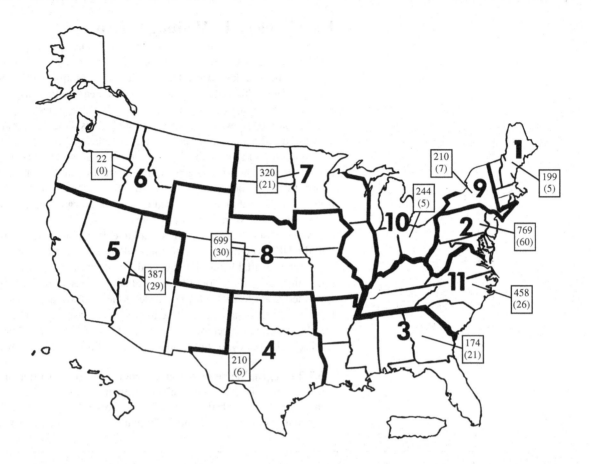

Figure 1. *The number of candidates listed for lung and heart-lung (in parenthesis) transplants by UNOS region as of Jan. 31, 2001 (these figures are updated monthly by UNOS), including the 11 different regions divided for administrative purposes only. Region 1 includes Connecticut, Maine, Massachusetts, New Hampshire, Rhode Island and Vermont. Region 2 includes Delaware, District of Columbia, Maryland, New Jersey, Pennsylvania and West Virginia. Region 3 includes Alabama, Arkansas, Florida, Georgia, Louisiana, Mississippi and Puerto Rico. Region 4 includes Oklahoma and Texas. Region 5 includes Arizona, California, Nevada, New Mexico and Utah. Region 6 includes Alaska, Hawaii, Idaho, Oregon, Montana and Washington. Region 7 includes Illinois, Minnesota, North Dakota, South Dakota and Wisconsin. Region 8 includes Colorado, Iowa, Kansas, Missouri, Nebraska and Wyoming. Region 9 includes New York. Region 10 includes Indiana, Michigan and Ohio. Region 11 includes Kentucky, North Carolina, South Carolina, Tennessee and Virginia.*

hospital at the center. Zone A will extend to all transplant centers which are within 500 miles from the donor hospital but which are not in the local area of the donor hospital. Zone B will extend to all transplant centers that are at least 500 miles from the donor hospital but not more than 1,000 miles from the donor hospital. Zone C will extend to all transplant centers that are located beyond 1,000 miles from the donor hospital.

3.7.11 Allocation of Lungs.

Lungs will be allocated locally first, then to patients in Zone A, then to patients in Zone B, and finally to patients in Zone C. In each of those four geographic areas, patients will be grouped so that patients who have an ABO blood type that is identical to that of the donor are ranked according to time waiting; the lungs will be allocated in descending order to patients in that ABO identical type. If the lungs are not allocated to patients in that ABO identical type, they will be allocated in descending order according to time waiting to the remaining patients in that geographic area who have a blood type that is compatible (but not identical) with that of the donor.

Changes made in heart-lung allocation now require that organs are allocated the same way to patients requiring isolated heart or lung transplants. This will make organ allocation more equitable for this group of patients who generally wait longer for transplants. This change requires patients awaiting a heart-lung transplant be listed on both the heart and the lung list. The patient accumulates waiting time and advances on the heart and lung waiting lists based only on the allocation criteria for that organ. In the past, heart-lung patients were not assigned a status but were ranked according to time accumulated on the waiting list. Under the new proposal, it is possible for these patients to be listed as Status 1A on the heart list. According to UNOS policy, heart-lung allocation is as follows:

3.7.7 Allocation of Thoracic Organs to Heart-Lung Candidates. Candidates for a heart-lung transplant shall be registered on the individual UNOS Patient Waiting list for each organ. When the patient is eligible to receive a heart in accordance with Policy 3.7, or an approved variance to this policy, the lung shall be allocated to the heart-lung candidate from the same donor. When the patient is eligible to receive a lung in accordance with Policy 3.7, or an approved variance to this policy, the heart shall be allocated to the heart-lung candidate from the same donor if no suitable Status 1A isolated heart candidates are eligible to receive the heart.

Multiple Listing:

Some patients feel it is to their advantage to be listed at more than one transplant hospital. This is only true if the two hospitals are in different organ procurement areas. Being on more than one list is allowed by UNOS, however this policy may change in the near future. To multiple list, most transplant centers require a personal visit from you and a separate evaluation, which is both timely and expensive. In some cases, the tests performed at one center can be forwarded to the other center. Some centers ask all or part of the tests be repeated using their staff and equipment. However, some centers may not allow you to be listed at more than one center.

Transferring Waiting Time:

Currently, UNOS' policy on transferring waiting time from one center to another states:

3.2.2.1 Waiting Time Transferral. A patient may transfer his/her primary waiting time from one transplant center (Initial Primary Center) to another center (New Primary Center) upon listing of the patient as a transplant candidate by the patient. After receipt of a written request from the New Primary Center which states the patient's intention to transfer his/her waiting time, the patient's listing date (the date from which primary waiting time will be calculated) at the New Primary Center will be entered into the computer system by the UNOS Organ Center as the date the patient was listed at the Initial Primary Center. This request must be signed by the patient, a legal guardian, or other individual having the power of attorney to act on the patient's behalf.

If you transfer wait time from your Initial Primary Center to a New Primary Center, but remain listed at the Initial Primary Center, "a new listing date" is assigned. In other words, waiting time at the original center starts again at zero, while the new center would show accrued waiting time since you were originally listed.

Inactive vs. Active Status:

According to UNOS, you are either ACTIVE or INACTIVE on the waiting list. If you are active, that means you are ready to go at any time. Being inactive means you aren't ready for a transplant. This could be due to an infection that may render you inactive for several days or weeks, or to the fact that your condition has improved and you want to postpone your transplant. UNOS policy states:

3.2.5 Waiting Time for Patients in an Inactive Status. Unless otherwise stipulated in each organ specific allocation policy, waiting time beyond 30 days shall not be accrued by patients while they are registered on the UNOS Patient Waiting List as being inactive.

PRE-TRANSPLANT PREPARATIONS:

"I confess I had become a real 'couch potato.' The less I DID, the less I COULD do. I started pulmonary rehab and can already feel a difference."
– JoAnn Davies

While you are waiting for your transplant, there are many things that you can do to prepare yourself physically, emotionally and financially. In addition, there are a number of practical things you will want to put in place well before your transplant, such as arranging for transportation or housing close to the hospital.

Beepers:

As mentioned earlier, you will be given a beeper, free of charge. Carry it with you at all times when you leave home. The transplant center will first try to reach you by phone, so double-check to make sure they have your correct phone number. If they cannot reach you at home, they will then try your beeper. Make sure the batteries are always fresh. If your beeper has a vibration function, you may want to use it when in a noisy environment.

If you are away from home for any length of time, it is very important you leave a number where your transplant center can reach you. If you are traveling out of range of your beeper, you may want to ask your beeper company to extend its service area.

Medical Appointments:

Although you are placed on the transplant waiting list, you should continue being seen by your local doctor. You will also need to be seen by the transplant clinic at three-month intervals. Make sure to contact your transplant team whenever there is a significant change in your health, such as when you develop an infection, are started on antibiotics or have a change in medications (including being started on prednisone), as well as whenever you are admitted into the hospital.

Dental Care:

It is important to plan ahead for any necessary dental work PRIOR to transplantation. When you are immune suppressed, you will have to wait at least six months before having any work done due to the risk of infection.

Vaccinations:

All of your vaccinations should be brought up to date before you are transplanted. Also, depending on your center, you may be asked to get the Hepatitis B vaccine, pneumovax (once in a lifetime), and a tetanus shot every 10 years.

Transfused Blood:

Sometimes during thoracic surgery there is the need for transfused blood. However, it is more commonly needed during a bilateral-lung or heart-lung transplant than a single-lung transplant operation.

Despite rigorous screening and testing methods in place at blood banks across the country, the risk of contracting an infection through a blood transfusion still exists. According to the American Association of Blood Banks, approximately one in 676,000 units of blood contains the HIV virus. One in 66,000 is contaminated with hepatitis B, and one in 1,000,000 is contaminated with hepatitis C. These risks are quite low, even for patients who receive multiple units of blood. Nevertheless, doctors and patients are wary of transfusions unless absolutely necessary.

One way to reduce the need for blood transfusions during your surgery is to make sure that your center uses blood-saving surgical techniques. The process, known as cell-salvage, collects and then re-transfuses blood from the patient's surgical incision. This requires the use of sophisticated equipment not found in every operating room.

Another precaution you may want to take is to bank your own blood, called autologous blood donation. With this technique, you will receive blood NOT from an anonymous donor but from your own previously donated blood. Ask your transplant center for information. You should know that banked blood is only good in liquid form for about 42 days. Depending on your wait, you may need to make additional donations. For more information, contact your local blood bank or:

The American Association of Blood Banks
Phone: 301-907-6977, Fax: 301-907-6895, E-mail: aabb@aabb.org
8101 Glenbrook Road, Bethesda, MD 20814-2749
Website: http://www.aabb.org

Getting Your Legal Affairs in Order:

As with any major illness, it is a good idea to get your legal affairs in order. This includes updating or executing a will, completing a Living Will or Advance Directive, and appointing a health care surrogate.

PREPARING A WILL: A last will and testament is a written document that stipulates how your estate is to be disposed of in the event of your death. For the simplest estates, you can pick up pre-printed forms that are available from office supply stores, but make sure that the form you use is recognized and approved by the courts in your state. For more complicated estates, one in which you have specific wishes and/or bequests, you may find hiring a lawyer is the best solution.

You can get referrals to estate lawyers from your local Bar Association, but the best way is to get a recommendation from a friend. Most lawyers charge $125 to $175 an hour. You should request an estimate up front, but most simple wills cost anywhere from $150 to $225. When you visit a lawyer, it is best to be prepared and know what you want done since you will be paying for their time. If you die without a will, the courts will dictate how your estate will be settled. They will appoint an administrator to work

THE VOICE OF EXPERIENCE

The Keys to Life

It has been over 13 years since I was first diagnosed with emphysema. I was 43 years old at the time and had smoked two packs of cigarettes a day for 30 years. I was living in the home of my dreams: a 225-square-foot cabin I built myself at 9,000 feet elevation in the mountains of Colorado. I supported myself by taking temporary engineering jobs in whatever part of the country there was work.

I wasn't able to quit smoking cigarettes until eight years after I was diagnosed. I had started smoking at age 13, and tried to quit at age 15, but failed. So, I know what it is like to be so addicted to a habit that it becomes the most important thing in your life.

While I waited the final months to transplantation, exercise was one of the keys to maintaining my health. I have written extensively on that subject and will not discuss it further except to say I was an exercise fanatic many years before I was able to quit smoking. Additionally, I believe exercise was instrumental in allowing me to quit cigarettes in the first place.

The use of supplemental oxygen has also helped me to stay healthy and minimize the damage this disease could do to my heart. During my wait for a lung transplant, oximeters became available to the public and this allowed me to monitor my oxygen levels during every physical activity I did; I have had lots of surprises. Many times when I thought I was adequately oxygenated, the oximeter told me I wasn't. This was especially true early in the disease process.

My father taught me that "Service to others is the rent we pay to live on this earth." It is that helping others that has been very helpful to me. For instance, in 1998, I produced a video of advice from emphysema superstars. The lessons I learned in the process have helped me much more than I believe those who see the video because so much had to be edited out. I have also produced videos for young teens to prevent them from starting to smoke cigarettes. I have a dream that some day we will be able to eliminate cigarettes from our society.

Another thing that helped me during the wait for my lung transplant is the synergy I felt from the online lung disease support groups. Every time I made a point to one of the lists, I learned so much more from the responses I got.

Now that I am transplanted, I find that these skills continue to come to my aid. God has helped me often in my walk with this disease. I am thankful I have had the opportunity to obtain a lung transplant so I can continue to help teens make the right decision about smoking.

– Ron Peterson, single-lung transplant recipient,
Dec. 27, 2000

out the details and report back to the courts. Your assets will be disposed of in lineal descent according to the laws of your state.

LIVING WILLS/ADVANCE DIRECTIVES: A living will or advance directive is a written document in which individuals give directions, in advance, about their medical care and designate who they want to make medical decisions for them if they lose the ability to make such decisions themselves. There are two types of advance directives: 1) treatment directives, the most common example being the living will; and 2) proxy directives, the most common example being the health care surrogate, or power of attorney.

A treatment directive, such as a living will, is a written statement expressing the forms of medical treatment a person wishes to receive or forego if he or she is unable to communicate directly with their doctors. A living will can be activated when an individual has irreversible unconsciousness, terminal illness or severe and irreversible brain damage. It also contains statements about any treatment you wish to avoid, such as cardiopulmonary resuscitation (CPR), artificial respiration or nutrition.

You should discuss your living will with your family and your doctor, and you should ask that it be made a part of your medical record. Most states have their own living will form, each somewhat different. You can usually obtain a copy of the form from your doctor's office or local hospital.

PROXY DIRECTIVES/HEALTH CARE SURROGATE: A proxy directive, such as a designated health care surrogate, is a person's written statement naming another person to make medical decisions for them if they become unable to make such decisions for themselves. Your surrogate should be someone who knows your wishes and will make decisions based on what he or she believes you would want.

A health care surrogate is usually a family member or close friend who can be readily available to your physician. It is important to appoint a health care surrogate even if you have made a living will, since it is difficult to address every possible situation. In the absence of a designated health care surrogate, most states have statutes stipulating who can make such medical decisions for patients.

POWER OF ATTORNEY: Executing a power of attorney for financial purposes may be advisable prior to transplantation, so that someone can write checks, pay the bills or take care of other business while you are in the hospital. A power of attorney is a document by which you give another person – your agent – the authority to make decisions about the financial aspects of your life. You can revoke or change your power of attorney at any time before you become incapacitated.

These documents need to be signed, dated and witnessed by two people. One of the witnesses must be someone who is not your spouse, blood relative, heir or person responsible for paying your medical bills. Once you have completed a living will, appointed a health care surrogate and/or a power of attorney, you should give a copy to your physician, minister, family members, close friends and your health care surrogate or power of attorney. Discuss with them the details of your living will, and ask that they keep a copy, and to make it available only if needed.

"If I only knew years ago what I know now, I never would have smoked and I'd be enjoying life now instead of watching it ebb out of me everyday."
– Karen Hoelzel

Nutrition:

Maintaining or achieving a healthy weight can improve your changes of being accepted for transplantation and reduce your risk of complications after surgery, such as diabetes. In addition, once you are on the anti-rejection medications, it will be difficult to lose any weight after the transplant. If you are overweight or underweight, consult with a dietician to help you find a diet that works for you.

Exercise:

It is beneficial, and often required by the transplant center, that you get into some kind of physical rehabilitation program prior to transplantation. However, while exercise will not alter your basic disease process, it will maximize your available muscle function. There are three basic types of programs. The one that is most appropriate for you depends on the severity of your impairment.

An at-home exercise program is most suitable for patients whose impairment is minimal or who have problems participating in a hospital-based program. An outpatient program is suitable for those patients who have moderate impairment and are reasonably mobile. An in-hospital program is suitable for those patients who are very disabled and require medical supervision.

A balanced program of exercise includes activities to improve cardiovascular endurance, muscular strength, flexibility and relaxation. If possible, the primary type of training should be aerobic in nature and task-specific; aerobic to improve the oxygen transport system and task-specific to ensure maximal application to functional activity in daily life.

For people with minor levels of disability, low-intensity exercises, such as walking and stationary bicycling, are better than exercises with high intensity, such as calisthenics or recreational games, like tennis. For those with severe impairment, the focus of the exercise should be on adaptation to the disability, energy conservation in everyday tasks, and should be carefully monitored by a therapist. Patients with pulmonary hypertension may not be required to participate in pulmonary rehabilitation because of the risk of cardiac failure.

It is important to exercise as much as possible to maintain or improve your current functional abilities, however limited they might be. Inactivity produces fatigue and loss of muscle tone. And, as the saying goes . . . "If you don't use it, you lose it." Studies have shown that the better shape you are in going into surgery, the easier your recovery will be after.

Some of the benefits of exercise include: improved exercise tolerance, better oxygen utilization by the body, increased endurance, improved joint range of motion and muscle tone, and decreased fatigue, insomnia and stress. *(Turn to page 266 and copy the worksheet provided to help you keep track of your progress.)*

GENERAL GUIDELINES ON HOW TO EXERCISE SAFELY:

- Before starting any exercise program on your own, you should first consult with your doctor.
- In general, a minimum of three or four days per week is recommended for healthy individuals.
- 30-minute sessions are recommend for healthy people; however, for those with pulmonary disease it may be easier to exercise for shorter periods during the day, rather than doing one long exercise session that may

leave you exhausted. This technique is called interval training.
- How hard you exercise depends on a variety of factors, including your overall conditioning, extent of disease, environmental conditions, etc. A good rule of thumb is to use the Borg Scale of "Perceived Rate of Exertion," which ranges from zero to 10. Zero is how you feel at rest, and 10 is how you feel working at your hardest for five minutes. For people with pulmonary disease it is recommended that you exercise between five and seven on that scale.
- Patients with large amounts of sputum may find postural drainage before exercise helps to improve airflow. For some, using an inhaled bronchodilator may be helpful as well.
- Every exercise session should begin and end with very low level exercise; a warm-up and cool-down period of about two to three minutes, followed by gentle stretching.
- Start slowly and progress gradually. Problems with exercise typically result when people do too much too soon, not allowing their muscles to adapt adequately to the exercise. Pace yourself.
- Listen to your body. If you feel pain or fatigue, you have done too much. It is important to remember that exercise should not cause discomfort. You should stop if you experience pain or pressure in your chest, unusual shortness of breath, dizziness or lightheadedness, persistent rapid or irregular heart rate during or after exercise.
- Before starting any exercise, take a slow, deep breath. Inhale through your nose and exhale through your mouth. Never hold your breath. For people with obstructive lung disease, practicing pursed-lip breathing while exercising may be helpful. To do pursed-lipped breathing, start by slowly inhaling through your nose, then breathe out while you purse your lips as if you are blowing on hot soup, and exhale slowly. Take twice as long to breathe out as you took to breathe in. Pursed-lip breathing helps to keep your airways open longer as you exhale.
- Drink plenty of water. The body's need for water is second in importance only to its need for oxygen. Start drinking before you feel thirsty.
- Schedule your exercise session into your daily routine. Keep a record as a reminder of your progress.
- Make it something you enjoy.

Travel Preparations:

Generally, you will have to live within a two-hour drive of the transplant center to accommodate the short ischemic times. Lungs and hearts must be in the body and working within four to six hours after they were removed from the donor. If you live farther than two to three hours by car, there are organizations available that can help you make arrangements, in advance, for air transportation. Your transplant coordinator or social worker will discuss this with you at the time you are listed.

It is important to designate a person who can be responsible to drive you to the hospital. It will make things easier if that person is given a beeper so you can contact THEM in the event that YOU get "the call." Once you get called by your transplant center, you will have very little time to get to the hospital, it is important to have your bags already packed. You may want to put together a phone list. This way you won't have to think who needs to be called when the time arrives, it will be all written down.

In addition, it is advisable to map out your travel route to the hospital in advance and do a test-drive so you will know exactly how to get there and where to park when the time arrives. It is also a good idea to have an alternate route in case of traffic problems.

You may also want an ambulance lined up to get you to the hospital instead of using a passenger car. Approval for ambulance transportation must be made in advance, as it is not always covered by insurance. For those patients who must travel considerable distances for evaluation, diagnosis, treatment, rehabilitation, there are organizations available that can help. For more information, contact:

The National Patient Travel HELPLINE
Phone: 800-296-1217 (available 24 hours)
c/o Mercy Medical Airlift, 4620 Haygood Road, Suite One,
Virginia Beach, VA 23455

The National Patient Travel HELPLINE provides information about all forms of charitable, long-distance medical air transportation. They also provide referrals to all appropriate sources of help available through the Angel Flight America Network. *Website:* http://www.npath.org

The American Organ Transplant Association
Phone: 281-261-2682, Fax: 281-499-2315
3335 Cartright Road, Missouri City, TX 77459-2548

The American Organ Transplant Association provides reduced or free airfare (Continental) and bus tickets (Greyhound) to transplant recipients and their families for hospital consultations and visits. Depending on availability, hotel accommodations for the first few days after patient's surgery can be arranged through the Sheraton Hotels. To be eligible, you must be referred by your transplant social worker.

They also advise on fund-raising locally or nationally, and will help you set up and administer transplant trust funds. No administrative fees are charged. *Website:* http://www.a-o-t-a.org

Flying With Oxygen:

For security reasons, most commercial airlines don't allow you to fly with your own oxygen tank. Instead, they provide, for a fee, tanks that fit under your seat. If you need oxygen to fly, most airlines require advance notice. Though policies vary among airlines, they all require some type of verification from your physician stating your oxygen needs, how many liters per minute, and whether it should be delivered by mask or nasal cannula.

It is a good idea to contact your airline a couple of days before you leave for your trip to confirm they have your oxygen ordered. When you arrive for your flight, they will require that you empty your portable tank at the gate before you board the plane. Allow for possible delays. Usually your oxygen supplier will arrange your oxygen needs while away from home. Fortunately, oxygen is reimbursed by most health insurance policies. For more information on traveling with oxygen check out these resources:

Breathin' Easy Travel Guide
Phone: 888-699-4360 or 707-252-9333, Fax: 707-252-3028
225 Daisy Drive, Napa, CA 94558

Breathin' Easy is a guide to traveling for people with pulmonary disease. It lists more than 2,000 places worldwide where patients can refill oxygen containers, in addition to regulations for the different airlines, cruise ships, railroads and other public transportation systems. It

Angels on Earth

I got "the call" at 2:00 a.m. on a Friday morning. I rushed to get my bag, called my daughter and called the charter service to have the plane ready. I was told I needed to be at Barnes within two hours, and I had arranged for a charter service through Sky King Airport, which is about five minutes from my home. Once there I tried to call Barnes with my ETA but the number they had given me wouldn't go through. Finally, I got through to the paging operator who, although she was supposed to, had no idea what I was talking about. I insisted she page the coordinator and finally got everything taken care of. By that time I was a nervous wreck, but when I climbed aboard that plane, this wonderful sense of euphoria came over me, and I knew everything was going to be all right.

We made it to the Spirit of St. Louis Airport in an hour and 45 minutes. The ambulance that met us at the airport didn't seem to be in a hurry to get to the hospital. Now, I realize that they were probably driving the speed limit, but it seemed to take forever.

I was admitted through the ER at 4.30 a.m., and was then brought to a room where the usual pre-transplant procedures are done. At 7:30 a.m., they came in and told me the away team had called to say there might be a problem with the lung. My surgeon didn't want me sedated until they knew for sure. Despite this news, I was feeling very calm and euphoric. At 9:00 a.m. all the necessary IVs, epidural, etc. were done and at 9:30 a.m. I was taken to OR. The nurse in the OR was trying hard to keep me calm, but I was totally relaxed, knowing that I was in the best possible hands.

I had a feeling that the angels were with me, and she was one of them. I lay in there until 11:30 a.m. when they finally walked through the door with the little red and white Playmate cooler. I thought this is just like it is on TV. My surgeon took one look at the lungs, and said, "It's a go!" and that's the last thing I remember.

– Judy L. Amerman, single-lung transplant recipient,
Oct. 25, 1997

---

also contains articles, tips and advice for the traveler who carries oxygen. *Websites:* http://www.breathineasy.com or http://www.oxygen4travel.com

Travel for the Patient with Chronic Obstructive Pulmonary Disease
c/o Harold Silver, 8029 Herb Farm Drive, Bethesda, M.D. 20817
  Travel for the Patient with Chronic Obtrusive Pulmonary Disease, written by Harold M. Silver, M.D., provides guidelines on how to travel safely and comfortably, how to cope with jet lag and fatigue, and how to deal with special problems with cruise, plane and car travel. It lists services available to travelers, such as National Oxygen Travel Service.

Handicapped Parking Permits:

If you haven't gotten one already, most transplant candidates for lung transplantation qualify for a handicapped license plate or placards. Usually a doctor will need to sign the application. These permits can be of real help in finding parking in congested areas. Also, in most states, you are allowed to park in metered parking spaces, for free, for as long as needed, while displaying your permit. Contact your local Department of Motor Vehicles for more information.

Housing:

For some patients, it may be necessary to move from home to a location closer to the hospital while waiting for transplant. Some centers provide for transplant housing in apartments or homes. Contact your transplant social worker for help making those arrangements. If no housing is available, most hospitals get special discounts for patients at participating hotels. To take advantage of them, you must ask. Sometimes, your health insurance will cover expenses for housing, so check with them, too.

You may also want to contact your local Bed and Breakfast Association, or short-term rental agency, to find temporary housing. It is a good idea to find a place that is on the first floor and comes fully furnished. Having family and friends close by when you are hospitalized can be one of the most effective medicines you can get. The following organization offers help in obtaining housing before and after transplantation:

National Association of Hospital Hospitality Houses Inc. (NAHHH)
Phone: 800-542-9730 or 828-253-1188, Fax: 828-253-8082,
E-mail: helpinghomes@nahhh.org
P.O. Box 18087, Asheville, NC 28814-0087

NAHHH is a membership organization of hospital hospitality house programs which provide lodging for families of hospital patients and/or outpatients who need to receive medical treatment far from home. The NAHHH can make referrals to registered lodging, which is provided free of charge or at a very discounted rate. They have more than 125 member organizations, including some Ronald McDonald Houses, American Cancer Society's Hope Lodges and the U.S. Military Fisher Houses. *Website:* http://www.nahhh.org

What to Bring to the Hospital:

When it comes to packing for your hospital stay, think in terms of comfort. Here are some suggestions on how to make your stay more enjoyable:
- Bring ear plugs to help filter out unwanted noises; at some large centers, you may be sharing a room with another transplant recipient.
- Bring a dark eye mask to help cut down on unwanted light; it helps to get some sleep when the lights are turned on in the hallways, or when you're in a semiprivate room.
- Bring a reusable ice pack to help with pain relief or other side effects.
- Bring a tape recorder, radio or books on tape to listen to. In the beginning it is hard to concentrate with all the medications and distractions, so don't plan on doing a lot of reading.
- If you plan to bring a portable radio or computer, you need to check with the hospital first. They can cause problems if they are not properly shielded.
- Bring an empty spiral notebook to keep a diary or have a place to write down questions for your doctor.
- Bring your own slippers or warm socks (rubber bottoms are best) to keep your feet warm. All hospitals provide nightgowns, which makes it easier for you to use the bathroom and for your doctors and nurses to examine you. However, you may want to bring your own clothes since this can make a big difference in your attitude.
- Bring your own toothbrush and toiletries; these are often nicer than what the hospital will provide.
- Since it is difficult to get your hair washed after surgery, you may want to

bring along some hair ties, a scarf or hat. However, most hospitals have some kind of dry shampoo available.
- Make up some flash cards so you can communicate easily while on the ventilator such as "Yes," "No," "I Hurt Here," "Close Door," "Get Nurse," etc. Some hospitals have an alphabet board that you can use.
- Most hospital rooms have televisions in them, but some charge a daily fee for their use (approximately $3 to $5 per day). If you plan to bring your own, you will have to have the device approved by the hospital first.
- Bring some board or card games. These are a great way to keep your mind occupied when television gets too boring.
- Bring pictures of close friends and family to decorate your room.
- Bring some of your own clothes, so you have something to go home in when you are discharged.

In addition, most hospitals do not permit the use of cellular phones, as these radiate unwanted frequencies and can cause problems for hospital equipment, especially for patients on telemetry equipment.

FINANCING TRANSPLANTATION:

"It took over four months for my insurance company to approve my transplant. They were very arrogant and I had to call them frequently to remind them I was still waiting."
– Andrea L. Aulbert

Transplantation is a very expensive procedure. The average cost of a lung or heart-lung transplant (including the evaluation, surgery and post-op care) for the first year can be more than $250,000. In addition, the costs can quickly add up if you have complications that require a lengthy stay in the intensive care unit ($1,000,000 or more).

Few patients are able to pay all the costs themselves, and most obtain funding through a variety of sources, including insurance, state and federal programs, charitable organizations, fund-raising campaigns and private funds. If you are travelling any distance to receive your transplant, remember to include the cost of food, lodging and transportation.

(Turn to page 267 and copy the worksheet provided to help you evaluate the differences among various health insurance policies.)

Health Insurance:
According to UNOS, approximately 70% of commercial insurers and 92% of Blue Cross/Blue Shield plans offer coverage for transplants. Medicaid programs in approximately 20 states also reimburse for transplants. In 1995, Medicare began covering lung and heart-lung transplants for Medicare-eligible beneficiaries, but only if the operation is performed at an approved center. *(For more information about Medicare, see page 46.)*

In the case of living-lobar lung donor transplantation, given the relative newness of the procedure and the limited number of centers performing it, most insurers may not have a defined policy for it. The best method is to seek approval for cadaveric lung transplantation. Once approved, then a new approval for living-lobar lung donor transplantation should be sought. Although the surgical technique and donor acquisition differs, the rest of the transplant procedure is the same. If the insurer is willing to provide benefits for cadaveric lung transplantation, the same benefits should be made available for living-lobar lung donor transplantation.

Most lung transplant centers have a transplant social worker and/or a financial counselor who can assist you. Usually you can ask for, and receive a case manager from your health insurance company. This person can be of great help in sorting through the process. In addition, UNOS has a free booklet, called "What Every Patient Needs to Know," that provides extensive information about financing transplantation. To obtain a copy, contact UNOS at 888-TX INFO-1 (888-894-6361).

MAJOR MEDICAL INSURANCE: Major medical policies were the original health insurance prior to managed care. These polices generally have a deductible and usually pay 75% to 90% of the bill. If you have this type of insurance, you need to contact your insurance representative to find out if lung transplantation is a covered service under their policy. If so, they may require that you go to one of their "centers of excellence." Some plans may help pay for the cost of travel to one of those centers if it is not nearby.

Most plans require that transplantation be pre-authorized. You should also find out what percentage of the cost is paid for by your insurance company, what deductibles or co-payments exist, and if there is a lifetime cap on coverage, or a cap on your annual out-of-pocket expenses. Since the transplant medications are expensive, you need to find out if prescription drugs are covered, and if, so, what, if any, limitations there are.

MANAGED CARE ORGANIZATIONS: Managed care organizations (or Health Management Organizations/HMOs) are similar to major medical insurance, except they restrict your choice of doctors and hospitals in order to make health care less costly. However, some plans have a PPO (Preferred Provider Organization) option through which you can go to providers outside the network, but you must pay an additional fee.

If you have an HMO, you will have to contact it to determine if it will cover lung transplantation. Some of these plans contract with a center located in another area of the country and will transport you to that center when the organ becomes available. Usually, you are permitted to take one person from your family with you.

Average First-Year Costs for Lung and Heart-Lung Transplantation

	Lung	*Heart-Lung*
Pre-Transplant Evaluation:	16,100	16,100
Organ Procurement:	24,000	24,000
Transplant Episode/Hospital Charge:	143,300	210,800
Transplant Episode/Physicians' Charges:	13,800	29,700
One-Year Followup Care:	43,000	43,000
Out-Patient Drugs:	12,800	12,300
GRAND TOTAL:	$253,000	$335,900

Table 2. *Average first-year costs for lung and heart-lung transplantation in year 2001 dollars. (Data provided by Millman and Robertson Inc.)*

EXTENDING INSURANCE COVERAGE THROUGH COBRA: If you are insured by a group health plan at work and leave your job or have your working hours reduced because of a medical condition or disability, you and your family may qualify for extended coverage through COBRA.

COBRA stands for the Consolidated Omnibus Reconciliation Act of 1985. This is a federal law that requires certain group health plans to allow participating employees and their dependents to extend their insurance coverage up to 18 months. This requirement is limited to companies employing 20 or more people.

While you may receive extended coverage through COBRA, you will be fully responsible for the full cost of your group health plan, which can be expensive. In addition, special rules exist for individuals who are disabled when their employment terminated or hours were reduced; the 18-month period is extended to 29 months. For more information about COBRA, contact the personnel department where you work.

HOSPITALIZATION OR INDEMNITY POLICIES: This type of coverage is designed to provide a fixed daily benefit regardless of your expenses, but only when you need treatment for a covered accident or sickness. Hospitalization policies are not Medicare Supplemental Insurance.

Federal Health Insurance Plans:

If you do not have private insurance, there are several federal and state programs in place which may be able to help you obtain the necessary funds for transplantation.

CHAMPUS: Government funding for qualified families of active duty, retired or deceased military personnel may be available through the Civilian Health and Medical Program of the Uniformed Services (CHAMPUS). CHAMPUS shares the cost of heart, lung, heart-lung, liver, kidney and combined liver-kidney transplants for patients. Patients must receive pre-authorization from the CHAMPUS medical director and meet CHAMPUS selection criteria. In addition, the transplant procedure must be performed at a CHAMPUS- or Medicare-certified transplantation center.

For more information regarding CHAMPUS transplantation benefits, contact a patient representative at your nearest VA health care facility, or call the CHAMPUS Benefits Service branch at 303-361-1126 (for active duty or retired veterans) or the U.S. Department of Veterans Affairs at 800-827-1000. For dependants of deceased veterans, call the Department of Veterans Affairs Health Administration Center at 800-733-8387 or check out their website at: http://www.va.gov

Veterans of the Armed Forces who first become ill while in service or who are indigent as defined by the Veterans Administration (VA), may be eligible to receive a transplant at a VA Medical Center. Some veterans may also receive medications funded by the VA. For more information, contact your local VA office or your nearest VA Medical Center.

CHAMPVA: The Civilian Health and Medical Program of VA (CHAMPVA) is available to certain dependents and survivors of veterans. The VA shares with eligible beneficiaries the cost of certain health care services and supplies. For more information, contact the CHAMPVA Center at 800-538-9552.

TRICARE: TRICARE, administered by the Department of Defense, is available to military retirees whose income or assets make them ineligible for VA health care benefits and to dependents of active duty military or retired military personnel, age 17 and older. For more information, call the Veterans Administration TRICARE at 800-470-8262 or 520-629-4728, or the TriWest Health Care Finders at 888-TRIWEST (888-874-9378).

MEDICAID: Medicaid is a federal and state health insurance program for certain low-income and needy individuals. It is administered by the Health Care Financing Administration and is designed to provide access to quality health care for elders, disabled individuals and their families who cannot otherwise afford health care. Within national guidelines, each state establishes its own standards of eligibility.

Each program varies considerably from state to state. However, some states have what is called a "spend-down" program. Medicaid spend-down is for individuals whose income exceeds the regular Medicaid income limits but who meet all the other requirements. Most Medicaid programs cover inpatient and outpatient hospital services, physician services, medical services, laboratory and x-ray services and prescribed drugs. However, some states do not cover the cost of lung or heart-lung transplants.

Signed into law is the "Ticket to Work and Work Incentives Improvement Act of 1999" (H.R. 1180), which eliminates income, assets and resource limitations for disabled individuals who return to work. It also provides the opportunity for employed individuals with a medically improved disability to buy into Medicaid.

Applications for Medicaid can be picked up or mailed to you from your local Department of Public Welfare office. To find out who you should contact in your state call 410-786-3000 or check out Medicaid's website at: http://www.hcfa.gov/medicaid/medicaid.htm

MEDICARE: Medicare is a federally funded health insurance program. It currently covers lung and heart-lung transplants for Medicare-eligible patients, but only if the operation is performed at approved centers. You may qualify for Medicare as part of Social Security benefits if you are 65 or older, if you have been receiving Social Security disability benefits for 24 months or as a dependent of a Medicare beneficiary.

The Balanced Budget Act of 1997 created the "Medicare+Choice" program to expand the range of health care options available to Medicare beneficiaries. This new plan allows beneficiaries to choose from five Medicare-provider options. Each of the options are summarized below.

In addition, information about Medicare managed care options can be obtained from the "Medicare Compare" database on their website at: http://www.medicare.gov. This database allows beneficiaries to compare Medicare health plan providers, benefits, premiums and costs and is searchable by state and zip code. For more information, contact Medicare at 800-MEDICARE (800-633-4227).

Original Medicare Plan (Fee-For-Service): The original Medicare Plan is the traditional pay-per-visit arrangement. You can go to any doctor, hospital or provider who accepts Medicare. You must pay the deductible, then Medicare pays its share, 80%, and you pay your share, 20%. The original Medicare Plan has two basic components: Part A and Part B. Part A (Hospital Insurance) helps pay for care in hospitals and skilled nursing facilities, and for home health and hospice care. If you are eligible, Part A is free and you don't have to pay a premium because you or your spouse paid Medicare taxes while you were working. Part B (Medical Insurance) helps pay for doctors, outpatient hospital care and some other medical services that Part A doesn't cover, such as physical and occupational therapists.

You are automatically eligible for Part B if you are eligible for Part A, however Part B is voluntary. If you choose Part B, the monthly premium is deducted from your Social Security payment. Part A and B only pay 80% of approved charges and do not cover outpatient prescription drugs. However, an exception is made for immunosuppressant drugs.

Medicare provides coverage of prescription drugs used in immunosuppressive therapy provided for by The Omnibus Budget Reconciliation Act (OBRA) of 1993. This act authorized phased in extensions of immunosuppressive medications for 36 months, provided the surgery occurs at a Medicare-approved facility and the individual had Medicare at the time of transplantation.

However, over the last two years, revisions to this coverage has been approved. In 1999, coverage of anti-rejection medications was extended 44 months under the Medicare Balanced Budget Refinement Act. Then on Dec. 15, 2000, Congress extended immunosuppressive medications for certain Medicare patients for the life of their transplant as part of a broad spending and Medicare bill.

Original Medicare Plan with a Supplemental Policy:* With the original Medicare Plan, Medicare pays its share of the bill and you pay the balance. However, you may purchase one of 10 standard Supplemental Insurance Policies (Medigap or Medicare SELECT) for extra benefits. You pay the Part B premium and an additional premium for your Supplemental Policy.

These policies may pay for some or all of the Medicare co-insurance amounts, some or all deductibles, and certain services not covered by the original Medicare Plan. These may include outpatient prescription drugs, some preventative screenings, some care in your home, and emergency medical care for travel outside the United States. Medicare subscribers who apply for a Supplemental Policy within six months of signing up for Medicare Part B must be accepted, regardless of health.

Medicare Managed Care:* A Managed Care Plan involves a group of doctors, hospitals and other health care providers who have agreed to provide care to Medicare beneficiaries in exchange for a fixed amount of money from Medicare every month. Managed Care Plans include HMOs, HMOs with a POS option (Point of Service) or a PPO option (Preferred Provider Organizations).

HMO subscribers receive the benefits of Medicare and Medigap coverage in one plan but are limited to the use of approved plan doctors and services. Under the PPO option, individuals use in plan doctors, hospitals and other services (much like the HMO option) but have the option to use health care services and providers outside the plan at a higher rate.

With an HMO Managed Care plan, you receive all Medicare covered services in addition to other benefits, such as prescription drug coverage. You pay the Medicare premium for Part B, plus you may pay a monthly premium and a co-payment per visit or service. However, most of these plans have instituted a annual limit on how much prescription drug coverage they will provide.

continued on page 49

HEALTH PLAN PURCHASING COOPERATIVES:

Another solution to finding health insurance is to opt for a health plan purchasing cooperative or alliance. These organizations help small employers obtain health insurance using the combined buying power of its member employers to obtain employee health insurance at a competitive rate. The Institute for Health Policy Solutions in Washington (http://www.ihps.org) suggests calling one of the following programs. If your state is not listed here, contact your state's insurance department. To obtain the phone number, call the National Insurance Consumer Helpline at 800-942-4242.

STATE:	PLAN:	NO. of EMPLOYEES:	REGION:	PHONE:
California	Pacific Health Advantage (PacAdvantage), http://www.pacadvantage.org	2 to 50	statewide	877-472-2238
Colorado	The Cooperative for Health Insurance Purchasing, http://www.alliance-chip.com	any size	statewide	800-996-2447 or 303-333-6767
Connecticut	Connecticut Business and Industry Association/ Health Connections, http://www.cbia.com	3 to 50	statewide	860-244-1900
Illinois	Illinois Manufacturers Association/ Health Options	2 to 50	Chicago area	800-482-0462
Kansas	Alliance Employee Health Access Inc., http://www.alliancehealth.org	2 to 50	statewide	785-266-1970
Michigan	Detroit Regional Chamber/Insurance Division	n. a.	Detroit Metro area	313-596-0368
Montana	Community Health Options	2 or more	n. a.	406-721-6275
New York	Long Island Association Health Alliance, http://www.liassoc.com	2 to 50	Long Island, Brooklyn, Queens, Nassau and Suffolk Counties	800-542-5513 or 516-493-3007
New York	HealthPass, http://www.healthpass.com	2 to 50	5 boroughs of NYC	888-313-7277
N. Carolina	Caroliance, http://www.caroliance.com	less than 50	statewide	800-873-6464
Ohio	Council of Smaller Enterprises (COSE), http://www.clevelandgrowth.com	1 to 250	N.E. Ohio	888-304-4769 or 216-621-3300
Oregon	Associated Oregon Industries - Healthchoice, http://www.aoi.org	2 to 50	statewide	800-390-3807
Utah	Care of Utah	2 to 50	statewide	801-355-2273
Washington	Association of Washington Businesses/ HealthChoice	3 or more	statewide	800-521-9325 or 206-943-1600

continued from page 47

* Some Medicare supplemental policies and managed care plans do not count the costs of lifesaving drugs, such as immunosuppressants like cyclosporine, Prograf and azathioprine, as part of the plan's prescription drug limitation. Rather they "carve out" those costs from the medical part of the plan. You pay the co-payment price and the insurance company pays the remainder.

Private Fee-for-Service Plan: You can choose a private insurance plan that accepts Medicare beneficiaries. You may go to any doctor or hospital you want. The insurance plan, rather than the Medicare program, decides how much to reimburse for the services you receive. You may have extra benefits the original Medicare Plan doesn't cover. You pay the Medicare premium for Part B, plus the Private Fee-for-Service Plan charges and an amount per visit or service. Providers are allowed to bill beyond what the plan pays, and you will be responsible for paying whatever the plan doesn't.

Medicare Medical Savings Account Plan (MSA): This is a test program for 390,000 eligible Medicare beneficiaries. Medicare pays the premium for the Medical MSA Plan and makes a deposit in your Medicare MSA to pay for medical expenses. If you don't use all the money in your Medicare MSA, next year's deposit will be added to your balance.

Money can be withdrawn from a Medicare MSA for nonmedicare expenses, but that money will be taxed. If you enroll in a Medicare MSA Plan, you must stay in it for a full year. You can only sign up for a Medicare MSA Plan in November of each year or during special enrollment periods. You pay the Part B premium, and you use the money in your Medicare MSA to pay for medical expenses.

Unlike other Medicare health plans, there are no limits on what providers can charge you above the amount paid by your Medicare MSA Plan. If you use all of your Medicare MSA money, you are still responsible for paying all of your medical expenses until you meet the deductible for your Medicare MSA Plan.

The following are some of the many publications available to Medicare beneficiaries from any Social Security office or by calling 800-MEDICARE (800-633-4227) or TDD at 877-486-2048.

Medicare & You 2000 (Publication No. HCFA-10050) is a summary of Medicare benefits, rights and obligations and answers to the most frequently asked questions about Medicare.

Guide to Health Insurance for People with Medicare discusses what Medicare pays and does not pay, and types of health insurance to supplement Medicare and gives hints on shopping for private insurance.

Medicare Questions and Answers (Publication No. HCFA-10117) provides answers to the most frequently asked questions about Medicare.

Medicare Supplemental Insurance/Medigap Policies and Protections (Publication No. 10139) is a booklet explaining Medigap policies and what they cover, your rights to buy a Medigap policy when your health coverage changes and where to get help.

> *"Lung transplantation is a modern miracle. My son was near death five years ago, but now is a living, breathing, productive member of society and a joy to his mother."*
> *– Marie Barry*

Other Types of Health Insurance:

Many trade groups offer group health plans. Also, check with your local Chamber of Commerce. Statewide small business associations are another possible source for health insurance. To find out if your state has such a group, contact:

The National Small Business United
Phone: 800-345-6728 or 202-293-8830, Fax 202-872-8543,
E-mail: nsbu@nsbu.org
1156 15th St., N.W., Suite 1100, Washington, D.C. 20005
Website: http://www.nsbu.org

If you are self-employed, you may want to try contact:

The Home Office Association of America
Phone: 800-809-4622 (in NYC 212-588-9097), Fax 212-588-9156
133 E. 58th St., Suite 711, New York, NY 10022
Website: http://www.hoaa.com

The National Association for the Self-Employed
Phone: 800-232-NASE (800-232-6273)
P.O. Box 612067, DFW Airport, Dallas TX 75261-2067
Website: http://www.nase.org

HIGH RISK INSURANCE POOLS: Some insurance companies provide coverage to state residents with serious medical conditions who can't find a company to insure them. These companies open enrollment during certain times of the year or on a year-round basis. These policies are rather expensive and not available in all states. However, when available, they may be an excellent way to obtain necessary health coverage. To see if your state has a high-risk insurance pool, contact your state's Department of Insurance or Insurance Commissioner.

Other Sources of Funding:

CHARITABLE ORGANIZATIONS: Some charitable organizations provide financial assistance through grants and direct funding. However, it is unlikely that one group can cover all costs associated with transplantation. For more information on charitable organizations check your local library.

FUNDRAISING CAMPAIGNS: Patients and families often use fundraising to help cover expenses not paid by medical insurance, such as childcare, transportation, food and lodging. This may, in fact, be a key source for financing transplantation. Proceed with caution and plan carefully before you begin; there are many legal and financial issues to consider. If you and your family have received Medicaid benefits, and funds are raised for you, the donated money may be counted as income.

Questions You Might Ask:
- How are donated funds kept? How are they released?
- How can I find out the status of my funds?
- Are there any fees deducted from actual funds?
- If I don't receive a transplant, what will happen to the funds raised?

- What if the funds exceed the cost of the operation?
- How many patients and families have you worked with?
- Can you offer references from other patients you have helped?
- Whom should I call if I have any questions or problems?
- Are you a 501C (3) organization, so that money raised on my behalf is tax-deductible by those who contribute?

Before you begin accepting donations, you need to have a place to put the money you receive, such as a trust fund or a special account. Public donations should never be mixed with personal funds. Check with your local government for legal requirements. *(For information about organizations that assist with fundraising, see page 211.)*

SOCIAL SECURITY: The Social Security Administration provides general financial assistance and medication grants to transplant patients through Supplemental Security Income (SSI), Medicare, and Social Security Disability Income (SSDI). Most transplant patients qualify for some kind of Social Security payments.

If your medical condition keeps you from doing any work for which you are qualified, and your disability is expected to last at least a year or to result in death, you should apply for Social Security. Unlike other disability policies, Social Security does not recognize partial or short-term disability.

To qualify, you must have earned enough work credits from the time you were able to work. You may receive benefits at any age. Other members of your family may also qualify for benefits. They include unmarried dependent children (including stepchildren, adopted children or, in some cases, grandchildren); unmarried children with a disability; or your spouse (if he or she is age 62 or older, disabled or caring for a child).

You should apply as soon as you become disabled since the claims process takes 60 to 90 days. You can apply by phone or mail or visit any Social Security office. If you are working part-time and make more than $740/month (adjusted annually) you will be automatically disqualified. If you are considered disabled, you will begin receiving SSDI benefits in the sixth month after the date you became totally disabled. You may qualify for SSI instead of, or in addition to, your SSDI benefits.

Social Security also publishes a large selection of free informational pamphlets and factsheets on its benefit programs, including Disability, Medicare, Supplemental Security Income and Survivors benefits. You can get copies at your local Social Security office or by calling 800-772-1213. For more information, check out their website at: http://www.ssa.gov

Understanding the Benefits (Publication Number 05-10024) tells you what you need to know about Social Security while you're still working and what you need to know when it's your turn to collect benefits.

Disability Benefits (Publication No. 05-10029) is a guide to Social Security disability benefits.

SSI (Publication No. 05-11000) explains the Supplemental Security Income program, which provides a basic income to people who are 65 or older, disabled or blind who have limited income and resources.

What You Need to Know When You Get Disability Benefits (Publication No. 05-10153) is a guide to your disability benefits.

KEEPING YOUR SANITY:

"Life throws you curve balls, you just have to dodge them and go on."
– Beth Davenport

Support and Counseling:

Most transplant programs offer support group meetings for patients and their family members. These meetings can be informal or may include speakers. At these meetings, participants get a chance to meet patients who have had successful transplants, as well as those patients whose transplants have failed. Patients often learn from and find hope from each other's struggles and triumphs. In addition, strong ties and a sense of community usually develops between members for what can be a lonely process.

Since there are many stresses associated with transplantation, it is helpful to discuss these with a counselor. A professional psychologist, psychiatrist or social worker is often a member of the transplant team, and is available for individual or family counseling. This can help individuals and/ or families to communicate, and best prepare for, and cope with the many adjustments and uncertainties that go along with transplantation.

Relaxation Techniques:

Learning simple relaxation techniques can greatly improve your ability to get through the period before, during and after your transplant. Many types of relaxation techniques exist that induce what Harvard researcher Herbert Benson, M.D., has termed the "relaxation response," a state of mental and physical calm elicited through focused concentration. The resulting physiological state is characterized by a slowing of heart and respiratory rates and a decrease in blood pressure. Practiced regularly, focused relaxation can increase mental awareness and produce a healthy detachment from daily anxieties.

There are quite a number of different relaxation techniques available; some may work for you, but not for others. For example, meditation that focuses on breathing may NOT be good for people with respiratory disease; guided imagery may work better. You can find instruction in relaxation techniques through libraries, books, stress management clinics, holistic education centers and some hospitals and medical centers. The most common types of relaxation techniques include:

GUIDED IMAGERY or VISUALIZATION helps to guide and focus your thoughts on pleasurable and calming images through the use of audiotapes or a therapist.

MEDITATION can be a spiritual as well as physical, practice designed to produce a shift in consciousness from an external focus of attention to an internal one. Forms range from the use of breathing, mantras, visual images, sounds, repetitive movement (Tai Chi), prayers, chants or affirmations.

PROGRESSIVE MUSCLE RELAXATION involves the tensing and relaxing of muscle groups in a progressive format, focusing on the sensations experienced, and recognizing the difference between tense and relaxed.

BIOFEEDBACK refers to a group of computer assisted procedures in which an external sensor is used to provide the participant with an indication of the state of bodily relaxation, usually in an attempt to effect a change in a measured quantity, such as heart rate or blood pressure. This technique is often done in a clinical setting.

HYPNOSIS uses a state of trance, with or without a therapist, that creates a relaxed state of awareness. Suggestions are given that the subconscious mind will accept, and then act on in a positive and helpful way.

MASSAGE THERAPY is a practice in which a trained practitioner uses hands to manipulate or otherwise affect soft and superficial tissue.

Coping Skills:

Things you can do to help you cope through a difficult situation include:
- Spending time alone
- Adding structure to your days
- Developing a new hobby
- Adopting a new pet

THE VOICE OF EXPERIENCE

Strength in Numbers

In 1990, lung transplantation was not being offered in any of the hospitals near where I lived in Cincinnati, Ohio. So, when the decision was made to have a lung transplant, I chose Barnes/Jewish in St. Louis, Mo., which was a six-hour drive away. Needless to say this move was extremely difficult to accept. Leaving family, home and friends for an unknown specified time, in a strange city, and facing the most important decision of my life, was beyond anything I could imagine. At that time, lung transplantation was borderline experimental surgery without long-term data available, so it was like going into battle, not knowing if you would ever return.

At Barnes, we had weekly support group meetings, where we dealt with financial issues, and what to expect in the OR and after transplantation. We also had a patient and caregiver support group once a week where we discussed mutual concerns and fears. There we learned how the post-transplant patients were doing, which always inspired us. However, I was shocked to see how many families began to unravel under the stress of the situation. We had sister leaving sister, spouse leaving spouse. Other family members would come in to help and we had picnics, ballgames and dinners together. A very close-knit, family atmosphere was formed, which has continued to this day.

Going through this experience I learned so much not only about my strengths, but also of the strengths of others. There was always someone worse off than I was, which helped to put everything in perspective. It filled me with compassion and I counted my blessings. But the most important thing I got from these meetings was the camaraderie between the 30 to 40 patients that attended. We were people with different backgrounds, different lung diseases, and of all ages, but we were all united by the same goal: Make it to transplantation. I certainly didn't expect to receive as much as I did by going to these support groups, but it was truly a memorable experience – and one I'll never regret.

– Janet Kolish, single-lung transplant recipient,
Sept. 15, 1991

- Learning new skills
- Keeping a diary or journal
- Attending religious groups
- Making time for play, humor and laughter; laughter stimulates the brain's production of endorphins, which decreases the body's perception of pain, and lowers blood pressure,
- Exercising
- Socializing with family and friends; stay connected to the outside world
- Prioritizing your time and energy
- Indulging yourself, e.g., take a bubble bath or get a massage
- Learning what you can and can't control
- Accepting the good with the bad
- Staying open to change
- Relaxing your standards; the world will not end if your house is not cleaned this weekend.
- Counting your blessings; for every one thing that goes wrong, there are probably ten blessings.
- Believing in yourself and adopting a positive attitude
- Concentrating on what you can still do, not on what you can't
- Stating your needs and wants; accepting support from others
- Learning to say no
- Learning to live one day at a time
- Showing and sharing your feelings
- Trusting others.

Negative coping skills, which may offer some short-term relief, but can create additional problems if repeated over a long period of time, include:
- Drug and alcohol use
- Passivity and procrastination
- Denial, pretending nothing's wrong, ignoring the problem
- Fault-finding, stubbornness, demanding your way
- Tantrums, pouting, withdrawal from friends and family
- Keeping your feelings to yourself
- Worrying or imagining the worst.

Your Support Network:

The importance of having at least one very good support person to assist you, before and after the transplant, cannot be stressed enough. However, some patients have had success going through the process alone by planning ahead for home health services, etc. In creating your support network, you may find that some people are good for emotional support, while others are not. You will find some people have their own way of expressing their support for you, but it might not be the type that you want or need. Be very clear when talking to people about what your needs are. If you don't ask, they may not know how to help.

A mistake often made by patients living with a chronic illness is to expect ALL their needs to be meet by one person. It is not only unrealistic, but often impossible. Support can come from a variety of sources, such as physicians, psychologists, social workers, clergy, friends, social workers, etc. Spread the load among as many people as possible and learn how to delegate. Often, people whom you never expected would come through for you will. Also, people whom you thought you could rely on, won't be there for you. Many people find providing support for chronically ill people a

Through Thick and Thin

In 1974, my husband, Richard, was diagnosed with alpha-$_1$ antitrypsin deficiency. Richard was 28 at the time and had 30% lung function. During the early days after his diagnosis, denial was the easiest coping mechanism I could muster. Although it may not have been the most productive, it was easier to concentrate on our two young children than on Richard's condition.

As Richard became increasingly ill and had more and more hospitalizations, my focus turned more toward him, but I was determined the children have as "normal" a life as possible. They participated in all the activities they wanted; I didn't want them to miss out because Dad was sick.

20 years later, Richard was accepted on the waiting list for a single-lung transplant, which he received on Jan. 11, 1995. Once Richard recuperated from the transplant surgery, I quit my job to begin a home-based business so we could spend more time together. It was important to me that he could do anything he wanted now that he had a new life!

He did extremely well for the first three years. He went from being confined to a wheelchair for 15 years – to walking everywhere! But in December 1997, he was diagnosed with chronic rejection. After living most of my life "waiting for the other shoe to drop," it seemed as though the shoe was now closer to the floor. It was devastating to watch him lose lung function again, get back on oxygen, and finally, get back into a wheelchair! All I could do was hope and pray that a second transplant would take place and be successful.

He was listed for a retransplant in March 1998, but was diagnosed with liver cancer in March 1999 and died on June 7, 1999. After Richard's death it became painfully obvious to me that I had no healthy friends. I had spent most of my married life caring for a chronically ill husband and our children. Yes, I had friends, but most of them were from the alpha-$_1$ and lung transplant community.

I have since learned that, as a caregiver, one MUST take care of your own needs, in addition to the ones of those you care for. It is very important to maintain your own circle of friends and hobbies, and have ways to get away to rejuvenate your strength, confidence and spirit. Through all the ups and downs, I always took care of Richard and my family, but never myself. Now I know better, and understand that thinking of oneself is not selfish – it is the only way to stay healthy, and ultimately, be the best caregiver for your loved one.

– Evelyn Heering, wife of Richard Heering, single-lung transplant recipient, Jan. 11, 1995

---

scary and a demanding task, and some may not be up to the challenge.

The impact declining health can have on marital relations can be traumatic. Much of the discord comes from changes in your financial circumstances, shifts in the division of household labor and a decline in the kinds of relations and activities shared. Marital discord is often felt somewhat greater by the spouses, rather than the afflicted person. This is why is it important to recognize the signs of stress in yourself and in your caregiver. Too much stress can be damaging to both you and the person who is caring for you. The following are stress indicators to watch out for:

TEN SIGNS OF CAREGIVER STRESS:
1) Denial about the disease and its effect on the person diagnosed

2) Anger at the person with the disease or others that no effective treatments or cures currently exist and that people don't understand
3) Withdrawal from friends and activities that once brought pleasure
4) Anxiety about facing another day and what the future holds
5) Depression begins to break your spirit and affects your ability to cope
6) Exhaustion makes it nearly impossible to complete daily tasks
7) Sleeplessness caused by a never-ending list of concerns
8) Irritability leads to moodiness and triggers negative reactions
9) Lack of concentration makes it difficult to perform familiar tasks
10) Health problems begin to take their toll physically.

If your caregiver experiences several of these symptoms on a regular basis, consult a physician, or use some of the following steps to help manage the stress in your life:

MANAGING STRESS FOR CAREGIVERS:
- Get help. Trying to do everything yourself will leave you exhausted. The support of family, friends and community resources can be enormous. If assistance is not offered, ask for it! And if you have difficulty asking for assistance, have someone close to you advocate for you. If stress becomes overwhelming, don't be afraid to seek professional help.
- Know what resources are available in your community. Adult day care, visiting nurses, delivery services and meals-on-wheels are just a few of the community resources available that can help.
- Accept changes as they occur. People with chronic illness change and so do their needs. They often require care beyond what you can provide.
- Become educated and involved in treatment options, care techniques and suggestions from your health care team. Ask questions and don't let up until you understand ALL the options.
- Be realistic. Until a cure is found, progression is inevitable. The care you provide does make a difference. Give yourself permission to GRIEVE for the losses you experience, but also focus on the positive moments as they occur and enjoy your good memories.
- Do legal and financial planning. Consult an attorney and discuss issues related to durable power of attorney, living wills and trusts. Planning now can alleviate stress later.
- Manage your own level of stress. Stress can cause physical problems (stomach irritation, high blood pressure, etc.) and changes in behavior (irritability, lack of concentration, loss of appetite, etc.). Use relaxation techniques that work for you, and, if these don't help, consult a physician.

Give yourself CREDIT, not guilt. Occasionally, you may lose patience and at times be unable to provide all the care the way you'd like. Remember that you are only human and doing the best you can. Your loved one needs you and you ARE there. That's something to be proud of.

BIBLIOGRAPHY:

Alzheimer's Association. "Caregivers Stress: Signs to Watch Out For . . . and Steps to Take," brochure 1995.

American College of Sports Medicine. "ASCM's Guidelines for Exercise Testing and Prescription." 5th Edition, 1995, Williams and Wilkins publishers.

American Thoracic Society (ATS). "Lung Transplantation: Report of the ATS Workshop on Lung Transplantation." *American Review of Respiratory Disease* 1993; 147: 772 - 776.

Arcasoy, Selim M., and Kotloff, Robert M. "Lung Transplantation." *The New England Journal of Medicine* 1999; 340 (14): 1081 - 90.

Barr, M., Schenkel, F., Cohen, R., Barbers, R., Fuller, C., Hagen, J., Wells, W., and Starnes, V. "Recipient and Donor Outcomes in Living Related and Unrelated Lobar Transplantation." *Transplant Proceedings* 1998; 30: 2261 - 2263.

Booth, Alan, and Johnson, David R. "Declining Health and Marital Quality." *The Journal of Marriage and the Family* 1994, 56: 218 - 223.

Boucek, M., Faro, A., Novick, R., Bennett, L., Fiol, B., Keck, B., and Hosenpud, J. "The Registry of the International Society of Heart and Lung Transplantation: Third Official Pediatric Report – 1999." *The Journal of Heart and Lung Transplantation* 1999; 18: 1151 - 72.

Boucek, M., Novick, R., Bennett, L., Fiol, B., Keck, B., and Hosenpud, J. "The Registry of the International Society of Heart and Lung Transplantation: Second Official Pediatric Report – 1998." *The Journal of Heart and Lung Transplantation* 1998; 17: 1141 - 60.

Bridges, Nancy D. "Lung Transplantation in Children." *Current Opinion in Cardiology* 1998; 13: 73 - 7.

Culp, Larry. "Flying With Oxygen," *Cystic Fibrosis Network* newsletter, Vol. 5 (3), January 1997, 5.

Davis, R. D., and Pasque, M. "Pulmonary Transplantation: Review Article." *Annuals of Surgery* 1995, 221: 14 - 28.

Gammie, J., Stukus, D., Pham, S., Hattler, B., McGrath, M., McCurry, K., Griffith, B., and Keenan, R. "Effect of Ischemia Time on Survival in Clinical Lung Transplantation." 35th Annual Meeting of the Society of Thoracic Surgeons 1999, Abstracts.

Health Care Financing Administration. "Medicare Program: Criteria for Medicare Coverage of Lung Transplants." Federal Register 1995; 60 (22): 6537 - 47.

International Society for Heart and Lung Transplantation. "17th Annual Data Report." April 2000.

Jones, N., Berman, L., Bartkiewicz, P., and Oldridge, N. "Chronic Obstructive Respiratory Disorders." *Exercise Testing and Exercise Prescription for Special Cases: Theoretical Basis and Clinical Application* (2nd Edition), James S. Skinner, Lea & Febiger, Philadelphia, 1993, 229 - 240.

Keller, Cesar A. "The Donor Lung: Conservation of a Precious Resource." *Thorax* 1998; 53: 506 - 13.

Meyers, B., Lynch, J., Trulock, E., Guthrie, T., Cooper, J., and Patterson, G. A. "Lung Transplantation: A Decade of Experience." *Annals of Surgery* 1999; 230 (3): 362 - 71.

Novick, Richard J. "Heart and Lung Retransplantation: Should It Be Done?" *The Journal of Heart and Lung Transplantation* 1998; 17: 635 - 42.

Novick, R., Stitt, L., Al-Kattan, K., Klepetko, W., Schäfers, H., Duchatelle, J., Khaghini, A., Hardesty, R., Patterson, G. A., and Yacoub, M. for the Pulmonary Retransplant Registry. "Pulmonary Retransplantation: Predictors of Graft Function and Survival in 230 Patients." *Annals of Thoracic Surgery* 1998; 65: 227 - 234.

Patterson, Alexander G. "Indications: Unilateral, Bilateral, Heart-Lung, and Lobar Transplant Procedures." *Clinics in Chest Medicine* 1997; 18 (2): 225 - 30.

Smolin, Tracey L., and Aguiar, Laura J. "Psychosocial and Financial Aspects of Lung Transplantation." *Critical Care Nursing Clinics of North America* 1996; Vol. 8 (3): 293 - 303.

Starnes, Vaughn A., et al. "Living-Donor Lobar Lung Transplantation Experience: Intermediate Results." *The Journal of Thoracic and Cardiovascular Surgery* 1996; 112: 1284 - 91.

Starnes, V., Barr, M., Schenkel, F., Horn, M., Cohen, R., Hagen, J., Wells, W. "Experience with Living-Donor Lobar Transplantation for Indications Other Than Cystic Fibrosis." *The Journal of Thoracic and Cardiovascular Surgery* 1997; 114: 917 - 922.

Stillwell, Paul C., and Mallory, Jr., George B. "Pediatric Lung Transplantation." *Clinics in Chest Medicine* 1997; 18 (2): 405 - 14.

Thoracic Organ Transplantation Committee. "Recommended Guidelines for Listing Candidates for Lung and Heart-Lung Transplantation." Modified November 1997. A Report of the United Network for Organ Sharing Board of Directors Meeting, June 25 - 26, 1998.

Trulock, Elbert P. "Lung Transplantation." *The American Journal of Respiratory and Critical Care Medicine* 1997, 155: 789 - 818.

United Network for Organ Sharing. "1997 Report of the OPTN: Waiting List Activity and Donor Procurement: Lung Volume." 1a.

United Network for Organ Sharing. "UNOS Policies, By-Laws and Articles." Nov. 19, 1999.

United Network for Organ Sharing. "The Scientific Registry and Organ Procurement and Transplantation Network Annual Report." 1998.

United Network for Organ Sharing. "The Scientific Registry and Organ Procurement and Transplantation Network Annual Report." 1999.

United Network for Organ Sharing. The Scientific Registry and Organ Procurement and Transplantation Network, 2000.

Weinberger, Steven E. *Principles of Pulmonary Medicine* 1996: 51 - 61.

Williams, Trevor J., and Snell, Gregory I. "Early and Long-Term Functional Outcomes in Unilateral, Bilateral, and Living-Related Transplant Recipients." *Clinics in Chest Medicine* 1997; 18 (2): 245 - 57.

2 During Transplantation

WHAT TO EXPECT THE DAY OF THE TRANSPLANT:

"This operation scares the hell out of me – but the alternative scares me even more."
– Gary Shields

The day or night that you receive the call from your transplant center that your donor lung(s) or heart are available will be a very exciting time. You will experience a wide variety of emotions including happiness, sadness, anxiety and fear. When a suitable donor is found, the transplant coordinator on duty will notify you. Once contacted, you will be instructed not to eat or drink anything. Usually, patients are admitted to the hospital through the emergency room, unless they are already an inpatient. The transplant coordinator will prepare you for the surgery. Generally, he or she will be available to update your family on the progress of your operation.

Depending on the time available, the following tests and procedures may be performed BEFORE you go to the operating room:
- Short history and physical exam
- Preoperative blood work
- Chest x-ray and electrocardiogram (EKG)
- Urine sample
- Betadine scrub
- Administration of the first dose of anti-rejection medication
- Aerosol/nebulizer treatment or chest physiotherapy treatment, if indicated
- Sinus irrigation, if indicated
- Placement of an IV catheter in your arm
- Meetings with the surgeon and the anesthesiologist to explain the procedure and answer any last minute questions you might have
- You will be asked to sign a form giving consent to the surgeons and anesthesiologists to perform your surgery.

Dry Runs:

A dry run is the ordeal of getting to the hospital, and getting prepped for surgery, only to find out that the organ was unsuitable for transplant. Roughly one-third of the trips by the "away team" to inspect the donor lungs turn out to be dry runs. Don't get discouraged if you get all the way to the transplant center and are told the organs were too marginal to be accepted. Every effort is made to ensure only the best organs are used for transplantation. But, due to unforeseen complications with the donor organs, the surgery may be called off at the last minute.

WHERE DO THE DONORS COME FROM?

"When we found out that the lungs they had for my Mom were infected with pneumonia, it was disappointing, but also encouraging. It means the real thing could be any day."
– Dani Bednar

Donors are hospital patients that have died and have notified their next of kin they want to be organ donors. In the United States, death is defined as the irreversible cessation of cardiopulmonary function or irreversible cessation of all function of the brain, including the brain stem. Brain death can be a result of severe brain injury, such as a gunshot wound, motor vehicle accident, cerebrovascular accident or other insult to the brain. Cerebrovascular accident is a term that includes strokes or bleeding from ruptured blood vessels in the brain.

Contrary to popular belief, the most common circumstance surrounding brain death is not motor vehicle accidents, but strokes and ruptured aneurysms. In 1998, males represented 58% of all cadaveric donors and females represented 42%. Donors with blood type O represented 48% of cadaveric donors, while those with blood type A accounted for 38%. Minority donors increased from 18% in 1989 to 24% in 1998.

Defining Brain Death:

State laws recognize both cardiac death and brain death criteria in determining death. Brain death is the complete and irreversible cessation of all brain function. Brain death occurs when some sort of brain injury causes the brain to swell. When the brain swells, it pokes through a small hole at the base of the skull (the only place it has to swell) and literally strangles its own blood supply. The brain cannot survive without blood flow. Brain function ceases about four to eight minutes after this occurs.

A physician conducts the required medical tests to make the diagnosis of brain death. These tests are based on sound and accepted medical guidelines and include a clinical examination to show that a person has no brain reflexes and cannot breathe on his or her own. In most cases, the tests are performed twice, with several hours in between to ensure an accurate result. Additionally, other testing may include a blood flow test (cerebral angiogram) or an EEG (electroencephalogram) to confirm the absence of blood flow or brain activity. Any level of brain function does not meet the criteria for brain death, and organs cannot be removed from such patients.

Brain death should not be confused with coma or vegetative state. A patient in a coma is medically and legally alive and may breathe when the ventilator is removed. A patient in vegetative state retains motor reflexes, and has a natural sleep-wake cycle, but is not aware of the activity.

Organ Recovery:

Surgical recovery of organs occurs only after a declaration of death has been made, which can only be done by a licensed physician. In the case of brain death, most states require two licensed physicians, preferably one being a neurosurgeon or neurologist. There is a deliberate and clear separation between the medical team that treats the patient until death and the organ recovery team that removes and preserves the organs after death. Therefore, the doctors who work to save the life of the patient have nothing to do with organ recovery by law.

People who are brain dead can donate tissue and whole organs, including two kidneys, two lungs, heart, liver, pancreas and intestines. Before the organs can be recovered for transplantation, the patient must be formally declared brain dead and consent must be obtained from the next of kin. Most states have passed "required request" laws, which make it mandatory for the hospital to offer the family the option of donating their deceased loved one's organs and tissues.

Organ donors who are brain dead have cardio-respiratory function maintained artificially by a mechanical ventilator. Organs continue to function because the circulation of oxygenated blood is supplied artificially. Special medications help maintain blood pressure and other bodily functions. Organs of brain dead patients can be maintained approximately 24 hours after the insult to the brain. However, depending upon the health of the individual and the extent of injury, they can be kept up to five days, but the sooner the organs are recovered the better.

The Role of the Organ Procurement Organization:

When someone dies or is near death, the hospital contacts the local organ procurement organization (OPO). OPOs are nonprofit organizations that

ORGAN PROCUREMENT AND PLACEMENT

Insult to the Brain
Patient Admitted to the Hospital
↓
If Brain Death Candidate,
Call Made to Organ Procurement Organization (OPO)
↓
OPO Evaluates Potential Donor
↓
Brain Death Declared
OPO Approaches Family for Consent
↓
If Yes, Medical Management of Donor Begins
Tests Performed
↓
Organ Match Run
OPO Contacts Transplant Program to Place Organs
↓
If Accepted,
Transplant Program Calls
↙   ↘

Medical Recovery Team In	Recipient to Transplant Center
↓	↓
Away Team Flies to Donor Hospital to Evaluate Organs	Preparation of Recipient Begins
↓	↓
If Good, Procurement Surgery Proceeds	↓
↓	Recipient to Operating Room
Return to Recipient	↓
↘	Hospital Surgery Begins
	↙

Patient Receives Organ Transplant

coordinate activities related to organ procurement. They are certified by the Health Care Financing Administration for a designated service area. OPOs work with hospitals to identify potential organ donors and to procure medically suitable organs for transplantation. Some OPOs' service area includes a single state or several states, while some states have several OPOs operating within their borders. There are 51 independent OPOs, and 10 in-house OPOs servicing 261 transplant centers.

The OPO is responsible for identifying and evaluating donors and obtaining consent from the family for the recovery of organs. They are also responsible for medically maintaining the donor and making arrangements for their distribution according to national organ sharing policies established by UNOS.

Once a family agrees to donation, a complex series of events take place. The local OPO enters information about the donor organ into the UNOS

THE VOICE OF EXPERIENCE

Dress Rehearsal for "THE CALL"

"THE CALL!" Those words no longer have any power over me. Waiting for that call had been the central focus of my life for a long time. Since I might have to leave at a moment's notice, I abandoned my fledgling career as a freelance artist; I relinquished the Girl Scout troop I had led for eight years; and I no longer volunteered at my daughters' schools. I spent hours watching the telephone, willing it to ring, my heart freezing when it did.

I had, in fact, stopped fearing "THE CALL" even before my son phoned me at midnight to tell me that he would get his new lungs that day. "Hello?" "Mom? You need to come, Dr. Neimeier has some lungs that look good." "OK. I'll be there in 45 minutes. Are you OK?" "Fine, you?" "Fine."

This wasn't the conversation I had envisioned during our 22-month wait. But I had already had rehearsals. The first came when I was at a concert. I told Jasen to call only in the event of "THE CALL" since I didn't want to interrupt the program. When my phone rang, I ran out of the auditorium only to find the battery dead. I turned to get the spare one, ramming into the "Doors Locked During Performances" sign. I paced and swore and hyperventilated for the final ten minutes of the show. When the doors burst open, an avalanche of parents came pouring out. I maneuvered my way through the crowd like a salmon swimming upstream until I was just four rows from my husband. I frantically waved and shouted "Battery!" He launched the battery to me, I jammed it in and speed-dialed Jasen, only to hear, "Could you bring me a box of tissues on your way home?"

The second rehearsal was when Jasen was hospitalized with pneumonia, and feeling healthy enough to get restless and bored. Since he couldn't be transplanted while sick, I took two hours to pamper myself. I slathered on a green, gooey facial mask, wrapped my hair in hot oil and plastic, and relaxed into a tubful of bubbles. I was tempted to ignore the phone when it rang, but hauled myself out, threw on a towel, dripped down the hall and grumpily answered, "Hello?" "Mom, you need to come right now! They're getting ready to transplant me!" "NOW? You're still sick! I'm all wet! How? What? How? U-u-h-h, NOW?" This was followed by a string of gibberish and "APRIL FOOL!" I still can't believe I fell for that one.

– Susan M. Johnson, mother of Jasen T. Shore, bilateral-lung transplant recipient, April 23, 1999

Organ Preservation Time Limits

Lungs ....4 to 6 hours
Heart ....4 to 6 hours
Heart-Lung.....4 to 6 hours
Liver ....12 to 24 hours
Pancreas........12 to 24 hours
Kidney ....48 to 72 hours

Table 3. Organ preservation time limits. (Data provided by the Living Bank.)

computer and obtains a match run sheet – a list of potential recipients ranked according to objective medical criteria (e.g., blood type, size of the donor verses the recipient, time spent on the waiting list and geographical distance between donor and recipient). Each donor organ will generate a differently ranked list of patients.

After printing the list of potential recipients, the OPO coordinator contacts the transplant surgeon caring for the top ranked patient to offer the organ. If the organ is turned down, the next center on the potential recipient list is contacted, and so on until the organ is placed. Once the organ is accepted for a patient, transportation arrangements are made and the transplant surgery is scheduled. This process is quite time consuming and can take approximately 24 hours.

Thoracic Organ Procurement:

The lungs of brain dead donors are much harder to come by than any other organ. Lungs are very sensitive and may rapidly deteriorate due to fluid buildup, chest trauma or injury and infection from being mechanically ventilated. Therefore, the number of donor lungs available for transplant are much lower than the number of donor kidneys, livers or hearts.

Organ donors are evaluated very carefully to ensure they can be safely transplanted and no diseases are transmitted to the recipient. However, medical problems that may prevent organ donation are quite few. These include a few infections and communicable diseases (e.g., HIV infection, encephalitis of unknown cause, malaria, disseminated tuberculosis, Jakob-Creutzfeldt disease, active viral hepatitis infection and malignancy). The following is a list of the type of information a donor center must provide to the recipient center for thoracic organ transplantation according to UNOS' policy.

3.7.12 Minimum Information for Thoracic Organ Offers.
3.7.12.1 Essential Information. The Host OPO or donor center must provide the following donor information to the recipient center with each thoracic organ offer:

(i)   The cause of brain death;
(ii)   The details of any documented cardiac arrest or hypotensive episodes;
(iii)   Vital signs including blood pressure, heart rate and temperature;
(iv)   Cardiopulmonary, social, and drug activity histories;
(v)   Serologies for HIV, hepatitis B and C, and CMV;
(vi)   Accurate height, weight, age and sex;
(vii)   ABO type;
(viii)   Interpreted electrocardiogram and chest radiograph;
(ix)   History of treatment in hospital including vasopressors and hydration;
(x)   Arterial blood gas results and ventilator settings; and
(xi)   Echocardiogram, if the donor hospital has the facilities.

The thoracic organ procurement team must have the opportunity to speak directly with responsible ICU personnel or the on-site donor coordinator in order to obtain current firsthand information about the donor physiology.

3.7.12.3 Essential Information for Lung Offers. In addition to the essential information specified above for a thoracic organ offer, the Host

OPO or donor center shall provide the following specific information with each lung offer:

(i) Arterial blood gases on 5 cm/H_2O/PEEP including PO_2/FiO_2 ratio and preferably 100% FiO_2 within 2 hours prior to the offer;

(ii) Measurement of chest circumference in inches or centimeters at the level of the nipples and X-ray measurement vertically from the apex of the chest to the apex of the diaphragm and transverse at the level of the diaphragm;

(iii) Chest radiograph interpreted by a radiologist or qualified physician within 3 hours prior to the offer;

(iv) Sputum gram stain with a description of the sputum character;

(v) Smoking history.

THE TRANSPLANT PROCEDURE:

"I am thankful for the past 5½ years I've been able to live and for this reason I don't take anything for granted. But, most of all, I will never forget how I got them, where they came from, and how I fought for my life.
– Carolyn Boyd

A lung or heart-lung transplant involves the removal of one or both of the diseased organ(s), and the surgical placement of a healthy organ(s) in its place. The surgical technique used has not changed dramatically in the past 10 years, and can last anywhere from four to 10 hours. The median length of stay in the hospital for a single-lung transplant is 14 days, and 18 days for a bilateral-lung transplant.

Operative Procedure for Single-Lung Transplantation:

An incision is made below the shoulder blade, and along the side of the chest. If your blood pressure and oxygen saturation fall while the blood vessels to the lung on that side are temporarily clamped, tubes will be inserted to connect you to the heart-lung machine, which will support your circulation until the new lung is ready to take over. Your old lung is then removed, and the new lung is sewn in place connecting the blood vessels to and from the lung (via the pulmonary artery and pulmonary vein) and the main airway (bronchus). At the end of the operation the ribs are brought back together, and the incision is closed.

Operative Procedure for Bilateral-Lung Transplantation:

An incision is made across the middle of the chest from your underarm, under your breasts, to the other underarm (otherwise known as a "clamshell" incision). The breastbone is partially divided and the chest cavity is entered between the ribs. The heart-lung machine may be used to support the circulation during the operation. This machine allows surgeons to bypass the blood flow to the heart and lungs. The machine pumps the blood throughout the rest of the body, removing carbon dioxide and replacing it with oxygen needed by body tissues.

The lung on one side is removed, and the new lung is sewn in place. The opposite lung is then removed, and the second lung is sewn in place. At the end of the operation the breastbone is wired back together, the ribs are brought back in place, and the incision is closed.

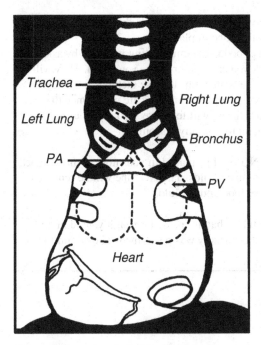

Figure 2. *Posterior view of the lungs, heart, pulmonary arteries (PA) and pulmonary veins (PV). Dashed lines indicate the site of the surgical connection between left and right mainstem bronchi, pulmonary arteries and veins, and cuff of the atrium (the upper chamber of the heart) in the case of heart-lung transplantation.*

Operative Procedure for Heart-Lung Transplantation:

An incision is made down the middle of your chest. Tubes are placed to connect you to the heart-lung machine, which will support your circulation until the new heart is ready to take over. When the donor heart-lung block has arrived, the transplant surgeon removes your old heart and lungs leaving a "cuff" of the atrium (the upper chamber of your heart) and the end of the main airway. This is what they will sew your new heart onto. In addition, they sew the main blood vessel to your body (the aorta) to the aorta of the donor heart. At the end of the operation the breastbone is wired together, and the incision is closed.

Operative Procedure for Living-Lobar Lung Donor Transplantation:

This type of surgery is often considered high-risk because the recipient is often very ill. With this type of operation, there are two donors who match the recipient's blood type. They each give a lobe (small portion) of their lungs to the recipient. The right lung has three lobes, and the left lung has two. The donor should be larger than the recipient so that the donor lobes fill each chest cavity. The three operations are performed simultaneously and typically involve the removal of both lungs in the recipient, and replacing each with the lower lobes from the donors. Patients are put on cardiopulmonary bypass during the operation.

Operative Procedure for Retransplantation:

The operative procedure for retransplantation is virtually the same as the first lung transplant. However, these surgeries are often more difficult because scarring from the original transplant can make the lungs harder to remove, causing more blood loss and the use of transfusions. Because of these problems, some patients are put on a pulmonary bypass machine.

WHAT TO EXPECT DURING YOUR HOSPITAL STAY:

"After an initial rough start getting off the vent, I have not looked back."
– Kathryn Flynn

Most likely, you will recover in the Cardiovascular Intensive Care Unit (CICU) where specially trained nurses will be available to you 24 hours a day. Length of stay in the CICU varies from patient to patient, but the usual stay is between three and seven days.

When You Wake Up:

Most patients wake up two to 10 hours after their surgery is finished. In addition to the following tubes and catheters that will be in place when you wake up, you will be attached to various monitors to track your heart rate (EKG), respiration rate, etc.

BREATHING TUBE (ventilator/respirator) will be placed through your mouth and into your trachea (the main airway). The ventilator breathes for you during surgery and while you are in the CICU until you are strong enough to breathe on your own. Patients remain mechanically ventilated for approximately one to three days, or as long as your body requires. You will not be able to talk or eat with this tube in place.

The CICU nurses are very good at communicating with you by asking yes and no questions, to which you can nod or shake your head. They will also give you paper and pencil to write with. If these methods fail, they often have a spelling board for patients to communicate with. Once the breathing tube is removed, your throat will feel sore. Usually, your nurse will give you ice chips to suck on to ease any discomfort.

NASAL/GASTRIC TUBE (NG) will be placed in your nose to the stomach to allow for the excretion of stomach fluids. The NG tube will be removed as soon as you are ready to take food and/or fluids.

CHEST TUBES are flexible tubes that are passed through your skin and placed around the area where the surgery was performed. They drain the

---

THE VOICE OF EXPERIENCE

A Prophesy Fulfilled

It had been 10 years since Mom died. So long in fact, that I couldn't visualize a clear picture of her. I had been on the waiting list for a lung transplant for five months. I knew it could be another five to 10 months before I would get the call, and even then, it might be a dry run. So, I was just taking life as it came, using my O_2, getting joy from my family and friends, my cat, my books and music. My days were pretty well contained inside the radius of my 50' concentrator hose.

On April 2, 1993, I awoke at 7:45 a.m. feeling breathless, sweating and with tears in my eyes. What a dream! My Mom was there, and I saw her face clearly. I didn't recall everything, but what remained was so vivid I was unable to move for awhile. I had just been with my mother and she was telling me something. The dream concluded by her wrapping me up in a huge hug. Then she pushed me away with a deliberateness that said, "You have something important to do." It stuck with me all that day.

That evening, I was about to settle down in front of the tube with a plateful of pizza to enjoy my favorite show when the phone rang. A voice said, "This is the Transplant Center. We think we have some lungs for you." I froze. I felt like a deer caught in the headlights of a fast moving car. For five minutes I quietly collected my thoughts. Then I replayed the memory of that morning's visit from Mom and I knew I everything would be okay.

I was the beneficiary of two new lungs that night. It was like rising from the dead. The work of rehab was a joy. I tried everything, swimming, walking, cycling, weight-lifting, racquetball. It was all fun. I trained for the 1994 Transplant Games and competed in cycling each year after that, winning a gold medal in 1995. I founded a bike team called "Team Alpha" to increase awareness and detection of alpha-$_1$ antitrypsin deficiency and to increase awareness of organ donation. Since inception, it has raised over $60,000. In 1999, I rode in the American Lung Association's "Big Ride Across America" from Seattle to Washington, D.C. in 48 days.

Life is precious. I am grateful for every day that I can give something back. I thank my donor every morning for this "Gift of Life."

– Mary Pierce, bilateral-lung transplant recipient,
April 2, 1993

---

blood and fluids in the chest cavity, which naturally occurs following surgery. These tubes are removed when the drainage stops. You may have two to four chest tubes when you wake up, and they usually stay in place for several days. The removal can be painful, but it is swift. You may want to ask your nurse for some pain medication before these are pulled out.

FOLEY CATHETER will be placed in your bladder to track how much urine you produce. This is generally removed within two to four days.

LARGE INTRAVENOUS CATHETERS (IVs) will be placed in your neck and arm. These will allow the nurses to draw most of the blood they need without needing to continually poke you in the arms. These IVs also allow for the administration of medications while you are on the ventilator.

WRIST RESTRAINTS will be gently tied as a precaution so you don't pull or dislodge your breathing tube or other monitoring lines as you wake up.

After Surgery:

After surgery, patients are cared for in an isolation room to protect against infection and to limit the number of people who come in contact with you. Most likely you will be in a private room, but some hospitals have semiprivate rooms in which the other patient is also a transplant recipient. It is common for patients to experience any or all of the following symptoms:

PAIN/DISCOMFORT: For the first 24 hours, pain is not usually a problem because the anesthesia works to knock you out. After 24 hours, when you begin to move and sit in a chair, you will feel pain from your incision. There will be plenty of pain medication available to you, so if you feel uncomfortable, don't feel bashful to ask for more.

In most cases, you will self-administer pain medication using a "pain pump;" whereby you press a button and the pain medication's scheduled dosage is released. Eventually, you will be removed from that and will receive pain medication through your IV, then in the form of pills. If you are experiencing adverse side effects from this medication, tell your nurse about them so that a substitute drug can be prescribed.

NAUSEA/POOR APPETITE: Medications, anesthesia and surgery will often make you feel nauseated. Medications are available that can help if you are experiencing this side effect.

DIFFICULTY AND PAIN WITH COUGHING: This is due to the incision and muscle weakness. One thing you can do to help make coughing easier is to splint your chest with a pillow or rolled up blanket. Simply hold or hug the pillow against your chest whenever you cough. Also, since the nerves to the new lung are severed, you will not be aware of secretions in your airways. You have lost your "cough reflex." Therefore, you must remember to purposefully cough each day to clear any secretions.

INCREASED HEART RATE (for heart-lung transplant recipients): A transplanted heart functions differently than your old one. A transplanted heart beats much faster (about 100 to 110 beats per minute) than a normal heart (70 beats per minute) since the nerves that regulate the heart are cut during the operation. In addition, your new heart will also respond more slowly to exercise and doesn't increase its rate as quickly as before.

"When I was in the ICU, I remember trying to use sign language to talk to my wife and family. I only know the alphabet, but I had forgotten that they could not understand any of it."
– Mitch Davey

LACK OF SLEEP: Since you are constantly being monitored, lack of good sleep is very common in the CICU. Often, your days and nights will get confused. If this becomes a problem, don't hesitate to ask your doctor for something to help you sleep.

STRANGE DREAMS/HALLUCINATIONS: Many patients experience strange dreams or hallucinations while in the CICU. This condition can be caused by a condition called, "ICU psychosis," which is a combination of sensory deprivation (not knowing if it is day or night, etc.), sensory overload (noises, TV, etc.), sleep disturbances and medication. If this becomes a problem, tell your nurse or transplant physician about it.

WEAK OR DIZZY: The first few times out of bed, your nurse or physical therapist will assist you until you are strong enough to walk on your own.

DIFFICULTY CONCENTRATING: This is temporary and will improve with time.

MOOD SWINGS/ALTERED PERSONALITY: Due to the effects of the medication and major surgery, you may experience unusual mood swings, such as excessive crying or anger. These side effects diminish as your medication is reduced.

Visitors:
When hospital personnel or family members come to see you, they need to wash their hands, and in some cases put on a gown, mask and gloves. Family members and any other visitors with a cold, illness or recent chicken pox exposure or vaccination should not visit the patient until they have recovered. Because recovery in the CICU is busy and tiring to the patient, it is recommended that visitors be limited to the most immediate family, and visitation be of short duration. Also, visitors should NOT bring flowers, plants or fruit to patients because of the risk of infections. Cards, balloons (foil, no latex) and stuffed toys are fine.

Diet:
In the beginning, your fluid intake will be restricted to maintain a state of relative dehydration to limit the extent of edema. Eventually, you will be on a diet of clear liquids and gradually progress to soft foods.

Exercise:
At first, your ability to exercise will be limited. However, walking is a must; although it may be difficult for you. This will increase circulation, speed healing, help keep your lungs clear, increase your leg strength and make you feel better, faster! Lying around, on the other hand, increases the risk of bedsores, pneumonia and blood clots. Exercise is also important after transplantation because the steroid drugs given to prevent organ rejection tend to reduce muscle and bone mass.

Most patients get out of bed by the second or third day after their transplant. Once out of bed, you will start with short walks (50' to 100') assisted by others or with a walker. During these walks, a physical therapist or nurse will monitor you. It is advisable to take your walks during low traffic hours (evening or early morning) to minimize the risk of infection. Remember you must wear your mask whenever you go outside your room.

A Dream Come True

"Mr. Heintz, it is 1:06 p.m., Halloween Day, and you have been transplanted." Who would have known those words would be the first words I would hear after starting my "new life." My transplant journey began Aug. 10, 1998, when I was officially put on the UNOS waiting list. 82 days later I was laying in Ochsner Foundation Hospital's Intensive Care Unit with the "Gift of Life."

Everyone wanted to know what it felt like to breathe for the first time in my life. I couldn't find a way to put it into words until my 10th day post-transplant. I was sitting in my room watching television, and I began to cry. My mother panicked and asked what was hurting me. Through all the tears, I couldn't speak. I had just laughed for the first time in my life without coughing, something most people take for granted. All I had been through had just become worth it with that one laugh.

My recovery seemed to move quickly from that point on. The chest tubes were removed 10 days after surgery. I had my first set of pulmonary function tests 11 days after surgery. For the first time in my life, I had PFTs that came close to those of a healthy person. Things began to fall into place; I was exercising, had energy, and could speak an entire sentence without having to stop in the middle to take a breath. I am now hyper.

On Nov. 13, I was released from Ochsner to begin my new life. My life had been turned upside down or maybe right side up depending on how you look at it. From my point of view, things had turned right side up. All I had to do now was stick to all the new medications, and take care of myself and I could have the life I had always dreamed of, a life without the limitations of cystic fibrosis.

– Franklin (Frankie) D. Heintz, Jr., bilateral-lung transplant recipient,
Oct. 31, 1998

Transferring to the Floor:

When you are extubated and stable on medications by mouth, you will be transferred to a room on the transplant unit. There is usually an adjustment period going from the CICU, where your nurse was always available, to being on the floor, where your nurse has three or four other patients to care for. You will be continuously monitored for oxygen saturation, pulse and blood pressure, and you will have frequent chest x-rays and blood tests.

Visitors and hospital personnel are required to wash their hands before entering your room, and in some cases put on a mask if they are sick. Even though you will be in an isolation room with necessary precautions posted on your door, some hospital personnel may not be aware of the danger they put you in if they are sick. Don't be afraid to ask them to wear a mask and gloves if they are sick.

Doctors and Nurses:

Typically you will be seen by quite a number of different doctors, but your primary doctor is your admitting physician; in most cases that will be your surgeon. They make rounds usually once a day in the early morning. You will also get visits from your transplant physician and your transplant coordinator, in addition to many other specialists. It is helpful to write down any questions you might have so that you will be prepared when your doctor visits. It may also be helpful to keep a journal of your hospital stay so you will remember key names, dates, procedures, etc.

Unlike in the CICU, you will have more than one nurse. RNs dispense your medication, and nurse's assistants take your vital signs. They both rotate shifts, usually at 7:00 a.m., 3:30 p.m. and 11:30 p.m. Shift changes are particularly busy times for nurses, so if you are due for pain medication soon, you may want to request it before they change shifts.

If you are having problems with your nurse, ask to see the head nurse or charge nurse. If that doesn't resolve the problem, ask to see the nursing supervisor. Some hospitals have a patient advocate who can also be of help.

Pulmonary Rehabilitation:

The first step in the recovery process involves a combination of chest physiotherapy, exercise and proper nutrition. Chest physiotherapy (CPT) is extremely important after a lung transplant. CPT involves a number of activities that are designed to keep your lungs clear of secretions, prevent lung collapse and pneumonia. Activities involved in CPT include deep breathing exercises, use of the incentive spirometer, chest percussion, coughing and the use of inhalation medicines (aerosols).

DEEP BREATHING EXERCISES are designed to expand your lungs to their fullest capacity. They also help to open up even the tiniest airways, and strengthen your breathing muscles, especially the diaphragm and muscles between your ribs.

INCENTIVE SPIROMETER (if over 4 to 6 years old) is a small, portable breathing exerciser that helps you to breathe more effectively. By setting the indicator on the incentive spirometer, you set the goal of how much air you want to breathe in. Next, you place your lips around the mouthpiece, and inhale until the blue disk moves to that mark. You should use the incentive spirometer as much as possible (i.e. every two hours or eight times a day).

CHEST PERCUSSION: is designed to help loosen secretions in your lungs, if necessary. A respiratory therapist usually performs chest percussion by placing you in various positions on your side, back and stomach, and placing a vibrator or tapping with their hands on the skin over your lungs.

COUGHING: Since the transplanted organ will not have the same nerve attachments, your ability to sense the need to cough will be impaired. In single-lung transplant recipients, your remaining lung will continue to signal the need to cough, but the new lung will not. In bilateral-lung transplant recipients, there may not be any signal to cough, so you should routinely make yourself cough to bring up any mucous or fluid that might be present.

Medications:

After your transplant surgery you will be receiving many different medications. Initially, the nurses will set up your medications for you. As soon as you are able, the nurses will teach you how to take your medications on your own. *(For more information about medications, see page 110.)*

COMPLICATIONS OF LUNG TRANSPLANTATION:

"I've started to learn to forget about looking too far ahead and worrying about what ain't happened yet."
– Damian Neuberger

Complications of lung transplantation can be divided into four main categories: 1) complications of the operation itself, 2) complications of rejection, and 3) complications of immunosuppression, and 4) complications of the medications.

Complications of the Operation:

General complications of thoracic surgery may include: pain, nerve dysfunction, pneumonia, collapsed lung, hemorrhage, persistent air leaks, respiratory failure and cardiac and hemodynamic complications (irregular heart rhythm and low blood pressure).

HEMORRHAGE can occur following the removal of the recipient's native lung due to pleural adhesions that can be attributed to the underlying disease. In addition, hemorrhage can be complicated by the use of anticoagulants used to thin the blood during cardiopulmonary bypass, which is required during some lung transplant operations.

REIMPLANTATION RESPONSE (or reperfusion edema) is not uncommon during the first few days after transplant and can occur in 15% to 35% of all patients. This can result from the length of time the organs are without blood flow, oxygen and nutrients; but it can also be exasperated by cardiopulmonary bypass.

This can cause very mild to very severe injury to the lungs. Most patients exhibit a complete resolution within several days or weeks. However, a minority of patients who develop reimplantation response go on to develop adult respiratory distress syndrome. Treatment includes inhaled nitric oxide and extracorporeal membrane oxygenation (ECMO).

AIRWAY COMPLICATIONS can occur in up to 5% to 10% of lung transplant recipients in their large airways (main bronchi). These consist mainly of bronchomalacia or bronchostenosis. Bronchomalacia represents airway collapse, or "floppy airways;" while bronchostenosis represents constriction of the airways or "bulky airways."

These usually occur in the first 100 days after the transplant, at or very close to where the old and new airways are stitched together. Most of these problems are relieved by balloon dilatation of the airways or a bronchial stent placement. Both of these procedures can be done through a bronchoscope, and sometimes as an outpatient.

GASTROINTESTINAL COMPLICATIONS include the development of intestinal obstruction due to the paralysis of the intestinal muscles. This may require intravenous feeding and a nasogastric tube, which is inserted through the nose into the stomach to suction out the stomach contents.

HYPERACUTE REJECTION occurs within minutes of transplantation due to antibodies in the recipient's blood stream that react with the new organ, and results in immediate organ failure. This doesn't occur very often; and it is quite rare since all patients are screened for antibodies and blood typing prior to transplantation.

PULMONARY INFECTION occurs in up to 80% of lung transplant recipients, commonly in the transplanted lung. Bacterial pneumonia represents the greatest threat in the early postoperative period, but fungal infections such as *Candida* or *Aspergillus* or viral infection with herpes or cytomegalovirus (CMV) can occur. Antibacterial antibiotics are routinely administered after the operation, and, if indicated, antifungal medications. *(For more information about reducing the chance of getting an infection, turn to page 90.)*

THE VOICE OF EXPERIENCE

Re-Listed for LIFE!

In 1992, I made the decision to have a lung transplant. Then, I had to make the same decision again. Serious complications developed during my first surgery. Originally, I was supposed to receive a double-lung transplant, but the lungs turned out to very damaged. At some point between their removal from the donor and the time they were to be transplanted in me, the lungs had filled with water and they had collapsed airways. My surgeon had to decide whether to go ahead with the surgery or re-implant the lung they had just taken out. So, instead of receiving a double-lung, I received a single-lung, along with a lung volume reduction surgery on the remaining lung. I had to be put on special life support, called ECMO. My surgeon did everything he could. But, I did survive, mainly because I fought with all I had and I still do today.

After surgery, I was still very compromised, but now in a different way. Eventually the lung began to work, but not after a lot of damage had occurred. My surgeon told me that I could have a second transplant. But I decided to wait to see if I would improve, but I didn't. Six months after my first transplant, I was re-listed again.

During the following year, I went inactive because my doctors thought I was doing too well. I have since been reactivated, but I was on internal hold. They wanted me to lose some weight before surgery. I can understand this, but it also makes me angry. All of this could have been avoided if only someone had checked the lungs before beginning the surgery.

But, I am dealing with it the best I can. I really believe that things happen for a reason because whatever is gonna happen is gonna happen! So now I must wait. Staying involved in life helps me deal with it. My husband and I just bought a new house and I got a new puppy.

Several months ago, I started to write the story of this part of my life, but that's just it, its only part. Life has many aspects to it and you can never really foresee or count on anything. I have finally gotten over what happened to me during my first transplant and moved on. You have to! Life is only as good as you make it! I work hard at keeping myself healthy, but its not always easy with only 26% lung function. Now, I am 54 pounds lighter and I placed myself on hold for the time being because I am doing so well. In life, things can suddenly change, and boy do I know that. I will never give up on my dreams, and with the help of God I will survive.

– Karen Fitchett, single-lung transplant recipient,
July 2, 1996, relisted Jan. 14, 1997

COMPLICATIONS OF REJECTION:

"My doctor was very clear before surgery that I was trading one disease for another. I had to keep reminding myself of that through several bouts of acute rejection and CMV."
– Andrea L. Aulbert

To understand the complications of rejection, it is first necessary to understand your body's natural defense system. Briefly, this system has two purposes: 1) to prevent and fight the spread of infections and 2) to rid your body of foreign substances. Such substances may include pollen, microorganisms, such as bacteria and viruses, or organs transplanted from someone else.

At the very heart of this system is the ability to distinguish between "self" and "nonself." Virtually every cell in the body carries distinctive molecules that identify it as "self." The body normally does not attack cells that carry a "self" marker. If your immune system sees a piece of tissue or cell that is not "self," or foreign, cells are called into action to destroy it. This is called an immune response.

Any substance capable of triggering an immune response is called an antigen. Antigens can be a protein, carbohydrate or fat, as well as a virus, bacteria, parasite or cells from another individual. An antigen announces it is not "self" via special protein substances which protrude from its surface. Everyone has his or her own unique mixture of them, and an organ from outside your body has its own mixture, which may be different from yours.

The success of this system relies on an elaborate and dynamic network of millions and millions of cells that pass information back and forth. The result is a sensitive system of checks and balances that produces a response that is prompt, appropriate, effective and self-limiting. When this system fails or is disabled, some devastating diseases can result such as cancer, rheumatoid arthritis and AIDS.

Nonspecific and Specific Defenses:

The body's natural defense system is a large, complex network of organs, tissues and specialized cells and chemicals, including both a nonspecific and specific defense system. The nonspecific defense system is the first line of defense and is capable of responding to ANY type of foreign substance. It is made up of the skin and mucous membranes, which form a mechanical and chemical barrier. Foreign substances that make it through this barrier are then confronted by destructive cells called phagocytes, natural killer cells and a variety of chemical substances that kill pathogens.

Phagocytes are present in nearly every organ of the body and include such cells as macrophages and neutrophils. These cells work by engulfing foreign particles, breaking down their contents and/or digesting them. Natural killer cells police the body in the blood and lymph. They are called "natural" because they do not need to recognize specific antigens before swinging into action. When they encounter a foreign cell, they attack the target cell's membrane and release several chemicals that disintegrates it.

The second line of defense is the inflammatory response, which prevents the spread of damaging agents, disposes of cell debris and pathogens, and sets the stage for repair. It is also a nonspecific response that begins when an injured cell sounds a chemical alarm which releases inflammatory chemicals including histamine. These chemicals cause the blood vessels involved to dilate (causing redness and heat) and capillaries to become leaky (causing local swelling), thus activating pain receptors.

This cascade of events attracts other cells to the area to clean up the damaged or dead cells and/or pathogens, which are eliminated from the body. If the area is not cleared of debris, pus is formed. The inflammatory response also releases clotting proteins that leak into the blood and seal off the area, beginning to form a scaffolding for permanent repair.

The Immune System:

The immune system, in contrast, acts like an army of protective cells and chemicals that are called into action against SPECIFIC targets. This system also recognizes and mounts an attack on previously encountered pathogens. It is also systemic, meaning it is not restricted to the initial site of infection.

The front-line soldiers involved in the immune system are the cells in your blood called lymphocytes, a type of white-blood cell, which originate in the bone marrow. There are two major classes of lymphocytes; T cells and B cells. T cells work chiefly by interacting directly with their targets and are live organisms, while B cells work chiefly by secreting chemical substances called antibodies, which are not living.

T cells:

T cells originate in the thymus, where they multiply and mature. This is also where T cells learn to distinguish between "self" and "nonself." From the thymus, some T cells congregate in the lymph nodes, while others travel continuously throughout the body using the blood and lymphatic vessels.

There are three subdivisions of T cells. The first group are the helper T cells, which carry the CD4 marker. Helper T cells are the cells that act as "directors" or "managers" of the immune system. Once activated, they circulate through the body, recruiting other cells to help fight the invader.

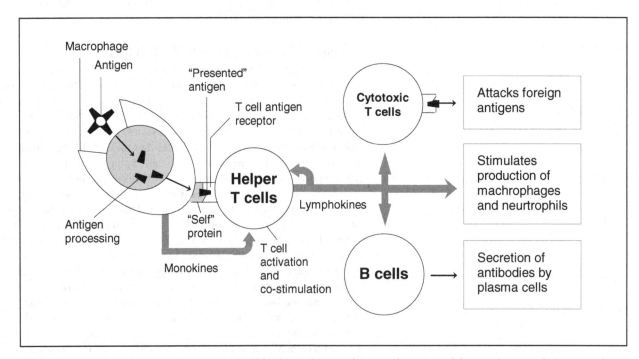

Figure 3. *A major role of macrophages is to engulf foreign antigens and present fragments of these antigens on their own surfaces, where they can be recognized by helper T cells. This, in turn, stimulates a variety of events that destroy the offending substance.*

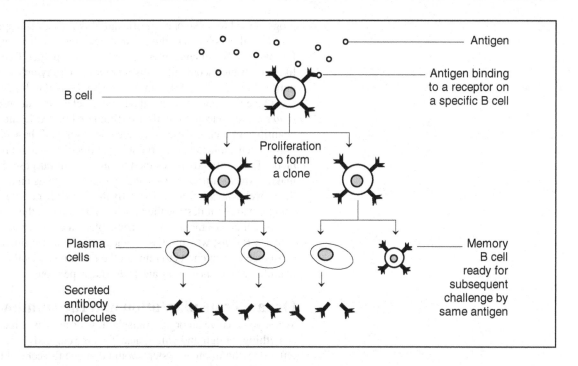

Antigen

Antigen binding
to a receptor on
a specific B cell

B cell

Proliferation
to form
a clone

Plasma
cells

Memory
B cell
ready for
subsequent
challenge by
same antigen

Secreted
antibody
molecules

Figure 4. An antigen binds to the antibody receptor, which stimulates the B cell to divide, producing clones that turn into plasma cells that secrete the necessary antibodies.

They are essential for activating B cells, T cells and more helper cells.

In addition to destroying pathogens, macrophages wandering throughout the body help T cells respond to specific antigens *(see figure 3)*. When a macrophage, or big-eater cell, encounters a substance it does not recognize, it ingests and processes the antigen. Then it "presents" parts of the antigen on its surface membrane. Now it can be recognized by a helper T cell bearing receptors for the same antigen.

During the binding process, the T cell binds simultaneously to the antigen and to the macrophage's "self" protein (major histocompatibility complexes or MHC) which then leads to T cell activation. The antigen "presenting" cell also displays a special molecule that engages specific receptor molecules on the T cell. This process is called co-stimulation. Macrophages also release special proteins, called monokines, which enhance this process.

Once helper T cells are activated, they release another protein called lymphokines, which stimulate production and activity of more helper cells, B cells and the second group of T cells, called the killer or cytotoxic T cells. The cytotoxic T cells, which carry the CD8 marker, are the cells that cause organ transplant rejection. They also specialize in killing virus-infected cells and cancer cells. Lymphokines also attract other types of protective white-blood cells, such as neutrophils, and enhance the ability of macrophages to engulf and destroy microorganisms.

As the released lymphokines call more and more cells into battle, the immune response gains momentum, and the antigens are overwhelmed by the shear number of elements acting against them. The third group of T cells are the suppressor T cells, which shut down the production of antibody-forming cells and draw the immune response to a close.

B Cells:

B cells arise from the bone marrow completely matured and are present in lymph nodes, blood, lymph fluid and connective tissue. Each B cell is programmed to make one specific antibody, which is a special, protective chemical that belongs to the group of molecules called immunoglobulin or Igs. When a B cell encounters an antigen, the helper T cell acts somewhat like an advance scout, and calls more and more lymphocytes into the battle until it finds the B cell that makes the antibody that binds to the antigen.

Once the appropriate antibody interlocks with the foreign antigen *(see figure 4)*, the selected B cells are stimulated to divide and make large quantities of themselves, forming clones. Some of these clones turn into plasma cells, a factory for producing antibodies that are released into the blood. Each antibody is destined for a different purpose. Some antibodies make antigens attractive to scavenger cells, such as phagocytes, that engulf the unwelcome microbe. Some activate a cascade of nine proteins, known as complement, that destroy the invaders and remove them from the body.

B cell clones that do not become plasma cells become long-lived memory B cells, which retain a blueprint of these antibodies. If the foreign substance ever attempts to reinfect the body, memory B cells can quickly manufacture the necessary antibody and wipe it out.

Organ Transplantation and the Immune System:

When you receive an organ transplant, your body will recognize it as something foreign and will attack. This is your body's normal reaction. If left alone, the immune system would damage the cells of the new organ and eventually destroy it. Your immune system is very good at finding and destroying trespassers. The problem is that it can't tell the difference between good guys and bad guys. Lymphocytes don't know the difference between a common cold and a helpful organ transplant. The lymphocytes just come to your defense, and, when they do, you have a rejection episode.

To prevent rejection, transplant recipients receive immunosuppressant drugs that suppress the immune system so the new organ is not damaged. The process of rejection involves many different cells, therefore centers use a variety of medications, such as cyclosporine (Sandimmune/Neoral or Gengraf), azathioprine (Imuran) and prednisone. The combination of these three medications is often referred to as "triple therapy" and results in a much more efficient immunosuppression. Matching donor and recipient HLA antigens (human leukocyte antigen) can also reduce the occurrence of rejection. However, the limited time the donor lungs can be preserved has precluded HLA matching in lung transplantation.

Since rejection can occur anytime after a transplant, these drugs are given to the patient the day of their transplant and thereafter for the rest of their life. Doctors must balance the dose of immunosuppressive drugs so that a patient's transplanted organ is protected, but his or her immune system is not completely shut down. Without an active immune system, a patient can easily develop infections. The most important thing patients can do to minimize the risk of rejection is to properly take their anti-rejection drugs and do everything possible to avoid infections and stay healthy.

If rejection does occur (and most everyone should expect to have at least one rejection episode in the first 100 days), it means that your body's immune system is fighting against the new organ. Unlike the other major organs, lungs are continuously exposed to the outside environment and have a large immune apparatus already established, which makes them more likely to reject. Plus, they are the largest transplantable organs, and the entire cardiac output is funneled through them. There are three basic types of rejection: hyperacute, acute and chronic.

Hyperacute Rejection:

Hyperacute rejection can occur within minutes of transplantation due to pre-existing antibodies in the recipient's blood stream that react with the new organ and result in organ failure. Such antibodies may be present in the recipient due to prior exposure through blood transfusion, pregnancy or previous transplantation. It may happen immediately or up to two weeks after transplantation. Fortunately, this type of rejection is very rare, and has been almost completely eliminated by blood group matching, and screening recipients for antibodies against the most commonly expressed antigens.

Acute Rejection:

Acute rejection is the most common type and frequently occurs in the first few weeks after surgery and remains a lifelong risk. It is caused by the recipient's immune response against the organ's antigens. Although the response is complex and involves multiple cell types and mediators, the key cell involved is the T lymphocyte. This type of rejection targets the cells that line the blood and lymphatic vessels of the transplanted organ. This is not cause for panic. When treated early, rejection can be stopped.

How Can I Tell If I Have Acute Rejection?

Sometimes when you experience a rejection episode you will feel just fine. Other times there may be clear signs and symptoms. In either case, several things can alert your transplant team to a problem. Symptoms of lung rejection include:
- Shortness of breath
- Persistent cough
- An unexplained decline of 10% or greater from baseline FEV_1
- Similar symptoms to an infection or flu, including fever.

Diagnosing Acute Lung Rejection:

The earlier any rejection problems are detected, the easier they are to treat. So it's very important to monitor your vital signs (temperature and heart rate), respiratory status (pulmonary function values) and get regular lab work done as directed. Sometimes you may not have any symptoms but still experience acute rejection. The diagnosis and treatment of acute lung rejection can be extremely difficult at times. The only way to show unequivocally that rejection is occurring is by biopsy. Some patients may never have any symptoms of rejection; therefore most centers recommend periodic surveillance bronchoscopies (or bronchs). However, some centers only perform biopsies when clinically indicated.

Lung Biopsy:

Bronchoscopies are done on an outpatient basis in a bronchoscopy suite. Bronchs consist of passing a flexible tube (a bronchoscope) through the nose or mouth into the trachea, and down into two main air passages of the lungs (bronchi). During the bronchoscopy at least eight to 10 tissue specimens are obtained for examination under a microscope (transbroncial biopsy). In addition, sputum samples will be collected and examined for the presence of bacteria or a virus (bronchoalveolar lavage).

This procedure is usually uncomfortable but not painful. Prior to the actual procedure, an IV is placed and medications are given to help you relax, and a local anesthesia is used to numb your throat. Most programs like to use a drug called midazolam hydrochloride (Versed), which acts by erasing your memory. However, you remain awake and can respond to commands. In preparation for a bronch, you should not eat anything by mouth the night before, and then only small amounts of clear liquids in the early morning.

The bronchoscopy usually takes approximately 20 to 30 minutes from preparation to finish. Following the procedure, the patient will be moved to a recovery room. After a bronch, your throat may be sore. You will also feel drowsy until the medications wear off. Therefore, you should not operate a car for at least 24 hours following a bronchoscopy.

Bronchs are a safe, diagnostic procedure and carry very little risk. Complications are infrequent, but when they do occur they include bleeding at the biopsy site, and possible pneumothorax (collapsed lung) in approximately 4% of all procedures. Results usually take several days to come back, at which point your coordinator will get in touch with you.

Stages of Rejection:

After a bronchoscopy, the biopsy specimens are examined under a microscope and the results are graded according to severity. Rejection is divided into five different stages:

Stage A0: No acute rejection
Stage A1: Minimal acute rejection
Stage A2: Mild acute rejection
Stage A3: Moderate acute rejection
Stage A4: Severe acute rejection.

Diagnosing acute rejection is a combination of examining the clinical symptoms in addition to the study of the miscroscopic nature of the tissue.

Treating Acute Rejection:

Acute rejection grades A2 or higher are usually an indication for intervention. The primary treatment for acute rejection is the addition to, or alteration of, your immunosuppressive medications. Currently, the use of immunosuppressants for lung transplant recipients is based upon experience with other organ transplants (e.g., kidneys, livers and hearts). The use of various agents that act on different parts of the immune system has evolved over time. Most centers employ "triple" immunosuppession, consisting of corticosteroids, azathioprine or CellCept, and cyclosporine or Prograf. Depending on the severity of rejection, your treatment may include:
- An increase in your daily immunosuppression dose
- Changes to your anti-rejection medications, e.g. switching from Neoral to Prograf, or azathioprine to CellCept
- Intravenous corticosteroids, such as Solumedrol, are given, also known as a "steroid pulse." The standard dose is 500 to 1,000 mg per day for three days followed by a tapered oral prednisone schedule. Approximately two weeks to one month later, a bronchoscopy may be repeated.

Recurrent Rejection:

For persistent or recurrent acute rejection, or when pulmonary function has not stabilized or improved with previous treatments, some centers use methotrexate or cytolytic therapy.

METHOTREXATE (Rheumatrex) has proven to be an effective alternative to high-dose corticosteroids in the treatment of heart transplant recipients with persistent acute rejection. In uncontrolled studies of lung transplant recipients, methotrexate helped to reduce the number of rejection episodes and slow the decline in lung function.

Methotrexate works by stopping the production of cells that are rapidly reproducing. Patients receive a total of six weeks of therapy unless side effects develop. Blood levels are monitored frequently and are followed by a repeat bronchoscopy. The effect of this short course of therapy has been a sustained reduction in the number of acute rejection episodes.

THE VOICE OF EXPERIENCE

Out of the Blue

I had a successful transplant of my right lung following 24 years of emphysema. I made a very speedy recovery and left the hospital on day nine. My check-ups were going fine and I was getting stronger as the months flew by. Then, out of the blue, I woke with a sore throat and a bad feeling in my chest. I started coughing up some putrid phlegm and promptly went to see my local pulmonary doctor who prescribed Cipro and a nebulizer. I really didn't have any trouble breathing and I expected the antibiotic to kick right in, but no such luck.

I returned to my doctor again and was prescribed Trovan, a newer antibiotic for chest infections. But by now my daily spirometry began dropping and I knew this to be a warning sign of possible rejection. After three weeks and little improvement, I agreed to a bronchoscopy, which showed no signs of rejection. Back home, I was put on another course of Cipro, but my FEV_1 continued to drop and I still had a productive cough. So, finally I made a date to return to my transplant center. The doctor there was sure I was going into chronic rejection even though there was no evidence of that from my bronchoscopy.

I had another bronch and still nothing showed up. But since my PFTs showed a considerable decline, I agreed to go through a course of Atgam infusions and was switched from Neoral to Prograf. The goal of the Atgam treatment was to completely knock out my lymphocytes and leave me with very little immune system activity. I checked into a private room and had a port installed. The plan was to hook me up to an infusion of Atgam every night for six hours, preceded by several meds to prevent side effects or reactions. I was amazed that my PFTs started to rise even before I left the hospital! I've heard so many horror stories about this treatment, but I tolerated it very well. Following my 10th infusion, I was discharged and went home.

Once back I had trouble understanding how this all began. I talked to my surgeon and he explained that I had caught a virus, which went untouched by the antibiotics. My defense system was then called into action and my own immune system just became too much for the immunosuppressants in its efforts to defeat the virus. Consequently, my own system began to attack the donor lung and this triggered the rejection.

The good news now is that one year later, I feel just fine. My PFTs are well within expected range and I am fit and active and having new adventures all the time. I look forward every day with excitement, although I still keep my daily logbook of indicators of anything amiss, and never hesitate to contact my transplant coordinator regarding any changes in my health.

– Joy Williamson, single-lung transplant recipient,
Aug. 12, 1997

CYTOLYTIC THERAPY with antihuman lymphocyte antibodies, produced in a variety of animal hosts, has been proven to slow, but not halt the rate of decline in the FEV_1. Cytolytic therapy is expensive to administer and hospitalization is required. There are several different types of antibodies that are used, such as OKT3, Atgam and Thymoglobulin. These agents may have serious side effects and further predispose the recipient to opportunistic infection (antimicrobial agents are employed when indicated). This treatment is considered experimental and, because of the risk to the patient, many centers no longer use cytolytic therapy or have never used it.

Diagnosing and Treating Heart Rejection:

For heart-lung transplant recipients, it is uncommon to have heart rejection. Therefore, frequent heart biopsies are not required. Usually, if rejection is present, it shows up in the lungs first. Consequently, heart-lung transplant recipients are followed with lung biopsies to check for the presence of rejection. However, the symptoms of acute heart rejection can vary from no symptoms at all, to palpitations, heart murmur or arrhythmia (irregular heartbeat), low blood pressure, edema, unexplained tiredness, and similar symptoms to an infection or flu. If it is suspected that you are undergoing heart rejection, an ECHO and heart biopsy may be performed.

A heart biopsy is performed by a doctor who does this as an outpatient in a biopsy suite. Heart biopsies consist of numbing the right side of your neck or groin, and passing a central line into your vein. Several small pieces of tissue are obtained for examination under a microscope. Heart biopsies are safe and carry little risk, but complications can occur. When they do, they include shortness of breath, bleeding at the biopsy site and perforation of the heart. The treatment of acute heart rejection depends on the severity and is similar to treatment of acute lung rejection.

Chronic Rejection:

Chronic rejection is a poorly understood process that affects all types of organ transplants. In the lungs, chronic rejection is called Obliterative Bronchiolitis Syndrome (OB). This form of rejection typically occurs more than a year after lung transplantation, but it has been reported as early as two months following the operation. The cause of OB is unclear, but its development is associated with the frequency of acute rejection episodes. There is also a suggestion that OB may be related to previous pulmonary infection, particularly cytomegalovirus infection (CMV). Sometimes, pneumonia-like reactions in airways and airspaces may induce OB.

Chronic rejection results in a gradual and progressive deterioration in lung function without explanation and is frequently accompanied by repetitive infections. The major difference between acute and chronic rejection, is chronic rejection is unlikely to respond to treatment. Chronic rejection involves your T cells and B cells and causes problems with air flow and oxygen exchange. It is thought this process is a result of airway injury that stimulates a reparative response leading to obliteration and scarring of the terminal bronchioles resulting in the presence of fibrosis.

As many as 50% of all lung transplant recipients will develop OB within five years. Although it is associated with significant mortality, it also can be clinically stable. Three patterns of progression of OB have been identified: 1) rapid onset with a relentless, progressive course; 2) rapid onset with initial decline, followed by stabilization; and 3) insidious onset and course.

Diagnosing Chronic Rejection:

The earliest manifestation of OB is a decrease in mid-expiratory flow rate (or FEV_{25-75}), although a decline in FEV_1 is the standard indicator of graft dysfunction. Clinical features also include cough, shortness of breath during exertion, progressive shortness of breath, irreversible airflow obstruction with moderate reduction of the DLCO, and decreased blood oxygenation and carbon dioxide in the blood. Pulmonary function testing and/or biopsy of the lung tissue can make the diagnosis of OB. Although, detecting OB by lung bronchoscopy is not as accurate or sensitive as it is when it is used to detect acute rejection.

In heart-lung transplantation, chronic rejection may also affect the heart. This is called, accelerated coronary artery disease; that is, narrowing of the arteries that supply blood, oxygen and nutrients to the heart. Chronic rejection in the heart can be detected by cardiac catheterization (shooting dye into the coronary arteries). Eventually, chronic rejection causes failure of the transplanted heart.

Treating Chronic Rejection:

Chronic rejection is hard to treat because the changes in the transplanted organ not only happen slowly but are irreversible. At this time, medications are not as effective in reversing chronic rejection as they are in reversing acute rejection. Therefore, every effort should be made to reduce the incidence of acute rejection since it is known to be a contributing factor in developing chronic rejection. To combat this chronic process, new therapies are currently being developed. Among them are immunosuppressive agents that are being studied to see if they have the potential to prevent and treat chronic rejection. However, most of these treatments are being studied in other organ transplants, the number of lung transplant recipients being studied has been very small.

METHOTREXATE (Rheumatrex): Some centers have tried methotrexate to slow the loss of lung function. A once-weekly dose of methotrexate is added to standard immunosuppressive therapy. The initial dose varies between five and 10 mg and is based on the patient's weight. The dose is gradually increased to between 10 to 15 mg once weekly. Patients undergo laboratory tests at least once monthly and more often if clinically indicated. The results so far have been encouraging. In one study, methotrexate reduced the episodes of rejection, and, in another, methotrexate slowed the rate of decline in FEV_1.

REGIONAL IMMUNOSUPPRESSION allows for the opportunity to administer drugs via the airways instead of systemically through the blood circulation.

Aerosolized Cyclosporine: Studies have shown that aerosolized cyclosporine can stabilize pulmonary function and reduce inflammation in patients with Obliterative Bronchiolitis Syndrome. Aerosolized cyclosporine is inhaled through a nebulizer for 10 consecutive days. Daily blood samples are drawn to determine lowest (or trough) levels of cyclosporine concentrations. After completion of the initial 10-day schedule, treatment is followed at home by a maintenance regimen of three days per week. The most frequent side effect consisted of cough and transient labored breathing.

High Dose Inhaled Steroids: Inhaled fluticasone (Flonase, Flovent) was used in one case report of a lung transplant recipient with OB that showed a significantly higher FEV_1 during the treatment period. The dose included two puffs by metered dose inhaler. In another study of seven heart-lung transplant recipients, the incidence of acute rejection episodes was lower in the nebulized steroid group than in the control group. The dose with budesonide (Pulmicort) was 2 mg twice daily for one year. The nebulized steroid seemed to have protective effect against long-term pulmonary dysfunction due to Obliterative Bronchiolitis Syndrome.

Rescue Therapy:

Once chronic rejection has been established, it can progress despite aggressive therapy. Multiple therapeutic approaches have been tried with variable success and frequent complications, leading some centers to seek experimental treatment for OB.

PHOTOPHERESIS: The documented use of photopheresis in lung transplantation has been very limited. In a study at the Cleveland Clinic, five patients with chronic rejection were treated with photopheresis. Four patients had a temporary stabilization or a slight improvement in their clinical status and FEV_1.

In photopheresis, a small number of infection-fighting cells (T cells) are taken from the patient and exposed to ultraviolet light and a chemical called methoxsalen (Oxsoralen) to deactivate the T cells. The cells are then re-infused into the patient where they begin to die. Other immune cells treat the dying T cells as waste. During a one- to two-week period, the dying T cells are cleared out of the immune system, which reduces the number of T cells that can attack the donated organ.

Treatment consists of one session of photopheresis per week for four weeks; followed by one session every two weeks for two months; then one session per month. Photopherisis is available but expensive, and may arrest the progression of OB but not reverse the scarring and fibrosis already established. Because the lungs are more susceptible to infection, the use of photopheresis in lung transplantation may prove to be difficult.

RETRANSPLANTATION: Another form of treatment for chronic rejection is retransplantation of the lung. However, this option depends largely on the availability of donor organs, which are scarce. In addition, the survival rates are not as successful as they are with the first transplant. The first year survival rate is roughly 48% vs. approximately 77% for the initial transplant. While figures for retransplantation are improving, this type of transplant remains controversial in the face of the organ donor shortage.

Preventing Rejection:

Obviously preventing rejection is much better than treating it. Here are some things you can do to keep your transplant as healthy as possible:
- Take your medications as prescribed by your doctor
- Maintain all lab and clinic appointments
- Avoid alcohol, recreational drugs and herbal supplements
- Follow dietary recommendations
- Maintain good communications with your transplant team
- Report any signs of rejection or infection promptly to your transplant coordinator.

COMPLICATIONS OF IMMUNOSUPPRESSION:

"Yes, the added years are great, but it is not 'Sit back and smell the roses.' One has to be on guard all the time."
– Monty Hughes

The immunosuppressive drugs used to prevent and treat rejection also suppress the recipient's ability to fight infection. Consequently, infections are a significant problem for transplant recipients. In addition, lung transplant recipients have a higher rate of infection than other recipients do. This can be attributed to a number of different factors.

First, all donor lungs are by definition intubated and mechanically ventilated, thereby exposing them to drawing in foreign bodies, colonization of bacteria and infection. Second, lung transplant recipients are commonly intubated for longer periods of time than other organ recipients, further increasing their risk of pneumonia. Third, the lungs are the only transplanted organ that is continuously exposed to the outside environment. Finally, the cough reflex and the ability to clear mucus are impaired in transplanted lungs due to cutting of the nerves during surgery. Eventually, some of these nerves may regenerate, but some may not.

Fortunately, the frequency of infections in lung transplant recipients has been reduced due to use of preventive therapies. However, after a lung transplant, infections caused by bacteria or viruses are of great concern. Sources of infection include not only other people and things, but your own body as well. For example, bacteria in your body live in places like your mouth and digestive system that help break down and process food.

Transplant recipients are at greater risk for unusual viral infections. These infections can cause rejection many years after a transplant. You need to watch carefully, report anything unusual to your transplant coordinator and treat infections immediately.

How Do You Know You Have an Infection?
Similar to the way rejection episodes are diagnosed, you will check for infections according to how you feel. Symptoms of infection may include:
- Fever above 100°F
- Scratchy or sore throat
- New cough, especially if it is producing sputum
- Shortness of breath, difficulty breathing, wheezing
- Drop in lung function values (FEV_1 and FVC)
- Chills, shaking episodes or night sweats
- Persistent cold or flu-like symptoms
- Redness, swelling or drainage around a cut or wound
- Nausea, vomiting, diarrhea lasting more than 24 hours
- Loss of appetite
- Burning on urination
- Earache.

In diagnosing infection, your sputum and blood may be analyzed for bacteria and viruses, and you may need a chest x-ray or bronchoscopy.

Bacterial Infections:
Upper and lower respiratory tract infections are the most common cause of bacterial infection after transplantation. *Pseudomonas aeruginosa* and *staphylococus* are the most common organisms involved.

BACTERIAL PNEUMONIA can occur in the early postoperative period after transplantation. Symptoms of pneumonia include, but are not limited to, nonproductive cough, shortness of breath and rapid breathing. Lung biopsy or sputum tests makes the diagnosis of pneumonia. If left untreated, the mortality is quite high, but pneumonia can be successfully treated with antibiotics. Infection with *Pneumocycstis carinii* pneumonia has been markedly reduced by the adoption of prophylactic therapy with oral trimethoprim-sulfamethoazole (Bactrim).

MYCOBACTERIUM TUBERCULOSIS infection may occur in lung transplant recipients due to immunosuppression, although the number of reported cases has been small. However, the recent resurgence of tuberculosis in the general population may make this a more common problem for transplant recipients. Transmission to transplant recipients can occur through reactivation of latent infection, transmission from donor lungs or exposures to people with active tuberculosis. However, testing recipients before and after transplant can prevent the infection. *M. tuberculosis* has responded well to antibiotics.

PSEUDOMONAS AERUGINOSA is a species of bacteria that is a serious complication of cystic fibrosis and lung transplantation. Cancer and burn patients also suffer from this organism. It is an opportunistic pathogen in humans who are immunocompromissed or have sputum sensitivities. *Pseudomonas* infections occur most often in hospitals where the organism is frequently found in moist areas and can be transmitted from patient to patient by hospital personnel. Patients requiring extensive stays in intensive care units are particularly at risk. Infection with *P. aeruginosa* is diagnosed by bronchoscopy and sputum samples. It is likely that antibiotics cannot effectively eradicate *Pseudomonas* from the lungs once established.

STAPHYLOCOCUS AUREUS: Patients receiving immunosuppressive treatment are at an increased risk for *staphylococus aureus* infection. Patients may acquire antibiotic resistant *staphylococci* from other colonized areas of their bodies or from infected hospital personnel who may be asymptomatic carriers. *Staphylococus* is highly contagious and can be passed on to others with close or routine contact. Diagnosis is made by bronchoscopy and sputum samples. Treatment consists of a combination of antibiotics. The choice of medication and dosage depend on the site of infection, the severity of illness and the sensitivity of the organism.

Viral Infections:

Cytomegalovirus (CMV) and reactivation of the herpes simplex virus are the most common causes of viral infection after lung transplantation.

CYTOMEGALOVIRUS (CMV) is one of the most frequent infections in lung transplant recipients. It belongs to a group of viruses called the herpes viruses. There are two types of CMV infection. The first is primary, which occurs in people who have never before been exposed to CMV. The second type is secondary, which develops in people who have been previously exposed to CMV. Contact between mucous membranes (the mouth and the genitals), mother to fetus exposure during pregnancy, blood transfusions and organ transplantation can transmit CMV. Live virus is present in the secretions of infected CMV patients. Patients with normal immune systems experience a "flu-like" illness of fever, malaise and cough, but may not know they have CMV. A blood test indicates whether a person has ever been infected with CMV and has developed an antibody to it. This is done as part of your transplant evaluation. Once a person is infected with CMV, they will always be "CMV positive." If a person has never been infected with CMV, they are called "CMV negative." The incidence of CMV varies by region of the country; in some regions greater than 50% of all adults are CMV positive. Once infected with CMV, the virus remains latent, and therefore can cause infection again in the future, particularly when the immune system is suppressed.

The mechanisms of getting CMV include: 1) Primary infection, this occurs if a CMV negative patient receives a CMV positive organ or is transfused with CMV positive blood. Roughly 60% to 80% of CMV negative patients will get CMV disease if they receive a CMV positive organ and no other treatment. 2) Reactivation, this occurs when a CMV positive patient receives a CMV positive or negative organ. The latent CMV infection the person had before the transplant can become active again and cause disease.

If it is known that CMV positive organs give CMV disease to CMV negative people, why is this type of transplant performed? CMV negative donors are usually that much fewer in number than CMV positive donors. For this reason, CMV negative persons might have to wait several times as long to get an organ. The risk of dying while awaiting a CMV negative donor is considered to be greater than the risk of contracting a known virus, for which known treatments exist. However, most centers attempt to match CMV negative donors with CMV negative recipients, and use only CMV negative blood products.

Fever tends to be the first sign of a CMV infection. Fatigue and low white-blood cell counts are also common. The symptoms can vary from very mild to severe. CMV can cause life-threatening disease if it gets out of control, especially in people with primary infection. It can infect just about any organ in your body. In the kidneys it is called CMV nephritis; in the lungs, CMV pneumonitis; in the liver, CMV hepatitis; in the heart, CMV myocarditis; in the retina, CMV chorio-retinitis; and in the brain, CMV encephpalitis. CMV pneumonitis may cause cough and shortness of breath. CMV gastritis and colitis may cause blood in the stools, nausea, vomiting and diarrhea. CMV encephalitis may cause seizures, headaches, confusion, and coma. Developing acute or chronic organ rejection is less common, but a potential danger of CMV as well.

The diagnosis of CMV may be difficult to make. Generally the history of the patient's transplant and illness must be considered together with all laboratory studies and tests. The symptoms are so broad and general that CMV can easily be mistaken for another problem. Probably the best evidence for CMV is evidence of CMV in the blood stream (CMV viremia) or on biopsy of an infected organ (inclusion bodies). However, even these tests are fallible. It is necessary that physicians caring for transplant patients keep a keen eye out for symptoms that may represent CMV infection and to repeat tests as necessary to detect CMV when it is present.

As explained above, the most likely circumstance of getting CMV infection is a CMV negative patient that receives a CMV positive organ. Immunosuppression also can make CMV disease more likely; especially antibodies like Orthoclone OKT3 and Atgam. Many efforts have been made to try and limit the number of patients that get CMV disease. Many transplant centers now use some sort of prophylactic treatment at the time of transplant to prevent future CMV infection, such as ganciclovir (Cytovene). Some studies have shown that these treatments may make the chance of developing CMV lower in some circumstances. Different transplant centers have different protocols for dealing with CMV since each center is faced with a different incidence of CMV, and they each use different amounts and types of immunosuppression.

Fortunately, new drugs have been developed that are effective treatment for CMV and have nearly eliminated CMV deaths among solid organ transplants. Ganciclovir (Cytovene), the first drug of choice, is given intravenously because it isn't absorbed through the intestines, and it causes white-blood cell suppression. In rare cases where ganciclovir is ineffective, foscarnet (Foscavir) is tried. It is equally potent, but has different side effects and toxicities. In addition, valacyclovir (Valtrex) is being investigated for the prevention of CMV in organ transplant recipients.

CMV disease is most common when immunosuppression is at its highest, which is usually the first few months after transplant, and with rejection episodes. CMV can be reactivated regardless of what one does, but washing your hands frequently throughout the day is perhaps the simplest way to help prevent infection. Do your best to avoid people with ANY type of infection, since CMV can resemble a cold. Also, keep in mind that CMV can be transmitted through blood or body fluids, so don't share personal items like toothbrushes, razors or silverware. If you are concerned about a possible infection, call your doctor immediately.

If the transplant recipient or the donor is CMV positive, you will be put on IV Cytovene for six weeks after transplant to help prevent infection.

COLDS AND INFLUENZA (flu) are viral infections of the bronchial tubes and lungs. They are spread most often by contaminated hands (e.g., by wiping your nose and not hand washing). Symptoms include fever, sore throat, cough, runny nose and muscle aches. Because a virus causes a cold, antibiotics cannot cure it. However, sometimes a bacterial infection will occur as a complication of a cold, which can be treated with antibiotics.

Ways to help prevent a cold or flu include eating and sleeping properly, getting plenty of exercise, washing your hands frequently, keeping your hands away from your nose, eyes and mouth, and using disposable tissues, not handkerchiefs, to reduce the spread of the virus.

Even though colds and flu have been around for years, scientists are still studying how they work. If you do get a cold or flu, contact your coordinator immediately. They will usually increase your antibiotics. Also, get extra rest, drink plenty of fluids (particularly warm fluids, which can help reduce congestion), check with your transplant coordinator before taking any over-the-counter cold medication and pay particular attention to any signs of lower respiratory tract infection signaled by chest cough and lowered FEV_1.

An annual flu vaccination is advisable after lung transplantation, but in some cases it does not always prevent the flu from developing.

HERPES SIMPLEX VIRUS has two different types infection. In the case of the first type, Type I or oral herpes, it is estimated 70% to 80% of all Americans have had prior infection with this virus. It is spread through direct contact with a person with herpes lesions. The symptoms are cold sores on lips, gums and mouth. The second type, Type II or genital herpes,

Life Outside The Bubble!

Before my transplant I worried if I got within a mile of someone with a virus, I would automatically get sick after I was transplanted. If someone coughed in my presence, I would catch that cough. I also thought germs would be waiting to attack whenever I set foot outside my door! But, my worst nightmare was if I got a virus, then I would be doomed.

It has now been two years since my double-lung transplant and I have had only one cold! Thinking I was going to die from it, I was in constant communication with my transplant coordinator. She reassured me it was a typical cold that any healthy person would experience. When I woke up on day four with no cold symptoms, I was sure I was done for! I called my coordinator and asked when I should expect to die. She laughed and said, "Your cold is gone Joanne. Congratulations, you've just experienced your first cold with healthy lungs!" Since then I've learned just how strong my immune system really is.

So, no I don't live in a bubble. As my surgeon says, "We gave you these lungs to go out and live." However, I am sensible. I wear my mask when in crowded areas especially during cold and flu season. I am careful around children. I also wear my mask when at the doctors, dentist, hospital or pharmacy. I avoid construction areas, dusty areas and where landscaping is in progress. When I garden, I mask and glove up. When I am on an airplane I wear a mask then too. I wipe surfaces clean with alcohol pads – such as phones, doorknobs, stair railings, grocery cart handles. I do carry a mask and Purell with me at all times, just in case. I also wash my hands constantly and have trained others to do so as well. But I certainly don't feel like I live in some sort of jail. I swim, bike, run, walk, hike and participated in the U.S. Transplant Games in 2000.

I love my healthy lungs and I will do whatever I need to do to keep them healthy. One of the best feelings I've had is to go through an entire day and realize, "I didn't even think about my lungs today." Then I take a deep breath and realize every breath I take is a miracle, and I wonder if people born with healthy lungs appreciate the fact that they can breath?

So, I refuse to live in a bubble! The only bubbles I like now are blowing soap bubbles and taking bubble baths! Oh yeah, and chewing bubble gum, too!

– Joanne Schum, bilateral-lung transplant recipient,
Sept. 13, 1997

---

occurs in only about 10% of all Americans. It is spread through sexual contact. Lesions appear in the genital areas and can be spread to other areas of the body. Symptoms involve itching, burning and painful, red lesions. However, the use of prophylactic acyclovir or ganciclovir in transplant recipients has made these infections uncommon.

Fortunately a new drug has been developed for genital herpes. Patients who have recurring episodes of these painful sores will get relief from famciclovir (Famvir), which only needs to be taken twice a day when symptoms develop. The older drug – acyclovir – will also stop outbreaks but doesn't relieve the pain.

EPSTEIN-BARR VIRUS is another virus that transplant patients need to avoid and is the cause of infectious mononucleosis. Like CMV, many people have this infection and never know it. With mononucleosis or "mono," the first line of defense is prevention. The virus is found in saliva and mucus, and can spread by coughing, sneezing or kissing. Stay away from people who have or are recovering from this infection. Recovery from mono is slow, even without a suppressed immune system, so be careful around people who say they had mono months ago. Mono in transplant recipients is rare because of the prophylactic use of acyclovir, which is effective against the virus. However, infection with the Epstein-Barr virus may cause a serious complication called post-transplant lymphoproliferative disease. *(For more information about this disease, see page 98.)*

RESPIRATORY SYNCYTIAL VIRUS (RSV) is one of the most common causes of lower respiratory illness in infants and young children and can be fatal. Immunosuppressed individuals are highly susceptible to RSV, and it can turn into bacterial pneumonia. RSV is associated with seasonal outbreaks of the flu in late autumn or in winter and can mimic the flu. Symptoms include difficulty breathing, cough, wheezing and fever. Infection requires hospitalization, and successful outcomes have been reported with aerosolized ribavirin (Virazole).

SHINGLES is a reactivation by the same virus that causes chicken pox (herpes zoster). Shingles only occurs in someone who has had chicken pox in the past. The chicken pox virus remains in your body for life, essentially asleep. But if the virus is reactivated, either by immunosuppression or stress, it can cause shingles. Shingles does not attack the lungs, but rather it is an acute disease of the central nervous system. Nerve cell bodies lying outside the brain and spinal column are usually the areas affected. These cells send severe pain along the course of the nerve down to the erupted skin areas. This is why shingles is rather uncomfortable.

It is rare for shingles to be very serious, but you are at risk if you have never had chicken pox (this can be checked by a blood test). Typical shingles begins with a general feeling of malaise accompanied by a slight fever and a tingling sensation or pain on one side of your body. Within days, a rash appears in that same area in a line along the affected nerve, and a group of small, fluid filled blisters crops up. Typically, this occurs along your chest, abdomen, back or face, but it may also affect other parts of your body. The area can be excruciatingly painful, itchy and tender. After one to two weeks the blisters heal and form scabs, although the pain continues.

Shingles is treated with anti-viral medications, such as acyclovir. There are a number of topical treatments or pain medications that can give you relief as well. The earlier you receive treatment, the better. If your child has not had chicken pox previously and is exposed to someone with shingles, the same procedure for chicken pox exposure must be followed. If the person's shingles are completely covered with clothing, then exposure has not occurred. *(For more information about chicken pox, see page 89.)*

Fungal Infections:

ASPERGILLUS is a fungal infection and is a potentially dangerous pathogen in immunocompromised patients. It is transmitted by inhalation of its spores. *Aspergillus* can develop into bronchitis, pneumonia and disseminated aspergillosis. Symptoms of aspergillosis include cough, productive sputum and difficulty breathing. Although infection itself has not always been the cause of death, mortality rates can be as high as 30% to 70%. A definitive diagnosis of *Aspergillus* bronchitis is usually made by biopsy. Various forms of bronchitis have responded well to treatment with itraconazole (Sporanox) or aerosolized amphotericin B (Fungizone). The standard treatment for pneumonia or disseminated aspergillosis is intravenous or inhaled amphotericin B and itraconazole. A new intravenous drug called, caspofungin acetate (Cancidas), was approved and is for those patients who did not respond to or were intolerant of other antifungal therapies.

CANDIDIASIS is a fungal infection, and is not uncommon in lung transplant recipients. Yeast infections of the genital tract are caused by *Candida albicans*. Symptoms include inflammation, redness, itching and whitish or yellowish discharge. Yeast infections can usually be effectively treated with drugs such as fluconazole (Diflucan) or ketoconazole (Nizoral). Oral candidiasis or thrush appears as creamy white film that can be scrapped off the tongue. Local agents such as clotrimazole lozenges are effective. *Candida* can also cause pneumonia, as well as disseminated infections in lung transplant recipients.

CRYPTOCOCCUS is caused by the fungus *fiobasidiella neoformans*. It has occasionally caused pulmonary or disseminated disease. Symptoms include meningitis with headache, blurred vision and mental disturbances, such as confusion, depression, agitation or inappropriate speech or dress. Depending on the incidence of infection in your area, prophlaxis should be considered for some recipients. In the United States, more cases occur in the Southeastern regions and in men 40 to 60 years old.

Childhood Diseases:

Pediatric recipients differ from adult recipients with regard to viral infections. Because your child is immunosuppressed, some common childhood illnesses can become a serious problem if your child hasn't developed an immunity to them. Before transplantation, your child's blood will be tested for the presence of antibodies that fight these illnesses.

Once discharged from the hospital, you will need to keep an eye out for these infections. Alert baby-sitters, parents of your child's friends and their schoolteachers about the risk of infection in your child. Ask them to notify you if ANY child is exposed to or develops one of them. Being exposed means having close physical contact with and/or sharing toys with another child who has the disease or who becomes ill with the disease soon after being with your child.

VARICELLA VIRUS (Chicken pox): If your child has not had chicken pox, it is extremely important for them to avoid contact with people who have it. Chicken pox is transmitted through the air or by close contact with an infected person. A person with chicken pox is contagious two days before the rash appears and until all lesions have formed scabs. Chicken pox usually occurs in children between the ages of three and eight years old. The first signs are fever, general discomfort and the appearance of a rash. The rash consists of small lesions surrounded by redness that eventually form crusted over scabs. The rash usually starts somewhere on the head and spreads down the trunk.

If your child has not had chicken pox and they have been with someone who breaks out with the disease within 24 to 48 hours after they have been together, call the transplant team immediately. Your child will need the varicella zoster-immune globulin (VZIG) injection within 72 hours of being exposed. The VZIG will decrease the severity of the chicken pox symptoms. In some cases, it may prevent your child from getting the disease.

If your child breaks out with chicken pox, he or she needs to be admitted to the hospital and given an intravenous medication called acyclovir. The medicine must be continued until no new chicken pox lesions appear and all old lesions are forming dry scabs; this may take up to 14 days.

In some cases, after a child develops chicken pox, the immunosuppressive medicines prevent their body from making enough antibodies to protect him or her from getting it again. After your child has recovered from chicken pox, your doctor will order a blood test to find out whether your child has developed enough antibodies to prevent them from getting chicken pox in the future.

RUBELLA (measles): If your child is not immune to measles and he or she is exposed to a child who breaks out with a measles rash within three to five days after being with that child, call your transplant coordinator. Your child will need an injection of immunoglobulin (Ig) within six days of being exposed.

Infection Prevention:

Prevention of infections is far better than treating them after they have developed. Your greatest chance of receiving an infection occurs immediately after your transplant, when your immunosuppressive drugs are at their highest level. Following are some suggestions on how to reduce your odds of getting an infection.

INFECTION PREVENTION IN THE HOSPITAL:
- Get a private room
- Limit the number of visitors and make sure they wash their hands before seeing you
- Ask anyone with a cold or an infection to refrain from seeing you until they are better
- Do not allow flowers, plants or fruits to be brought into your room
- Wash your hands often with antimicrobial soap, especially before meals
- Make sure all hospital personnel wash their hands before seeing you
- Ask that you receive your own blood pressure cuff, rather than use the one the nurses have been using on other patients
- Always wear a mask while outside your hospital room and walk in the hallways during low traffic hours; evenings and early mornings are best.

INFECTION PREVENTION AT HOME:
- Stay healthy, get plenty of sleep, drink enough fluids and eat a well-balanced diet
- Report any signs of infection to your transplant coordinator promptly
- Keep antimicrobial soap at all sinks; wash your hands often and keep your hands away from your mouth
- Avoid or take precautions around people with infections (e.g., colds, flu), including sick children
- Don't share dishes, glasses or eating utensils with people who are sick
- In the beginning, avoid areas were the likelihood of sick people is great
- Always wear a mask when flying on an airplane and when visiting the hospital, doctor's office or pharmacy
- Avoid smoke-filled environments
- When using a public restroom, once you've washed and dried your hands, use a paper towel to open the door to exit
- Clean and dress cuts or scraps immediately. If you need a tetanus shot, contact your transplant center first.

- Keep your house clean using antimicrobial cleaners
- Limit the use of humidifiers since high humidity levels indoors encourage the growth of microscopic dust mites, molds and mildew; if you use a humidifier, keep it clean and be sure to use distilled water or a demineralizing filter when filling.
- Use individually wrapped antimicrobial wipes to clean surfaces of things used by other people, such as public telephones
- Avoid areas under construction; such areas may carry fungal infections
- Wear gloves when gardening or stirring up dirt, and clean hands and nails well to help avoid fungal infections
- Don't clean cat litter boxes or birdcages
- Get the influenza (flu) vaccine each year. If anyone in your immediate family is getting a vaccine, make sure it does not contain the live virus. *(For more information about vaccinations, see page 145.)*

COMPLICATIONS OF THE MEDICATIONS:

"The only true disability in life is a bad attitude."
– Allan Shuford

Common Complications:

The following are some of the side effects you may experience from your medications. It is important to remember that you will not have every one of them. Most of these side effects will vary depending on your drug dosages.

ANXIETY DISORDERS are a group of disorders characterized by chronic, unrealistic anxiety, often punctuated by acute attacks of panic. This type of anxiety must be differentiated from normal anxiety, which occurs in realistically threatening situations.

Taking immunosuppressive drugs may make you more susceptible to anxiety disorders. Characteristics of anxiety disorders include a feeling of apprehension, excessive worry, uneasiness or dread of the future. It may also manifest as phobias of various types, accompanied by panic attacks.

Physical symptoms include heart palpitation; constriction of the throat; hyperventilation; cold, sweaty and trembling hands; painful digestion and pressure about the head. Psychotherapy, along with relaxation techniques and drugs, can help control anxiety.

DEPRESSION can result from a combination of genetic and psychological factors. In addition, certain drugs can contribute to depression, such as anti-hypertensives, alcohol, oral contraceptives, anti-anxiety drugs and steroid medications, such as prednisone. Many chronic medical conditions are considered risk factors for depression. If you are experiencing four or more of the following symptoms continually for more than two weeks you may be suffering from depression:
- Overwhelming feelings of sadness and grief
- Loss of interest and pleasure in activities you used to enjoy
- Unexplained tiredness, decreased energy or restlessness
- Significant loss or gain in weight, or changes in appetite
- Low self-esteem, helplessness or guilt
- Trouble concentrating or making decisions
- Thinking about death and suicide, or suicidal attempts.

Fortunately, with proper diagnosis and treatment, depression can be completely cured. Treatment with antidepressive medications along with therapy is usually recommended. However, the full effect of these drugs may not be seen for four to eight weeks. Some of the more common antidepressive medications include Prozac, Paxil and Zoloft.

DIABETES is a complication that may occur whether or not you had diabetes before your transplant. After transplantation, high blood sugar is mainly a side effect of prednisone. Symptoms of high blood sugar may include extreme thirst, weakness, dizziness, blurry vision and urinating in large amounts. Your blood sugar will be checked with each blood draw. If diabetes occurs, a patient may be required to go on a diabetic diet, take a pill or take insulin shots to regulate his or her blood sugar.

EDEMA is the accumulation of fluid in the body and may be the result of a chronic process such as hypertension or your immunosuppressive medication. Prednisone tends to cause edema in the face and legs as a result of sodium and water retention, whereas cyclosporine and Prograf cause edema in the legs and ankles due to reduced blood flow to the kidneys.

Edema can be treated by reducing salt intake, increasing physical activity, elevating feet and maintaining enough fluid in your body so it does not retain it if it doesn't have enough. Depending on the severity of your edema, your doctor may prescribe a diuretic or water pills.

HAND TREMORS are a frequent side effect of high levels of cyclosporine or Prograf in the blood stream. Low blood sugars or changes in electrolytes or organ function may cause tremors. Transplant recipients should notify their transplant physician if they are experiencing tremors so they can be evaluated for the cause and treated as needed.

HEADACHES are common complaints for as many as 40% of the all transplant recipients. This side effect is usually worse when levels of drugs, such as cyclosporine, Prograf or CellCept are high, and often disappear or improve once the level is lowered. Many headaches experienced by transplant recipients are sinus headaches, and can often be relieved by using acetaminophen (Tylenol) and/or diphenhydramine hydrochloride (Benedryl). Recipients should be careful not to exceed the recommended daily dose of acetaminophen due to a risk of liver damage.

A less-common side effect of cyclosporine is migraine headaches. People have a tendency to describe any bad headache as a migraine, but a migraine is a specific type of headache. It arrives with blinding pain (usually on one side of the head), nausea, vomiting and severe sensitivity to light and sometimes sound. Migraines range in severity from mild to severe. Unfortunately, researchers do not know why cyclosporine causes migraines. Some think the drug causes a constriction in the blood vessels of the brain.

If you are experiencing severe headaches since being on cyclosporine, you need to discuss this with your transplant team. Your cyclosporine level should be checked and your dose adjusted if the level is too high. If your headaches continue, some doctors may choose to treat the pain with another medication such as propranolol (Inderal), acetaminophen (Tylenol with or without codeine), sumatriptan (Imitrex) or zolmitriptan (Zomig). However, some doctors may switch you to another immunosuppressant.

Migraines can also be treated with muscle relaxation techniques, ice packs, resting in a quiet, dark room or by pressing on the bulging artery found in front of the ear on the painful side of the head. Sometimes just avoiding the things that trigger migraines is enough to prevent or reduce them for many people. Among suspected triggers are:

Foods: red wine; chocolate; nuts; aged cheese; nitraite/nitrite-preserved foods, such as hot dogs, pepperoni, salami; caffeinated foods and beverages; monosodium glutamate (MSG), which is used in Chinese food; and smoked or pickled fish/meat.

Sensory Stimuli: flickering/bright lights; sounds; sunlight; and odors such as perfume, chemicals and cigarette smoke.

Lifestyle Changes: times zones; sleep patterns and eating habits (getting enough sleep and eating regularly scheduled meals are important factors in helping avoid migraines); caffeine withdrawal; and stress.

Medications: antibiotics, tetracycline, griseofulvin (Fulvicin); anti-hypertensives (Procardia, Capoten); hormones (oral contraceptives, estrogens); histamine-2 blockers (Tagamet, Zantac); nonsteroidal anti-inflammatory drugs (Indocin); and vasodilators (nitroglycerin).

Others: menstrual cycle; weather/season changes; and high altitude.

HYPERTENSION is estimated to occur in 40% to 90% of all transplant recipients. Cyclosporine is most frequently associated with hypertension, followed by Prograf, prednisone, CellCept and Rapamune.

If you have high blood pressure, it is very important to make some lifestyle changes. A combination of weight control, regular walking or other exercise, eating a low-fat and low-salt diet and medication will keep your blood pressure within range. Generally speaking, the systolic (top number) should be less than 150 and the diastolic (bottom number) should be less than 90. Optimal blood pressure is defined as less than 120/80 mm Hg, while borderline is classified as between 135/85 and 139/89 mm Hg, and high is anything 150/90 and above.

HIGH CHOLESTEROL can occur in about 25% to 50% of all organ transplant recipients. Prednisone causes an increase in cholesterol production, while cyclosporine and Prograf decrease the body's ability to eliminate cholesterol.

To help control your cholesterol levels, exercise regularly, adopt a low-fat, low-cholesterol diet, and monitor your levels. If your cholesterol is still not under control, you may need to start taking medication. Some common medications used to control high cholesterol levels are pravastatin (Pravachol), simvastatin (Zocor) and atorvastatin (Lipitor).

INSOMNIA: Many transplant recipients experience sleeping problems or insomnia as a result of taking prednisone and/or cyclosporine. Fortunately, insomnia is very treatable. By making some simple lifestyle changes, insomnia can be controlled. For example, keep a regular bedtime and wake time schedule; avoid napping during the day; don't drink beverages containing caffeine after dinner time; avoid alcohol and nightcaps (it can help you fall asleep more quickly, but it disturbs the progress of natural sleep, and doesn't produce restful or restorative sleep). Avoid heavy

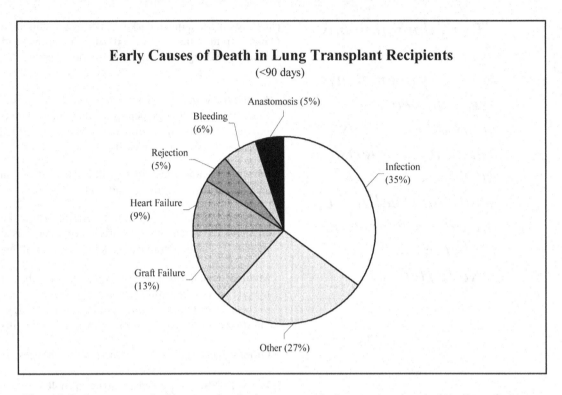

Early Causes of Death in Lung Transplant Recipients
(<90 days)

Anastomosis (5%)

Bleeding (6%)

Rejection (5%)

Heart Failure (9%)

Graft Failure (13%)

Infection (35%)

Other (27%)

Chart 11. Early causes of death (<90 days) in lung transplant recipients. (Data from St. Louis International Lung Transplant Registry Report, April 1996, Washington University School of Medicine, St. Louis, Mo.)

bedtime snacks; don't go to your bedroom or get into bed until you feel drowsy; and try a calcium supplement about 30 minutes before bedtime, or drink a glass of milk, which contains an amino acid (tryptophan) that can cause drowsiness. For more chronic problems, insomnia medication may be needed, such as zolpidem (Ambien) and temazepam (Restoril).

KIDNEY PROBLEMS: Taking immunosuppressant medications for a number of years, particularly cyclosporine, can cause mild to moderate kidney damage. Cyclosporine treatment can cause significant decreases in blood flow to the kidneys and creatinine clearance. Since you may not feel differently when your kidneys are not functioning normally, your creatinine level is monitored frequently. Watch for any increased swelling in your ankles, feet or hands or severe headaches. It is also important to drink plenty of water every day to help keep your kidneys healthy.

MOOD SWINGS/PERSONALITY CHANGES are a very common side effects of prednisone. When patients on prednisone feel down, they are really down, and when they are happy, they are bouncing off the walls with joy. This side effect is related to dose and tends to disappear when dosages are brought down to maintenance levels.

MUSCLE CRAMPS could be caused by a lack of magnesium or the side effects of your medications. Muscle cramps often subside when your dosages are reduced. Taking magnesium supplements may be warranted, but you should check this with your doctor. Perhaps the best medicine for muscle cramps is frequent exercise and muscle stretching at bedtime.

NUMBNESS AND TINGLING SENSATIONS: Some transplant recipients are prone to altered or tingling sensations in their fingers, lips

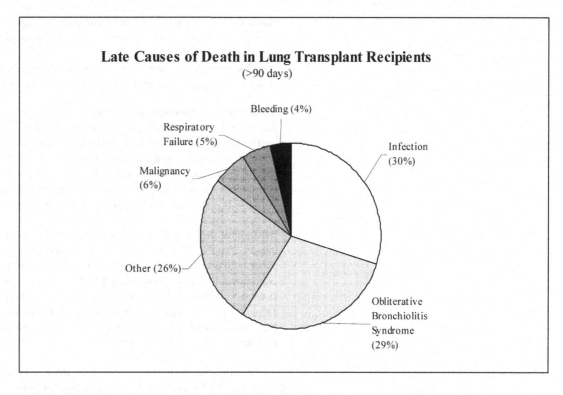

Late Causes of Death in Lung Transplant Recipients
(>90 days)

Bleeding (4%)

Respiratory
Failure (5%)

Malignancy
(6%)

Infection
(30%)

Other (26%)

Obliterative
Bronchiolitis
Syndrome
(29%)

Chart 12. Late causes of death (>90 days) in lung transplant recipients. (Data from St. Louis International Lung Transplant Registry Report, April 1996, Washington University School of Medicine, St. Louis, Mo.)

and feet. This is caused by a low blood magnesium level, which can occur with cyclosporine, and typically is especially prominent in the early transplant period. Cyclosporine does have an effect on the nerves, but the reasons for it are still unclear. Your magnesium levels will be monitored, and if low or borderline, it may be treated with supplemental magnesium. If this doesn't give relief, you may want to try over-the-counter medications containing capsacin, or the prescription drug amitriptyline (Elavil).

OVERGROWN OR BLEEDING GUMS (Gingival Hyperplasia): The tendency for gums to bleed and excess gum tissue to develop are all side effects of cyclosporine. Proper dental hygiene is the most effective form of prevention, which includes flossing, massaging the gums, brushing your teeth at least twice a day and seeing your dentist at least twice a year.

Some transplant centers have been trying an antibiotic called azithromycin (Zithromax) to decrease gum overgrowth. This antibiotic can increase your cyclosporine level, so check with your transplant team first. The last resort for overgrowth of gum tissue is dental surgery where the excess tissue is trimmed. This procedure is not a permanent solution and you must continue good hygiene to keep it from coming back.

SKIN CANCER: Organ transplant patients are more susceptible to developing skin cancer following surgery and need to take extra precautions to avoid prolonged sun exposure and monitor their skin for any signs of change. After transplantation, approximately 35% to 70% of organ transplant recipients will develop skin cancer depending on geographic location. While 80% of the estimated 1.3 million new cases of skin cancer diagnosed each year will be basal cell carcinoma, research finds that squamous cell carcinoma is much more prevalent in transplant recipients.

Skin cancer is divided into three categories:

Basal cell carcinoma is the most common and the least deadly form of skin cancer. The cure rate is better than 95% if caught early. Basal cell carcinoma looks like pearly growth or an area that won't heal. It can be translucent and gradually grow or can look like a sore that won't heal. Basal cell carcinomas can be removed by freezing or surgery.

Squamous cell carcinoma is the second most common form of skin cancer and like basal cell carcinoma, this disease is 95% curable if caught early. But, squamous cell carcinoma can spread and can be potentially lethal in immunosuppressed patients if left untreated. Squamous cell carcinoma looks like a crusty, scaly patch with a hard, thick surface. If caught early, squamous cell carcinomas can be removed by freezing or surgery. If it spreads, more aggressive treatments may be required.

Malignant melanoma is the least common, but most deadly form of skin cancer. People who have had several blistering sunburns when young or those with a family history of the disease are potential candidates. Melanoma looks like a pigmented mole, sometimes with an uneven border. In addition, the color and diameter may change over time. Depending on the tumor's thickness, it can be removed surgically. If it has spread, more aggressive treatments, such as radiation or chemotherapy, may be needed.

Preventing sun exposure is one of the main keys to steering away from skin cancer. The American Academy of Dermatology's sun protection guidelines include: avoiding outdoor activities between 10 a.m. and 4 p.m. when the sun's rays are their strongest; seeking shade whenever possible; wearing a broad spectrum sunscreen with a Sun Protection Factor (SPF) of

---

TIPS ON HOW TO COMMUNICATE WITH YOUR DOCTOR

- Put together a handout that briefly describes and dates your medical history, all the medications you are presently taking, any surgeries you've had, any allergies you might have, all your doctors names, addresses, phone and fax numbers. *(Turn to page 268 and fill out worksheet provided.)* Make copies of this sheet and bring it with you for all of your appointments. You may also want to include your vaccination schedule.
- Ask questions that are simple or narrowly focused.
- Compile a list of questions before your next clinic visit or before rounds take place.
- Take notes, or have a friend or family member do this for you, or bring a tape-recorder so you can recollect your discussion.
- Ask your doctor to write down his or her instructions for you.
- If the issue you want to discuss is complicated, it may be best to correspond with your doctor in writing first, then fax or e-mail it over, and ask them to call you back.
- If you don't understand your doctor's responses, ask questions until you do. You may want to start them with "Can you help me understand . . ."
- Talk to your nurse, coordinator or technician. They are good sources of information, too.
- If you still have trouble understanding your doctor's recommendations, ask your doctor for printed material about your condition or where you can go to get more information.

at least 15; and wearing sun protective clothing.

Skin cancer is most effectively treated with early detection. Transplant recipients should learn to perform frequent skin self-examinations and report any changes in moles or new lesions to their dermatologist. The signs to look for are any moles or patches that are:
- Larger than a pencil eraser
- Asymmetrical in shape
- Have irregular or jagged borders
- Uneven in color or have more than one color in the spot
- Or any sores that do not heal in a few weeks.

SKIN CHANGES can occur with steroids and cyclosporine. These include acne, excessive hair growth, and thin and fragile skin that bruise easily. It can also cause redistribution of body fat resulting in "moon face." Some transplant recipients develop skin warts. They usually occur on the hands or feet. You may need to see a dermatologist for treatment. *(For more information about how to care for your skin, see page 146.)*

ULCERS AND ABDOMINAL PAIN of the stomach and the small intestines is thought to be associated with prednisone use. For this reason, transplant physicians commonly prescribe drugs that reduce acid in the stomach to be taken along with prednisone. Some of the drugs that reduce stomach acid include nizatidine (Axid) and lansoprazole (Prevacid).

Rare Complications:

CANCER: Being a transplant recipient does NOT put you at a higher risk for common cancers such as breast, prostate, colon and lung cancer. However, you are at a higher risk for rare cancers, such as nonHodgkin's lymphomas, lip and skin cancer, Kaposi's sarcoma (cancerous skin lesions), and carcinomas between the genitals and the anus and the kidney and liver.

A number of variables come into play when determining the incidence of cancer in transplant recipient, among which include the length of time since transplantation, the intensity of your immunosuppression, and your ethnicity and geography. In a study of 219 lung transplant recipients, the prevalence of cancer was 4%. The incidence of lymphomas and nonmelanoma skin cancer in transplant recipients is approximately 1.9% and 4.3%, compared to 0.1% and 1.6% respectively in the general population.

Because of the increased risk for cancer, it is very important that you continue your clinic visits, perform breast or testicular self-examination, and have a mammogram, digital rectal exam and colonoscopy, etc. If a cancer is detected early, it can be treated with many different therapies, such as decreased immunosuppressive medications, acyclovir or chemotherapy.

UNOS, in cooperation with the American Cancer Society, is in the process of linking the Israel Penn Transplant Tumor Registry (IPTTR) with UNOS' Scientific Registry of Transplant Recipients in order to study the incidence of cancer among transplant recipients. The IPTTR contains records on more than 13,000 patients who have developed some type of cancer since their organ transplant. For questions about the registry, contact:

Israel Penn Transplant Tumor Registry
Phone: 513-558-6006
University of Cincinnati, 231 Bethesda Ave., ML 0558,
Cincinnati, OH 45267-0558

CATARACTS can occur while taking prednisone. It is important to have your eyes checked regularly by an ophthalmologist. If cataracts do occur they can be treated with corrective eyeglasses, contact lenses or with surgical removal and replacement of the lens.

CORONARY ARTERY DISEASE (atherosclerosis) is a problem that can develop in patients who have received a heart-lung transplant. Patients will usually experience chest pain and/or other symptoms. This is called angina and is an early warning sign of a blocked heart artery. However, transplant patients may not have any symptoms of a blockage building up because there is not any sensation in the heart.

OSTEOPOROSIS is a disease that gradually weakens bones, especially in the spine, wrists and hips. As the bones become more fragile, they are likely to break. Some bone loss is normal as we grow older. Transplant recipients are at a greater risk for developing osteoporosis since immunosuppressant medications, such as steroids, taken over a long period of time can weaken bones. In fact, individuals who take 7.5 mg per day or more of prednisone, for six months or more, risk rapid bone loss.

Osteoporosis can be difficult to detect, especially since people in the early stages often have no symptoms. This is why it is important to have a bone density test (DEXA scan). Bone density tests are the most practical way to accurately measure the density of your bones. These tests should be repeated every year, on the same machine if possible, to track any bone loss.

Fortunately, there are things you can do to help prevent or slow bone loss. One of the best ways is by participating in weight-bearing exercise, such as brisk walking or weight-lifting. Your doctor or healthcare professional can advise you on an exercise program that is right for you.

Another way to increase your bone strength is by taking calcium (approximately 1,500 mg per day), along with vitamin D (approximately 400 to 800 units per day). You may want to adopt a diet that contains adequate amounts of calcium and vitamin D, and reduce or eliminate risk factors of osteoporosis, such as smoking and alcohol consumption. Fortunately, there are medications on the market, such as alendronate (Fosamax), which are very effective in increasing bone density.

POST-TRANSPLANT LYMPHOPROLIFERATIVE DISEASE (PTLD) is believed to be associated with Epstein-Barr virus infection, the same virus that causes mononucleosis, and the net effect of a number of immunosuppressive agents employed simultaneously (e.g. cyclosporine, Orthoclone OKT3, etc.). The infection causes B cells to grow like a tumor. This first sign can be enlargement of lymph nodes, fever and tiredness, however, other problems can mimic similar symptoms.

Unlike other tumors, decreasing your daily dose of immunosuppressive medicine can often control PTLD, although surgery and/or radiation may be employed. Acyclovir and other antiviral agents can also be used. Fortunately, PTLD occurs in only a small number of lung transplant recipients (2 of 109 patients or 1.8%). To help prevent PTLD notify your doctor if you notice any unusual lump, especially in your neck, groin or armpit.

RECURRENCE OF PRIMARY DISEASE can occur after transplantation. However, it has only been documented in four diseases: sarcoidosis, lymphangioleiomyomatosis (LAM), giant cell interstitial pneumonitis and diffuse panbronchiolitis.

BIBLIOGRAPHY:

American Academy of Dermatology. "Look for Danger Signs in Pigmented Lesions of the Skin," fact sheet.

American Academy of Dermatology. "Sun Safety 101," 1999.

"American College of Rheumatology Issues Guidelines for Prevention and Treatment of Corticosteroid-Induced Osteoporosis." *The Journal of the American Medical Association*, Jan. 7, 1997.

Associated Press. "Special Proteins May Block Organ Rejection." *Wall Street Journal,* Aug. 6, 1997.

Barr, M. L. "Photopheresis in Transplantation: Future Research and Directions." *Transplant Proceedings* 1998; 30: 2248 - 50.

Barr, M., Meiser, B., Eisen, H., Roberts, R., Livi, U., Dall'Amico, R., Dorent, R., Rogers, J., Radovancevic, B., Taylor, D., Jeevanandam, V., and Marboe, C. for the Photopheresis Transplantation Study Group. "Photopheresis for the Prevention of Rejection in Cardiac Transplantation." *The New England Journal of Medicine* 1998; 339: 1744 - 51.

Bertin, D., Haverty, T., and Sander, M. "Post-transplant Development of Lymphoproliferative Disorders and Other Malignancies Following Orthoclone OKT3 Therapy." *Principles of Drug Development in Transplantation and Autoimmunity* 1996: 633 - 641.

Boland, Maureen. "Worried: Don't Let Anxiety Harm Your Health." *Family Circle* magazine, April 22, 1997, 72 - 6.

Brenier-Pinchart, M., Lebeau, B., Devouassoux, G., Mondon, P., Pison, C., Ambroise-Thomas, P., and Grillot R. "Aspergillus and Lung Transplant Recipients: A Mycologic and Molecular Epidemiologic Study." *The Journal of Heart and Lung Transplantation* 1998; 17: 972 - 9.

Cahill, B., O'Rourke, M., Strasburg, K., Savik, K., Jessurun, J., Bolman, R., and Hertz, M. "Methotrexate for Lung Transplant Recipients with Steroid-Resistant Acute Rejection." *The Journal of Heart and Lung Transplantation* 1996; 15: 1130-7.

Chaparro, C., and Kesten, S. "Infections in Lung Transplant Recipients." *Clinics in Chest Medicine* 1997; 18 (2): 339 - 51.

Date, H., Lynch, J., Sundaresan, S., Patterson, G. A., and Trulock, E. "The Impact of Cytolytic Therapy on Bronchiolitis Obliterans Syndrome." *The Journal of Heart and Lung Transplantation* 1998; 17: 869 - 75.

Dauber, James H. "Post-transplant Bronchiolitis Obliterans Syndrome: Where Have We Been and Where Are We Going? *Chest* 1996; 109(4): 857 - 9.

Dusmet, M., Maurer, J., Winton, T., and Kesten, S. "Methotrexate Can Halt the Progression of Bronchiolitis Obliterans Syndrome in Lung Transplant Recipients." *The Journal of Heart and Lung Transplantation* 1996; 15: 948 - 54.

Food and Drug Administration (FDA) Press Office. "FDA Approves Rapamune to Prevent Organ Rejection." Sept. 15, 1999.

Forman, Judy. "Inroads Being Made Against Osteoporosis." *The Boston Globe*, April 5, 1993, 29 - 33.

Gaber, A. Osama, et al. "Results of the Double-Blind, Randomized, Multicenter, Phase III Clinical Trial of Thymoglobulin versus Atgam in the Treatment of Acute Graft Rejection Episodes after Renal Transplantation." *Transplantation* 1998; 66 (1): 29 - 37.

Ghandour, Fadi Z., and Hricik, Donald E. "Hypertension in the Transplant Recipient." *Transplant Chronicles*, Vol. 5 (2): 16.

Hausen, B., and Morris, R. E. "Review of Immunosuppression for Lung Transplantation: Novel Drugs, New Uses for Conventional Immunosuppressants, and Alternative Strategies." *Clinics in Chest Medicine* 1997; 18 (2): 353 - 66.

Health Resources and Services Administration. "Organ Transplantation: Matching Donors and Recipients." January 1995.

Hoel, Donna. "Blue or Beyond Blue?" Chronimed Pharmacy's *Encore* magazine, Spring 1996, 15 - 6.

International Society of Heart and Lung Transplantation: Cooper, J., Billingham, M., Egan, T., Hertz, M., Higenbottam, T., Patterson, G. A., Smith, C., Trulock, E., Vreim, C., and Yousem, S. "A Working Formulation for the Standardization of Nomenclature and for Clinical Staging of Chronic Dysfunction in Lung Allografts." *The Journal of Heart and Lung Transplantation* 1993; 12: 713 - 6.

Kahan, Barry D. for the Rapamune U.S. Study Group, University of Texas School of Medicine, Houston, Texas. "A Phase III Comparative Efficacy Trial of Rapamune in Renal Allograft Recipients." XVII World Congress of the Transplantation Society, Abstract, 1998.

Keenan, R., Iacono, A., Dauder, J., Zeevi, A., Yousem, S., Ohori, N., Burckart, G., Kawai, A., Smaldone, G., and Griffith, B. "Treatment of Refractory Acute Allograft Rejection with Aerosolized Cyclosporine in Lung Transplant Recipients." *The Journal of Thoracic Cardiovascular Surgery* 1997; 113: 335 - 41.

Kelly, P., Gruber, S., Behbod, F., and Kahan, B. "Sirolimus, A New, Potent Immunosuppressive Agent." *Pharmacotherapy* 1997; 17 (6): 1148 - 56.

King-Biggs, Melissa B. "Acute Pulmonary Allograft Rejection: Mechanisms, Diagnosis, and Management." *Clinics in Chest Medicine* 1997; 18 (2): 301 - 10.

Kirk, A., Harlan, D., Armstrong, N., Davis, T., Dong, Y., Gray, G., Hong, X., Thomas, D., Fechner, Jr., J., and Knechtle, Stuart J. "CTLA4-Ig and Anti-CD40 Ligand Prevent Renal Allograft Rejection in Primates." *The Proceedings of the National Academy of Sciences*, USA 1997; 94: 8789 - 94.

Lemke, Gina. "Your Immune System and Immunosuppressants." TRIO's *LifeLines* newsletter, Sept./Oct. 1996, 6.

Levine, S., Angel, L., Anzueto, A., Susanto, I., Peters, J., Sako, E., and Bryan, C. "A Low Incidence of Post-transplant Lymphoproliferative Disorder in 109 Lung Transplant Recipients." *Chest* 1999; 116 (5): 1273 - 7.

Lindgren, D., and Christy, K. "The ABCs of CMV." Chronimed Pharmacy's *Encore* magazine, Spring 1996, 13.

Marieb, Elaine N. "Chapter 12: Body Defenses." *Essentials of Human Anatomy and Physiology*, Fifth Edition. (Addison Wesley Longman Inc., 1997, ISBN: 0805341854)

McGinn, L., and Harker, K. "Pediatric Lung Transplantation Program: Patient Handbook." Pediatric Lung Transplant Team, Children's Hospital at Shands, University of Florida, 1999.

Mize, Janet B. "Understanding Rejection in Solid Organ Transplantation." Stadtlanders' *LifeTIMES* magazine 1999; Vol. 1: 16 - 20.

"Monoclonal Antibody Approved for Renal Rejection." *American Journal of Health System Pharmacy* 1998; 55: 207 - 8.

Murray, J. F., and Nadel, J. A. "Disorders of the Intrathoracic Airways," and "Idiopathic Pulmonary Fibrosis and Other Interstitial Lung Diseases of Unknown Etiology." *Textbook of Respiratory Medicine*, 2nd Edition, Vol. 2 published by Saunders 1994.

National Cancer Institute and National Institute of Allergy and Infectious Diseases. "Understanding the Immune System." National Institutes of Health.

National Institute of Allergy and Infectious Diseases. "The Immune System." *NetNews*.

National Institutes of Health (NIH). "Facts about Heart and Heart/Lung Transplants." NIH Publication No. 90-2990, September 1990.

National Kidney Foundation and the American Association of Critical-Care Nurses. "A Quick Look at the Organ Procurement Process."

"New Monoclonal Antibodies to Prevent Transplant Rejection." *The Medical Letter* 1998; 40 (1036): 93 - 4.

Novick, Richard J. "Heart and Lung Retransplantation: Should it Be Done?" *The Journal of Heart and Lung Transplantation* 1998; 17: 635 - 42.

O'Hagen, A., Stillwell, P., Arroliga, A., and Koo, A. "Photopheresis in the Treatment of Refractory Bronchiolitis Obliterans Complicating Lung Transplantation." *Chest* 1999; 115 (5): 1459 - 62.

Pham, S., Rao, A., Zeevi, A., Fontes, P., McCurry, K., Keenan, R., Kormos, R., Hattler, B., Fung, J., Starzl, T., and Griffith, B. "Five Year Experience on Combined Donor Bone Marrow Infusion and Lung Transplantation." 1999 Abstracts presented at the 35th Annual Meeting of the Society of Thoracic Surgeons.

Punch, Jeffrey D. "Your Child and Prednisone: Answers to Parents' Questions about Prednisone." C.L.A.S.S., Children's Liver Association for Support Services, 1996.

Reichenspurner, H., Girgis, R., Robbins, R., Yun, K., Nitschke, M., Berry, G., Morris, R., Theodore, J., and Reitz, B. "Stanford Experience with Obliterative Bronchiolitis after Lung and Heart-Lung Transplantation." *Annals of Thoracic Surgery* 1996; 62: 1467 - 73.

Reinert-Lucas, Carole. "Depression." Stadtlanders *LifeTIMES* magazine 1997, (1): 25 - 7.

Roche Laboratories Inc. "Understanding Rejection: A Patient's Guide to Guarding Against Kidney Rejection." 1997.

Santus, Kristine. "Hypertension in Transplant Recipients." Stadtlanders *LifeTIMES* magazine 1998; (3): 22 - 5.

Schlesinger, C., Meyer, C., Veeraraghavan S., and Koss, M. "Constrictive (Obliterative) Bronchiolitis: Diagnosis, Etiology, and a Critical Review of the Literature." *Annals of Diagnostic Pathology* 1998; 2: 321 - 34.

Snell, G. I., Esmore, D. S., and Williams, T. J. "Cytolic Therapy for the Bronchiolitis Obliterans Syndrome Complicating Lung Transplantation." *Chest* 1996; 109 (4): 874 - 8.

Speich, R., Boehler, A., Russi, E., and Weder, W. "A Case Report of a Double-Blind, Randomized Trial of Inhaled Steroids in a Patient with Lung Transplant Bronchiolitis Obliterans." *Respiration* 1997; 64: 375 - 80.

Spiekerkoetter, E., Krug, N., Hoeper, M., Wiebe, K., Hamm, M., Harringer, W., Haverich, A., and Fabel, H. "Prevalence of Malignancies after Lung Transplantation." *Transplantation Proceedings* 1998; 30: 1523 - 4.

St. Petersburg Sleep Disorders Center. "Insomnia" and "Sleep Hygiene," fact sheet.

Sundaresan, Sudhir. "Bronchiolitis Obliterans." *Seminars in Thoracic and Cardiovascular Surgery* 1998; 10 (3): 221 - 6.

Tager, A. M., and Ginns, L. C. "Complications of Lung Transplantation." *Critical Care Nursing Clinics of North America* 1996; Vol. 8 (3): 273 - 92.

Takao, M., Higenbottam, T., Audley, T., Otulana, B., and Wallwork, J. "Effects of Inhaled Nebulized Steroids (Budesonide) on Acute and Chronic Lung Function in Heart-Lung Transplant Patients." *Transplant Proceedings* 1995; 27 (1): 1284 - 5.

Trulock, Elbert P. "Lung Transplantation." *American Journal of Respiratory and Critical Care Medicine* 1997; 155: 789 - 818.

United Network for Organ Sharing. "The Scientific Registry and Organ Procurement and Transplantation Network Annual Report." 1999.

Wagner, Teri. "Immunosuppressants of Tomorrow." Stadtlanders' *LifeTIMES* magazine insert, 1997.

Wain, J., Wright, C., Ryan, D., Zorb, S., Mathisen, D., and Ginns, L. "Induction Immunosuppression for Lung Transplantation with OKT3." *Annals of Thoracic Surgery* 1999; 67: 187 - 93.

Wekerle, T., Klepetko, W., Wisser, W., Senbaklavaci, O., Moidle, R., Hiesmayer, M., Tschernko, D., and Wolner, E. "Lung Retransplantation: Institutional Report on a Series of Twenty Patients." *The Journal of Heart and Lung Transplantation* 1996 February; 15 (2): 182 - 9.

"What is CMV" from Transweb's website at: http://www.transweb.org/qa/qa_txp/faq_cmv.html

Yousem, S., Berry, G., Cagle, P., Chamberlain, D., Husain, A., Hruban, R., Marchevsky, A., Ohori, N. P., Ritter, J., Stewart, S., and Tazelaar, H. "A Revision of the 1990 Working Formulation for the Classification of Pulmonary Allograft Rejection: Lung Rejection Study Group," *The Journal of Heart and Lung Transplantation* 1996; 15: 1 - 15.

3 After Transplantation

GOING HOME:

"I couldn't even think of all the pills one would have to take. Then I talked with my mentor, who helped me understand that it wasn't about taking a few pills, it was about living." – Ann Marie Benzinger

The transplant process is different for everyone. The length of time you stay in the hospital will vary depending on whether or not you've had any complications. Some people only stay a week or two, while others stay for months. After your transplant, you will require special medical care, which can only be met through frequent visits to the transplant clinic. In addition, the first few months after transplant surgery are when the most serious complications are likely to occur. Typically, you will have to continue to live near the transplant center so you can be closely monitored.

While most people look forward to leaving the hospital, the actual discharge may be met with mixed emotions. For several weeks you have had the support and care of 'round-the-clock nursing. You may feel overwhelmed by all the instructions, medications, etc. However, remember that you will be in close contact with your transplant team. You will be seen every week or two for the next couple of months. Blood work, chest x-rays and pulmonary function tests are usually required at these visits.

It is highly recommended that you arrange for a hospital bed BEFORE you get home, because it may be too difficult to sleep on a flat bed so soon after surgery. Everyone recovers at a different pace, and it is normal to have good days as well as bad days. Your body is going through many adjustments as it gets used to the medications and recovers from surgery.

Also, it is fairly common for family members to feel exhausted by the time you are discharged. They may feel some anxiety about their loved one leaving the hospital so soon. It is important to make sure family members take care of themselves, get plenty of sleep and eat a healthy diet.

Your family may also experience a shifting of roles within the family. The recipient may now be well enough to do tasks he or she couldn't do before the transplant. As you recover from surgery and your lung function improves, it is now time for caregivers to step aside and let you do things on your own, which is sometimes a lot easier said than done.

If the illness had a long duration, it is possible that the recipient may have forgotten how to be healthy and readjustment may be difficult. In addition, being on such high medication dosages is difficult to adjust to. It may take as long as 12 months to start to feel somewhat "normal" again. Discussing these issues with your family, transplant social worker and in support group meetings can be very helpful.

Restrictions and Instructions after Discharge:

- Do not lift anything greater than 10 pounds for six to eight weeks after surgery.
- Do not perform any strenuous activity for six to eight weeks after surgery.
- Do not drive for eight to 10 weeks after surgery. This is necessary to decrease the risk of accidental trauma to your chest.
- Clean your incision daily by showering with warm water and soap.
- Wear a mask when you are in the hospital, pharmacy, or when you are in crowded places (e.g., the grocery store, mall, movie theater, restaurant, airplane, etc.). When you are about six months post-transplant and your immunosuppression is reduced, you will not have to wear a mask as often, but you should always wear it when you go to the hospital or doctor's office or whenever you are likely to run into people who are ill.

Special Restrictions for Children:

- Do not lift your child under the arms.
- In older children, prohibit them from climbing, swinging or hanging by the arms; lifting, pushing or pulling objects that could cause strain; bike riding or other vigorous activities in which they may fall.
- School-aged children should avoid contact sports, such as football.

Your Daily Journal:

Routine monitoring after your lung transplantation is designed to detect and prevent complications as soon as possible. Although monitoring is most intensive in the first year, it must be continued for the rest of your life. You will be required to measure your vital signs, such as weight and pulmonary function, and record them in your journal twice a day. When you are further out from your transplant, you won't have to do this as often.

However, as you get three, four, even five years out, and aren't having any problems, it is only natural to feel you don't need to do this. However, there is great danger to your health if you let your guard down. *(Turn to page 269 and copy the worksheet provided to help you keep track of your vital signs and spirometry.)*

WEIGH YOURSELF: Do so in the morning after urinating and before you dress or eat breakfast.

TAKE YOUR BLOOD PRESSURE: Blood pressure is the measurement of the force or pressure of blood against the walls of the blood vessels as it circulates in the body. There are two pressures: the systolic pressure (top number) and the diastolic pressure (bottom number). Systolic pressure is the pressure against the walls of the arteries when the heart contracts (squeezes). Diastolic pressure is the pressure against the walls of the arteries when the heart is relaxed.

To take your blood pressure, do it the same time each day and after you have been sitting for a few minutes. Remove the clothing from your upper arm and wrap the cuff snugly around it. The lower edge should be one inch above the elbow. Inflate the cuff until you no longer feel a pulse. The cuff will slowly deflate, then give you a reading. Record this in your journal.

TAKE YOUR HEART RATE: To take your heart rate, locate the radial artery, which runs along your wrist. Place your index and middle finger on your wrist just below your thumb. Once you've located your pulse, count it by watching the second hand on a clock for 15 seconds, then multiply that number by four to get the number of beats per minute. If you prefer, you can use the main (carotid) artery on either side of your neck, which is sometimes easier to find.

TAKE YOUR TEMPERATURE: Remember not to have anything to eat or drink three minutes before taking your temperature or you may get a false reading. Use a digital thermometer to make it easier to read.

TRACK YOUR DAILY PFTs: Record your FEV_1 and FVC using your home spirometry. These hand-held devices are often provided to you by your transplant center before you leave the hospital. You will use the same breathing technique you would use as if you were at the pulmonary function lab. Repeat these tests until you get three sets that are fairly consistent, and record the highest number. Your transplant center will give you guidelines on when to call if your pulmonary function tests start to fall. Usually, a 15% drop is significant enough to warrant a call.

Some centers will have you send your PFT results via modem. The modem works with a hand-held sensor that is attached to a box, which in turn is attached to your telephone line. You blow into it and the other end receives the information. This is a great method to use because your transplant center can automatically tell if you forget to do it.

Incision Care:

When you return home, it is important that you keep an eye on your surgical incisions. As they heal, it may feel itchy, which is normal. Keep the area clean and dry. Paint incisions with Betadine swabs twice-a-day until completely healed. Do not use lotions or creams on incisions and don't use baby powder or talcum powder either. Report any redness, irritation, opening or leakage immediately.

Once all your stitches have been removed, you may want to apply aloe vera or vitamin E lotion to help reduce the redness of your scar.

Notify Your Transplant Coordinator If Any of the Following Occurs:

- Blood pressure upper number (systolic) is over 150 and lower number (diastolic) is over 90
- Temperature 100° F or above
- New cough, especially one that is producing discolored sputum
- Declining FEV_1 or FVC figures
- Nausea, vomiting or diarrhea lasting more than 24 hours
- Cold or flu-like symptoms, such as fever, sore throat or increased tiredness
- Inability to keep down immunosuppressive medicines
- Cuts that will not heal or that have drainage
- Pain in your chest
- Severe headaches
- Swelling of the ankles
- Loss of appetite
- Exposure to chicken pox or measles if you are not immune
- Anytime a new medication is prescribed for you.

LIFE AFTER TRANSPLANTATION:

"One needs to know one's disease, drugs and their complications, medical treatments, insurance rules and regulations, and a multitude of other things just to get the best that we can from this maze we find ourselves in."
– Gene Downey

It's an old joke . . . PATIENT: "Doc, will I be able to play the piano after my transplant?" DOC: "I don't know, could you play the piano before your transplant?" In other words, you can do just about anything after the transplant that you could do before, eventually. In the beginning, you will have to make some changes in your lifestyle to accommodate the medical and drug regimen. You will also have to learn how to take the necessary precautions against infection since you are now immunosuppressed.

Clinic Visits:

In the first months following your transplant, you will have many follow-up visits with your transplant team. These may include lab work, chest x-rays, pulmonary function tests and physical rehabilitation. As you get further out from your transplant and if you have an uncomplicated course, the frequency of these visits will decrease over time. However, they will need to see you if you experience any changes that might indicate the presence of infection or rejection. Remember to bring your list of medications and vital signs to each clinic appointment. Following is an example of the type of follow-up schedule you may have post-transplant:

FIRST SIX WEEKS:
- Clinic appointment every one or two weeks
- Blood tests every week (for Sandimmune, Neoral or Prograf, CBC, Basic Metabolic Panel and liver function)
- Physical therapy every day
- PFTs, chest x-ray and six-minute walk test every other week
- Lung bronchoscopy once a month.

SIX WEEKS TO THREE MONTHS:
- Clinic appointments every six weeks
- Blood tests every week (for Sandimmune, Neoral or Prograf, CBC, Basic Metabolic Panel and liver function)
- PFTs, chest x-ray and six-minute walk test every six weeks
- Lung bronchoscopy at three months.

THREE MONTHS TO ONE YEAR:
- Clinic appointment every six months
- Blood tests every week, then every other week at six months (for Sandimmune or Prograf, CBC, Basic Metabolic Panel and liver function)
- PFTs, chest x-ray and six-minute walk test every six weeks
- Lung bronchoscopy at six and 12 months
- Dental visit okay at six months, then twice yearly.

ONE YEAR TO TWO YEARS:
- Clinic appointment every six months
- Blood tests every month (for Sandimmune, Neoral or Prograf, CBC, Basic Metabolic Panel and liver function)
- PFTs, chest x-ray and six-minute walk test every six months
- Lung bronchoscopy every six months.

TWO YEARS AND UP:
- Clinic appointment once a year
- Blood tests every three months (for Sandimmune, Neoral or Prograf, CBC, Basic Metabolic Panel and liver function)
- PFTs, chest x-ray and six-minute walk test every six months
- Lung bronchoscopy once a year.

If indicated, heart-lung transplant recipients may also have an ECHO, heart biopsy, left and right heart catherization, angiogram and stress test.

Routine Health Maintenance:

After transplantation, it is sometimes easy to forget your nontransplant-related health care. Be sure you're doing all you can to stay at your healthiest. The following are suggested guidelines only:
- Flu shot once a year
- Dental visit minimum of twice a year for adults, three times a year for children. Some transplant centers may require to you take antibiotics prior to your dental visit.
- Eye exam once a year
- Skin cancer screening once a year (more if indicated)

THE VOICE OF EXPERIENCE

One Step at a Time

I was diagnosed with primary pulmonary hypertension in 1990. In 1995, my liver started to fail and I vomited almost everything I ate for four months. Meanwhile, I begged my doctor to find me a donor, resulting in three false alarms until the final call came. After being in the hospital for most of the year, I received a double-lung transplant on Oct. 6, 1995.

Immediately following the surgery, I began to hemorrhage. They took me back into the OR where I received 44 units of blood. They inserted another chest tube, and finally, the bleeding stopped. During my hospital stay, I was very weak. I couldn't stand by myself. Although once I could get to my feet, I could walk with assistance. When it was time to go home, I was terrified. My ability to concentrate was impaired by the all the meds. I was on prednisone along with Haldol for mood swings. I couldn't figure out how to give myself all those meds, or use the microspirometer. Even though I was a nurse, it just didn't "click." I left the hospital on Nov. 11 after 35 days.

Once home, my husband did my meds for me. I also had a friend stay with me to help me stand so that I could practice walking around the house. Even though my oxygenation was 98%, I had grown dependent on the supplemental oxygen. I managed to wean myself off it during the day, but at night it was hard. Finally, my husband shut the machine off to show me I was okay.

On Nov. 25, the day of my son's birthday, I felt that I could stand up. So, I grabbed my ankles and climbed up my legs to a standing position. My son happened to walk into the room and seeing no one around, he knew I had stood by myself for the very first time. He ran to me, hugged me and said, "Mom! That is the best birthday present you could ever give me." Since that first step, I haven't stopped moving forward ever since.

– Angie Eldam, bilateral-lung transplant recipient,
Oct. 6, 1995

- For female patients annual mammogram and PAP smear, in addition to a monthly breast exam
- For male patients annual testicular exam and PSA (prostrate specific antigen) level.

All transplant recipients should wear a medical identification bracelet or necklace so that their medical status can be identified easily. You may want to include the following information: Lung transplant recipient, immunosuppressed, transplant center and phone number, and any allergies you might have to medication. To order your ID bracelet, contact:

Medic-Alert
Phone: 800-ID-ALERT (800-432-5378)
2323 Colorado Ave., Turlock, CA 95380
Website: https://www.medicalert.org/signup2.asp

Lab Work:

Lab work is a very important part of taking care of yourself after a transplant, especially during the first six months, when you are most likely to have problems. Because the absorption of your immunosuppression varies by patient, you may need to have your medication dosage adjusted frequently until you can find your maintenance dose. The following information is meant to provide you with a better understanding of some of the lab work involved and how to interpret the results:

CYCLOSPORINE/PROGRAF:
Target range is patient-specific.
Shows how much cyclosporine or Prograf is in your blood. Low levels increase the risk of rejection. High levels can cause problems with the kidneys and increase the chance of infections. You should always have your blood drawn 12 hours after your last dose for the best results based on a twice-a-day regimen.

BUN AND CREATININE:
Normal Values: BUN, 10 to 20 mg/dl; Creatinine, 0.4 to 1.1 mg/dl
Indicates how well your kidneys are functioning. High levels may mean the kidneys are not functioning properly, which can result in kidney failure. A diet high in protein can increase the BUN.

WHITE BLOOD COUNT (CBC):
Normal Values: 4.5 to 11.0 thou/cu mm (4,500 - 11,000)
Shows how many infection-fighting cells (white-blood cells) are in your blood. Low levels can mean too few infection-fighting cells. High levels can mean you have an infection. Some medications, like azathioprine and intravenous acyclovir, can lower your white-blood cell count, while others, like prednisone, can elevate it.

HEMATOCRIT:
Normal Values: 36% to 46%
Indicates how many oxygen carrying red-blood cells are in your blood. Low levels can make you anemic, tired and short of breath. High levels can make your blood thicker and cause problems with clotting. Bleeding can make your hematocrit go down, blood transfusions can make it go up.

PLATELETS:
Normal Values: 150 to 450 thou/cu mm (150,000 - 450,000)

Shows how many platelets are in your blood. These cells make your blood clot. Low levels can make you bleed more easily. High levels can make your blood very thick and may require a blood thinner. Liver disease and some medications can cause problems with your platelet count.

POTASSIUM:
Normal Values: 3.5 to 5.0 meq/l

Indicates how much potassium is in your blood. Potassium helps the heart and other muscles work. High levels can cause problems with the heartbeat and too much acid in the blood. Low levels can cause problems with the heartbeat. Kidney failure and high levels of acid in the blood can increase the level, while diuretics can cause low levels. Sodium bicarbonate helps to lower this level.

MAGNESIUM:
Normal Values: 1.8 to 2.8 mg/dl

Shows how much magnesium is in your blood. Your body needs magnesium to carry out many of its daily functions. A low level can cause muscle weakness, sleepiness and problems with the heartbeat. Medicines like cyclosporine and Prograf can cause your magnesium level to go down. Magnesium oxide helps to keep the level normal.

GLUCOSE (blood sugar):
Normal Values: 65 to 110 mg/dl

Indicates how controlled your diabetes is. High levels can cause problems such as excessive thirst, fatigue, hunger and weight loss. Low levels can make you feel faint and cause sweating, nervousness, fast pulse and a headache. Acute stress, such as surgery or infection, can make glucose levels go up. While too much insulin can cause the glucose to be too low. Exercise, severe cold, high fever and a poor diet can lower blood sugar levels.

CHOLESTEROL:
Normal Values: <200 mg/dl

Shows whether there is a problem with your liver and whether you are at higher risk for having a heart attack. When the liver is not working well, the level may be low. Certain diseases, such as diabetes, medicines like prednisone and cyclosporine and bile tube problems, such as blockage, can cause high cholesterol levels. A high level can cause narrowing or blockage of the blood vessels, which may lead to a heart attack. Eating fatty foods up to 12 hours before the test may cause high levels; therefore a fasting state is often required for this test. Diet and exercise can usually lower high levels.

MEDICATIONS AFTER TRANSPLANTATION:

"Before my transplant I was concerned that I would be tied down to a horrendous schedule of taking pills at many different intervals. However, it is nowhere near the problem that I had anticipated."
– Dick Wyatt

One thing all transplant patients agree on that is there are a lot of pills to take. As a transplant recipient, it is important to understand what each medication is used for, how each should be taken and what side effects you should watch out for. In order to take an active role in your health care, you need to take responsibly for taking your medications properly for them to work as they were designed. The success of your transplant depends largely on you ability to take these medicines exactly as prescribed. Developing regular habits can be life-saving!

It is also helpful to keep in mind that most of the side effects are dose-related. These will decrease or go away when your dose is lowered. They can also be lessened with daily exercise, a careful diet or other medications. Remember, you will not experience ALL of the side effects listed here since each patient reacts differently.

Before you leave the hospital you will be taught how to administer your own medications. Unlike most drugs, your transplant drugs are ones that you MUST continue to take for the rest of your life, even though you may experience some troublesome side effects. However, alternative drugs can be used when more conventional drugs cannot be tolerated.

When your physician prescribes a new medication, here are some important questions to ask:

1) How does this medicine work?
2) Can I take this with other medications?
3) What side effects can I expect?
4) Should I avoid certain foods, beverages or other products?
5) What are the potential drug interactions?

Medication compliance (or adherence) is one of the strongest predictors of long-term survival after transplantation. The primary cause of organ failure and the development of chronic rejection can be due to patient noncompliance. Being a noncompliant patient includes making alterations in your medication usage (missing doses, premature discontinuation), changing dosage (taking more or less medication than prescribed) and changing the timing (taking doses erratically or at improper intervals). Transplant recipients are more prone to noncompliance issues because of the quantity and complexity of the medications they need to take. Some of the other reasons patients have trouble staying compliant include confusion about instructions, side effects, forgetfulness or inconvenience.

Improve Your Medication Compliance:
- Take your medications as directed; do not stop or make any changes on your own.
- Read the package insert.
- Medications have both brand and generic names, therefore, it is important to become familiar with both.
- Take your medications every day at the appointed time, do not skip a dose. Find times during the day that trigger you to remember to take your

Making the Transition

On July 9, 1994, I received a double-lung transplant for primary pulmonary hypertension at Duke University in Durham, N. Carolina. After I was discharged from the hospital, I stayed in Durham for an additional six weeks so I could participate in rehab. When in Durham, I felt safe knowing I was just minutes from the hospital. When I finally got to go home, I was shocked at how scared I was. My husband stayed home with me at first. He learned how to give me chest PT, and I maintained contact with many of my friends and family. I found being around others helped me feel a little safer. I also kept telling myself that I would be all right alone.

After my transplant I wasn't getting a whole lot of sleep and it was hard to remember all of my medications. So I started to get most of my medicines out the night before. Then, in the morning, I'd have them ready to go. And since I have to see so many doctors, I kept forgetting whom I was supposed to see when. Some of the offices would call the day before to remind me, but some wouldn't. So I started putting all of my doctors' appointments on my calendar as soon as I got them. I have also forgotten to check my blood pressure and temperature. As time goes by it has gotten easier to remember things, especially those important things.

Even though I've had three bouts of rejection, a stent placed in my lung, sepsis and pneumonia, I don't let it run my life. I have a 19-year-old daughter and a 12-year-old son and a husband, so I stay very busy. I clean house, take care of my family and make sure I have time for myself, too. I have adjusted to my new life as a transplant recipient and feel better now than I ever have before.

– Darelene (Dare) Reitz, bilateral-lung transplant recipient,
July 9, 1994

medicines, like meal times or brushing your teeth, or use tools to help you remember, such as an alarm clock, pillbox or calendar.
- Fit the medication into your schedule. If you are having difficulty taking your medications at the times prescribed, contact your transplant coordinator to see if other options exist.
- Report any side effects to your transplant team.
- If you miss a dose or vomit within one hour of taking your medications – notify your transplant coordinator immediately – do not double the dose without permission.
- Store medicines at room temperature, away from heat, direct light or moisture. Therefore, storing them in the bathroom with a shower in it may not be the best place.
- Never allow your medications to run out; if possible, keep an extra month's supply on hand.
- If your family doctor wants to change or add a new medication, have him or her check with your transplant team first. There are some medications you shouldn't take due to your transplant.
- Don't take any over-the-counter medications without the approval of your transplant physician.
- Don't drink alcohol with your medications.
- Throw away any expired medications.
- Store all medications out of reach of small children and pets.

Induction Therapy:

Some transplant centers take advantage of a concept called "induction therapy." This involves the intravenous administration of antibody medications, such as Orthoclone OKT3 and Atgam, in the early PRE- and post-operative periods of transplant surgery. These agents are very potent immunosuppressants that are given in an attempt to induce acceptance of the new organ in an attempt to reduce the chance of rejection. Two antibody preparations were approved by the Food and Drug Administration (FDA) in 1997 for induction therapy in kidney transplant recipients, basiliximab (Simulect) and daclizumab (Zenapax).

Immunosuppressive Agents:

These are medications that you will take to prevent rejection of your transplanted organ. Many different cells are involved in this process; therefore transplant centers use a variety of medications to interrupt rejection at various stages. Some immunosuppressants limit the number of lymphocytes that could attack your new organ. Others decrease the white-blood cell count by limiting the production of substances used in the formation of white-blood cells. Steroids lower inflammation, which is the body's natural response to an injury or invasion. The majority of all immunosuppressive drugs have been tested in kidney, liver and heart transplant recipients but are used "off-label" for all other organs.

CYCLOSPORINE USP: Sandimmune, Neoral (cyclosporine USP modified), Gengraf (generic equivalent of Neoral) and AB Rated cyclosporine (generic equivalent of Neoral)

DESCRIPTION: Cyclosporine is used primarily as an immunosuppressive agent to prevent rejection of kidney, liver and heart transplantation. This was the one drug that helped revolutionize transplantation by improving survival, reducing hospitalization and patient disease. Cyclosporine is also being used in various autoimmune diseases such as psoriasis, rheumatoid arthritis, Crohn's disease and lupus. Cyclosporine is normally used in combination with other medications, such as azathioprine and prednisone. The FDA originally approved cyclosporine in 1983.

Neoral, a mirco-emulsion oral formulation, was FDA approved in 1995. Neoral works the same way as Sandimmune, but is absorbed more completely and consistently from the gastrointestinal tract. It is especially useful in patients who appear to be poor absorbers of Sandimmune.

The patent for cyclosporine expired in September 1995. Not long after, SangStat Medical Corp. introduced SangCya as the first therapeutically equivalent alternative to cyclosporine USP modified oral solution in November 1998. However, SangCya was recalled in July 2000 because patients may not absorb enough if taken with apple juice. SangStat will need to be do additional studies before re-releasing the drug.

In January 2000, Eon Labs Manufacturing received marketing clearance for a generic equivalent of cyclosporine USP modified in capsule form. At about the same time, Abbott Laboratories and SangStat Medical Corp. received FDA approval to market Gengraf capsules as therapeutically equivalent to cyclosporine USP modified capsules in May 2000.

HOW TO USE THIS MEDICATION: This medication is divided into two doses, which should be taken 12 hours apart. The amount you take is calculated according to your weight, type of transplant and length of time since transplantation. Therefore, your physician will give you specific dosage instructions tailored especially for you and no one else.

Doses of cyclosporine are based on a target blood or serum concentrations. Therefore, your blood levels must be monitored to check to see if you have the right amount of the medication in your blood stream. To determine your serum concentration most transplant centers use the lowest level or trough blood level, which occurs just before you take your next dose of cyclosporine. In this case, DO NOT TAKE CYCLOSPORINE BEFORE HAVING YOUR BLOOD DRAWN. Another form of monitoring, but one that is not widely used, is to test for the "area under the curve," which measures the total drug exposure over a specific period of time.

Depending on the level of this drug in your blood stream, your transplant center will raise, lower or keep you at the same dosage. Bioavailability of cyclosporine is highly variable with only 20% to 50% of the drug being absorbed. Peak concentrations are reached in an hour and a half to two hours. In addition, cyclosporine has the potential to become toxic to your kidneys. Your doctor will carefully monitor your kidney function while you are on this medication.

Cyclosporine USP and cyclosporine USP modified are available in liquid form. It may be mixed with orange juice or almost any other liquid, except grapefruit juice. While you can mix it with milk, most patients find it unpalatable. You must use a glass container, not plastic or styrofoam, as they may absorb the medicine. Use the syringe provided and carefully measure your prescribed amount of cyclosporine. Dispense into the liquid and stir well. Drink immediately, do not allow diluted solutions to stand. After drinking all of the liquid, rinse the glass with more milk or juice and drink this as well to ensure that the entire dose is taken.

Cyclosporine liquid will remain stable for two months after the bottle is opened. DO NOT STORE CYCLOSPORINE LIQUID IN THE REFRIGERATOR or IN EXTREME HEAT or SUNLIGHT; store at room temperature below 86° F. If you need to be away from home, you can draw up the cyclosporine in a syringe one or two hours ahead of time. Wrap the syringe in a plastic bag AND brown paper bag (to protect it from light) so that it can be taken at the proper time.

Cyclosporine USP and cyclosporine USP modified also come in capsules and are available in two strengths: 100 mg and 25 mg. Sandimmune is also available in 50 mg capsules. Capsules come in a foil blister pack. Once an individual pack is opened, the capsule is stable for up to seven days. Make sure that you note the expiration date on the packet. Since cyclosporine gel-caps are sensitive to extreme heat, don't leave your medication in a hot car. If you miss a dose of this medication, contact your transplant coordinator for instructions.

POSSIBLE SIDE EFFECTS: *Most Common:* increase and/or darkening of body hair, especially around the face (hirsutism), acne, headache, tremors or shaking of the hands, increased growth of gum tissue (gingival hyperplasia). *Common:* kidney toxicity, high blood pressure, increased risk of infection. *Less Common:* brittle hair or fingernails, loss of appetite, nausea or vomiting, diarrhea, tingling in the hands or feet, heartburn, abdominal pain and nervousness. *Rare:* lymphomas.

CALL YOUR DOCTOR IF YOU EXPERIENCE: fever, sore throat, tiredness, weakness, nervousness, unusual bleeding or bruising, tender or swollen gums, convulsions, irregular heartbeat, confusion, numbness or tingling of your hands, feet or lips, difficulty breathing, severe stomach pains with nausea or bloody urine.

PRECAUTIONS:
- Cyclosporine USP and cyclosporine USP modified are not bio-equivalent and cannot be used interchangeably without physician supervision.
- Never take cyclosporine USP and cyclosporine USP modified at the same time since this would result in over medication.

Drug Interactions:
- Caution should be taken in using cyclosporine with drugs that are known to impair renal function.
- Never take any medication, prescription or over-the-counter, that has not been cleared by your transplant physician first.
- There are many drugs that have the potential to increase or decrease cyclosporine concentrations. For example, some antibiotics, such as erythromycin (Pediazole), can cause cyclosporine toxicity. Others medications that may INCREASE the level of cyclosporine in your blood include: clarithromycin (Biaxin), ciprofloxin (Cipro), ketoconazole (Nizoral), diltiazem (Cardizem), itraconzole (Sporanox), cimetidine (Tagamet), metoclopramide (Reglan), amphotericin B (Fungizone), fluconazole (Diflucan) and ranitidine (Zantac).
- Medications that may DECREASE the level of cyclosporine in your blood include: rifampin (Rifadin), phenytoin (Dilantin) and co-trimoxazole (Bactrim, Septra).
- Ibuprofen is often a problem for patients on cyclosporine since it causes a constrictive effect on the small blood vessels in the kidneys. Normally the kidneys respond by compensating for the cyclosporine effect. Ibuprofen can inhibit this process making the kidneys more vulnerable to the toxic effects of cyclosporine. Ibuprofen is available over-the-counter in many different drugs, including sinus medications and cold remedies. Furthermore, the entire class of drugs that ibuprofen belongs to, such as Advil and Motrin, can cause this problem. They are called NSAID, or nonsteroidal anti-inflammatory drugs. Other members of this class of drugs include naprosyn (Aleve) and many others.
- Cyclosporine increases blood potassium levels. Excessive potassium levels can be reached if cyclosporine is taken with a salt substitute, potassium supplements or high potassium foods.

Food Interactions:
- Patients should avoid grapefruit juice, since this can increase your cyclosporine levels.

For more information on Neoral and Sandimmune, contact:
Novartis Pharmaceutical Corp.
Patient Information: 888-NOW-NOVA (888-669-6682)
59 Route 10, East Hanover, NJ 07936
Novartis Patient Assistance Program: 800-257-3273 or 888-455-6655, Fax: 908-277-4399
P.O. Box 52052, Phoenix, AZ 85072-0170
Website: http://www.pharma.us.novartis.com

For more information on Gengraf, contact:
  Abbott Laboratories
  Patient Information: 800-633-9110
  100 Abbott Park Road, Abbott Park, IL 60064-6400
  Website: http://www.abbott.com

For more information on AB Rated cyclosporine capsules (USP modified), contact:
  Eon Laboratories Manufacturing Inc.
  Patient Information: 800-526-0225 or 718-276-8600, Fax: 718-949-3120
  227 - 15 N. Conduit Ave., Laurelton, NY 11413
  Website: http://www.eonlabs.com

TACROLIMUS: Prograf
DESCRIPTION: Prograf is a relatively new agent that is used in the prevention of organ rejection. The FDA approved it in 1994 for use in liver transplantation and in 1997 for kidney transplantation. Prograf works by inhibiting the activation of T cells, therefore producing immunosuppression. Research in the laboratory indicates that Prograf inhibits lymphocyte proliferation 50 to 100 times more potently than cyclosporine, consequently, the dosages needed while taking Prograf are significantly less than those associated with cyclosporine. Research has also demonstrated that Prograf is an effective approach to reducing the incidence of rejection compared to cyclosporine.

Prograf is considered a primary immunosuppressive agent or for patients having difficulty tolerating cyclosporine. It may also help reduce the risk of chronic rejection or Obliterative Bronchiolitis Syndrome (OB) in lung transplantation. In a randomized trial of 133 lung transplant recipients, the incidence of OB dropped from 35.8% in cyclosporine group, to 21.7% in the Prograf group. Unlike cyclosporine, Prograf does not cause excessive hair growth (hirsutism), increased growth of gum tissue (gingival hyperplasia) or high cholesterol. In addition, the cost of Prograf is less than cyclosporine therapy.

HOW TO USE THIS MEDICATION: Prograf is available as an injection or in capsule form (0.5 mg, 1 mg and 5 mg). You must take it exactly as directed by your transplant physician so your blood levels can be monitored. Since food interferes with the absorption of Prograf, take this drug either one hour before or two hours after meals. IF YOU MISS A DOSE OF THIS MEDICATION, take it as soon as possible. If it is almost time for your next dose, skip the missed dose and go back to your regular dosing schedule. Do NOT take two doses at once.

POSSIBLE SIDE EFFECTS: *Most Common:* headache, tremors, difficulty sleeping, tingling in hands or feet, stomach cramps, diarrhea and nausea. *Common:* hypertension, altered kidney function, anemia, itching or rash, reduced magnesium levels and changes in potassium levels. *Less Common:* diabetes and hair loss. *Rare:* lymphomas or other malignancies.

CALL YOUR DOCTOR IF YOU EXPERIENCE: constant hunger, continued thirst, frequent urination, vomiting, tingling or numbness of your hands or feet, diarrhea, fever or chills, unusual bleeding or bruising, swelling of feet or legs, rash or itching.

"I am post-transplant and use prednisone. Some days I get depressed when I look in the mirror. I don't even look like myself. But, I sure look better than any corpse I have ever seen."
– Suzanne Tierney

PRECAUTIONS:
Drug Interactions:
- Prograf should not be used simultaneously with cyclosporine.
- Prograf may cause more kidney damage when taken together with other drugs that also cause kidney problems, such as amphotericin B, ganciclovir and NSAIDs (nonsteroidal anti-inflammatory drugs).
- Never take any medication, prescription or over-the-counter, without checking with your transplant coordinator first.
- There are many drugs that may increase or decrease the amount of Prograf in your blood, such as antifungal drugs.
- Medications that may INCREASE the amount of Prograf in your blood include: erythromycin (ERY C, E.E.S./erythromycin ethylsuccinate, Pediazole, etc.), clarithromycin (Biaxin), ketoconazole (Nizoral), diltiazem (Cardizem), cimetidine (Tagamet), metoclopramide (Reglan), fluconazole (Diflucan), itraconzole (Sporanox) and ranitidine (Zantac).
- Medications that may DECREASE the level of Prograf in your blood include: rifampin (Rifadin), dexamethasone (Decadron), phenytoin (Dilantin), phenobarbital (Solfoton) and carbamazepine (Tegretol).

Food Interactions:
- Patients should avoid drinking grapefruit juice since it can increase levels of Prograf in your blood.
- Patients should avoid using salt substitutes or potassium supplements since Prograf has the potential to increase potassium levels. It is important that your potassium levels be checked regularly.
- For best absorption, take this drug either one hour before or two hours after meals.

For more information on Prograf, contact:
Fujisawa Healthcare Inc.
Customer Services: 800-888-7704
Three Parkway N., Deerfield, IL 60015-2548
Prograf Patient Assistance Program: 800-4-PROGRAF (800-477-6472)
c/o Medical Technology Hotlines, P.O. Box 7710,
Washington, DC 20044-7710
Website: http://www.Fujisawa.com

AZATHIOPRINE: Imuran, generic equivalent available
DESCRIPTION: Azathioprine is an immunosuppressive agent used to prevent rejection of your transplanted organ, and is used in combination with other medications, such as cyclosporine and prednisone. Azathioprine works by blocking the growth of white-blood cells. The FDA originally approved azathioprine in 1968 for the prevention of rejection in kidney transplantation. It is also useful in the treatment of rheumatoid arthritis, and lupus.

HOW TO USE THIS MEDICATION: Your physician will give you specific instructions for taking this medication. The dosage is determined, in part, by your weight and a blood test, which measures the number of white-blood cells in your system. If your white-blood cell count is low, the dose may change. Azathioprine is supplied in 50 mg tablets and is available in a less-expensive generic version. Azathioprine may be taken with food, since it has the potential to cause stomach upset. IF YOU FORGET A DOSE AND TAKE AZATHIOPRINE SEVERAL TIMES A DAY, take it as soon as you remember, then go back to your regular schedule. IF YOU TAKE AZATHIOPRINE ONCE A DAY AND YOU FORGET YOUR DOSE, do not take the missed dose, rather go back to your regular schedule. If you miss more than one dose, check with your transplant coordinator.

POSSIBLE SIDE EFFECTS: *Common:* low white-blood cell count and low platelet count (possible bleeding or bruising). *Rare:* rash, fever, sore throat, nausea, upset stomach, diarrhea, joint pain and temporary loss of hair.

CALL YOUR DOCTOR IF YOU EXPERIENCE: vomiting, diarrhea, rash, fever, sore throat, mouth sores, unusual bleeding or bruising, pale stools or darkened urine.

PRECAUTIONS:
- Azathioprine can decrease white-blood cells counts; therefore platelet counts and complete blood counts should be performed regularly.
Drug Interactions:
- If you are taking allopurinol (Zyloprim), which is used for gout, it may increase the levels of azathioprine in your body.
- If you are using warfarin (Coumadin), which is used as a blood thinner, azathioprine may decrease the effect of warfarin.
- If you are taking ACE inhibitors (such as Vasotec, Capoten, Lotensin), which are used for hypertension, in combination with azathioprine, this may cause a severe lowering of your white-blood cell counts.

For more information on Imuran, contact:
Faro Pharmaceuticals Inc.
Customer Service: 877-994-3276
10607 Haddington Drive, Houston, TX 77043
Faro Patient Access Program: 877-705-2630
P.O. Box 52030, Phoenix, AZ 85072

MYCOPHENOLATE MOFETIL: CellCept
DESCRIPTION: CellCept is used in the prevention of organ rejection. In 1995, the FDA approved it for use in kidney transplant recipients, and later approved it for heart and liver transplant recipients. It stops cells from multiplying, and, therefore, prevents lymphocytes from attacking your transplanted organ. CellCept takes the place of azathioprine and works in conjunction with cyclosporine and prednisone. Patients may be switched to CellCept if they have continuing bouts of acute rejection. Clinical trials in kidney transplant recipients have shown that CellCept reduced acute rejection by 50% to 70%, but there may be more incidences of infection. However, little evidence exists of CellCept's use in lung transplantation. In a trial of 13 lung recipients, pulmonary function stabilized in seven.

HOW TO USE THIS MEDICATION: CellCept comes in 250 mg capsules or 500 mg tablets. Swallow the tablets whole; do not break, crush or chew before swallowing. DO NOT OPEN CAPSULES. If capsules are opened accidentally, do not inhale or touch the powder contained inside the capsules. For best absorption, it should be taken on an empty stomach, one hour before or two hours after meals. CellCept is also available in liquid form and is usually taken twice a day. IF YOU MISS A DOSE OF THIS MEDICATION, take it as soon as possible. If it is almost time for your next dose, skip the missed dose and go back to your regular schedule. Do NOT take two doses at once. It is important for patients to receive regular laboratory tests while taking this medication.

POSSIBLE SIDE EFFECTS: *Most Common:* diarrhea, reduced white-blood cell count, infection and vomiting. *Common:* mild to moderate stomach pain, fever, headache, anemia, high blood pressure, edema, nausea and constipation. *Less Common:* rash, cough, shakiness and insomnia.

CALL YOUR DOCTOR IF YOU EXPERIENCE: rash, itching, any evidence of infection, such as fever or sore throat, swelling of hands, ankles, or feet, frequent urination, blood in urine, vomiting and stomach pain, bloody or black stools, or if you vomit blood or material that looks like coffee grounds.

THE VOICE OF EXPERIENCE

Life on High Octane Fuel

I received a double-lung transplant for cystic fibrosis on June 5, 1991. My life went from living in the hospital three out of four weeks a month to juggling a full-time job, a part-time business, teaching Sunday school, promoting organ donor education and putting together my support group's newsletter. I live with my husband and two teenage sons. Life is wonderful, but I still deal with the side effects of prednisone.

Before my transplant I learned about the possible side effects, but I never imagined having them all at once. While on high doses of prednisone I kept getting hot flashes then chills. First I'd turn on the air conditioning, then the heat. My husband thought it was a bad case of P.M.S. I said, "No, it's more like menopause!" I settled on 68° for hot flashes and a quilt for the chills.

Next came the mood swings. Happy one second and crying the next. I found noise confusing. Little things really bothered me. Before transplant, my family and I established a phrase they could use in case I got grouchy. When Dick or the boys told me I was on my "high octane broom," I knew it was time to chill out. It really saved a lot of hurt feelings and tears.

Then there's the hunger and weight gain. I keep a constant supply of rabbit food available and exercise. My hungry horrors are curbed with celery and carrot sticks, small salads and popcorn. For the weight gain, I walk a 15-minute mile three times a week around our beautiful lake. It's enough to keep me energized and maintain my weight. Besides, I always keep "emergency clothes" just in case things get a bit too tight!

Then my hair went from being baby-fine, straight and light, to thick, wavy and dark. Plus, I had hair, hair and more hair everywhere! I use a depilatory for the face, wax for the thick and dark eyebrows, and shave more often.

Diabetes developed while my prednisone doses were high, which necessitated taking insulin until my dose was lowered. Diet and exercise have controlled my sugar levels for the past four years, but whenever I get an infection and my prednisone dose is increased, the diabetes resurfaces.

After nine years of dealing with these things, I've become quite adaptable. I thank God each day for my precious gift. I enjoy every second of every day and no longer sweat "the small stuff."

– Betty Harrington, bilateral-lung transplant recipient,
June 5, 1991

PRECAUTIONS:
Drug Interactions:
- Do not take CellCept in conjunction with azathioprine.
- Do not take antacids containing aluminum or magnesium one hour before or two hours after taking CellCept, since they have the potential to decrease the amount of CellCept absorbed in your blood.
- When CellCept is taken together with acyclovir, an antiviral drug, the amount of both drugs in the blood rises. It is important that you be carefully monitored while taking these two medications.
- CellCept has the potential to increase concentrations of Cytovene.
- If you have diabetes, this medicine may affect your blood sugar. You must follow your blood sugar levels closely and ask your doctor before adjusting the dose of your diabetes medicine.

For more information about CellCept, contact:
Roche Pharmaceuticals
Patient Information: 800-526-6367
Medical Needs Program: 800-285-4484
340 Kingsland St., Nutley, NJ 07110-1199
Website: http://www.rocheusa.com

SIROLIMUS (rapamycin): Rapamune
DESCRIPTION: In September 1999, the FDA approved a new anti-rejection drug, called Rapamune. It is used for the prevention of organ rejection in kidney transplant recipients. The mechanism of Rapamune is somewhat unclear, but it is thought to inhibit the second phase of T cell proliferation. Results from clinical trials in kidney recipients demonstrate that taking Rapamune along with cyclosporine and corticosteroids reduced the incidence and severity of organ rejection up to 60%.

HOW TO USE THIS MEDICATION: Your physician will give you specific instructions for taking this medication. It is recommended that Rapamune be taken four hours after taking cyclosporine USP modified. Your dosage is determined, in part, by your weight and blood test, which measures the number of white-blood cells in your blood. Your renal function will be monitored for elevations in creatinine levels, along with the amount of fat in the blood. Rapamune is available as an oral solution and is also available in a pouche. It may be taken with food since it has the potential to cause stomach upset. Because of the variability of this drug, it is better to take it consistently with or without food.

IF YOU MISS A DOSE OF THIS MEDICATION, take it as soon as possible. If it is almost time for your next dose, skip the missed dose and go back to your regular dosing schedule. Do NOT take two doses at once.

POSSIBLE SIDE EFFECTS: increased cholesterol and triglycerides, increased fat in the blood, hypertension, rash, acne, anemia, joint pain, decreased potassium, diarrhea, decreased platelets (blood clotting substance), decreased white-blood cells, fever, headache, abdominal pain, decreased muscular strength, nausea or vomiting, peripheral edema and tremor.

PRECAUTIONS:
- Patients should minimize their exposure to sunlight because of the increased risk of skin cancer.

Drug Interactions:
- Rapamune should be used with caution with other agents that are known to impair kidney function.
- Drugs that may increase Rapamune blood concentrations include: calcium channel blockers such as nicardipine (Cardene) and verapamil; antifungal agents such as clotrimazole (Mycelex), fluconazole (Diflucan) and itraconazole (Sporanox); antibiotics such as clarithromycin (Biaxin) and erythromycin; gastrointestinal agents such as cisapride (Propulsid) and metoclopramide (Reglan); and cimetidine (Tagamet).
- Drugs that may decrease Rapamune levels include: anticonvulsants such as carbamazepine (Tegretol), phenobarbital (Solfoton) and phenytoin (Dilantin); and antibiotics such as rifabutin and rifapentine.
- Rapamune should not be administered along with ketoconazole (Nizoral).

Food Interactions:
- Avoid grapefruit juice since it may increase Rapamune levels.

For more information on Rapamune, contact:
Wyeth-Ayers Laboratories
Medical Affairs Drug Information: 800-934-5556
P.O. Box 8299, Philadelphia, PA 19101
Professional Services/Indigent Patient Program: 800-395-9938
Website: http://www.ahp.com/wyeth.htm

PREDNISONE: generic equivalent available

DESCRIPTION: Prednisone belongs to the family of medications known as corticosteroids or simply steroids. This class of drugs should not be confused with anabolic steroids, which some athletes abuse. Prednisone is used as a part of most immunosuppressive regimes for organ transplants. Steroids have anti-inflammatory properties and suppress activated macrophages (cells that ingest other substances). Prednisone is the most commonly prescribed steroid and is used in many conditions, including asthma, lupus and many other inflammatory conditions. The FDA first approved prednisone in 1955.

HOW TO USE THIS MEDICATION: Prednisone comes in varying strengths and forms. Tablets come in 1 mg, 2 mg, 5 mg, 10 mg, 20 mg and 50 mg. Prednisone is rapidly absorbed in the stomach and peak effects occur after one to two hours. You should take this medication with food to help prevent upset stomach. IF YOU MISS A DOSE OF THIS MEDICATION, take the dose as soon as you remember, then go back to your regular schedule. IF IT IS ALMOST TIME FOR YOUR NEXT DOSE, DOUBLE THE NEXT DOSE TO CATCH UP, so you take the total amount you should receive for that day. Prednisone is very inexpensive but has the reputation for having the worst side effects. Most of the side effects of prednisone are dose related and thus decrease as your dose is lowered.

POSSIBLE SIDE EFFECTS: *Most Common:* insomnia; mood changes; nervousness; increased appetite and weight gain; and stomach upset or indigestion. *Common:* salt and water retention or swelling of ankles, hands and face; headache; decreased ability to concentrate; depression; euphoria; and oily skin or acne, usually on face, back and chest. *With Prolonged Use:* slow healing wounds; thin or fragile skin that may bruise easily; fat deposits on the face (moon face), upper back and abdomen; muscle weakness, especially in the thigh and upper arm regions; osteoporosis; blurred vision or cataracts or glaucoma; diabetes; suppressed growth in children; hypertension; increased risk of skin cancer; and risk of pancreatitis.

CALL YOUR DOCTOR IF YOU EXPERIENCE: swelling of the feet or legs, unusual weight gain, black tarry stools, severe nausea or vomiting, vomiting material that looks like coffee grounds, changes in menstrual periods, headache, muscle weakness or prolonged sore throat, cold or fever.

PRECAUTIONS:
- Since prednisone can suppress your adrenal gland, you must never stop taking prednisone abruptly. Acute adrenal insufficiency and even death may occur following abrupt discontinuation. Withdrawal from long-term corticosteroid therapy should be gradual.
- Prednisone may slow or stop bone growth in children and teenagers, especially when they have used it for a long time. Your child should be followed carefully by a pediatrician, as well as your transplant physician.
- Prednisone should be used with caution in people with myocardial infarction, hypertension or heart failure, glaucoma or other visual disturbances, gastrointestinal disease such as diverticulitis, ulcerative colitis, and liver disease or cirrhosis.
- Prednisone should be used with extreme caution in patients with psychosis, emotional instability, herpes simplex ocular infections, renal disease, osteoporosis, diabetes, hyperthyroidism, Cushing's syndrome and seizure disorders because the drug may exacerbate these conditions.

Drug Interactions:
- Tell your doctor if you are taking any blood-thinning medications.
- Interactions with diuretics may cause loss of blood potassium. Signs of low potassium levels include: weakness, muscle cramps and tiredness. Report any of these symptoms to your physician.
- Drugs that may increase the effects of steroids increasing the chance of side effects include: oral contraceptives; estrogens; some antibiotics such as erythromycin; antifungals such as ketoconazole (Nizoral). Barbiturates and some anticonvulsants may reduce the effectiveness of steroids.

Agents Used for Recurrent or Resistant Rejection:

Sometimes when you've been treated for rejection with high-dose steroids, rejection is still present. This is often referred to as recurrent or steroid resistant rejection. In this situation various different drugs are used, such as methotrexate and Atgam.

METHOTREXATE: Rheumatrex, generic equivalent available
DESCRIPTION: Methotrexate is a chemotherapy agent used against rheumatoid arthritis, severe psoriasis and some types of cancers. FDA approval for methotrexate was given in 1953. Methotrexate works by stopping the production of cells that are rapidly reproducing.

In transplant recipients, it is being used to reverse rejection and has proven to be an effective alternative to high-dose steroids in the treatment of heart transplant recipients. However, experience with methotrexate in lung transplant recipients is limited. In a couple of small trials (only 10 and 12 patients) methotrexate helped reduce the number of rejection episodes and slow the decline in lung function. Like some of the other medications transplant recipients take, methotrexate is very expensive.

HOW TO USE THIS MEDICATION: Methotrexate is used in combination with your other immunosuppressive medications, such as cyclosporine and prednisone. Your physician will give you specific instructions for taking this medication that is tailored especially for you. Absorption of methotrexate is dose related. Therefore, your doctor will require periodic blood tests while you are on this medication. Methotrexate has the potential to cause serious toxicity and patients are closely monitored while on this drug.

Methotrexate comes in tablets of 2.5 mg. Food interferes with methotrexate's absorption into the blood. Therefore, it is best taken on an empty stomach, at least one hour before or two hours after meals. However, it may be taken with food if it upsets your stomach. The usual dose is 5 mg once a week. IF TAKEN ON A DAILY BASIS, METHOTREXATE CAN BE FATALLY TOXIC. Methotrexate takes time to work. Improvement in your symptoms is variable and may take several weeks. Adverse reactions to methotrexate are common, but are usually dose related. If you experience unwanted side effects, notify your transplant physician.

POSSIBLE SIDE EFFECTS: *Most Common:* stomach upset, nausea or vomiting, loss of appetite, low white-blood cell count and decreased resistance to infection. *Other:* diarrhea, chills and fever, unusual tiredness, respiratory infection, dizziness, diminished liver and kidney function and malignant lymphomas.

CALL YOUR DOCTOR IF YOU EXPERIENCE: cough, difficulty breathing, infection, severe diarrhea, stomach irritation and mouth or gum sores.

PRECAUTIONS:
- Caution should be taken when methotrexate is given to patients with impaired kidney function.
- Methotrexate can cause liver toxicity, fibrosis and cirrhosis, but generally only after prolonged use. Patients taking other drugs which are known to cause liver toxicity should be closely monitored.
- Methotrexate should be used with caution in patients with ulcer or colitis.
Drug Interactions:
- The entire class of NSAID, or nonsteroidal anti-inflammatory drugs, should be avoided while taking methotrexate. They have the ability to elevate methotrexate to dangerous levels. Members of this class include ibuprofen, Advil, Aleve, Nuprin, Motrin and many others.
- Certain antibiotics may decrease absorption of methotrexate such as tetracycline, chloramphenicol and nonabsorbable broad-spectrum antibiotics. Make sure to check with your transplant physician if a nontransplant physician wants to put you on antibiotics.
- Penicillins may increase concentrations of methotrexate and should be avoided.

For more information on Rheumatrex, contact:
Wyeth-Ayers Laboratories
Medical Affairs Drug Information: 800-934-5556
P.O. Box 8299, Philadelphia, PA 19101
Professional Services/Indigent Patient Program: 800-395-9938
Website: http://www.ahp.com/wyeth.htm

MUROMONAB-CD3: Orthoclone OKT3

DESCRIPTION: Orthoclone OKT3 is an immunosuppressant used for the treatment of acute rejection in patients who have undergone kidney, heart or liver transplantation. Administration of Orthoclone OKT3 interferes with the generation and function of cells that destroy T cells. The FDA approved Orthoclone OKT3 in 1986 for acute kidney transplant rejection, and subsequently approved Orthoclone OKT3 for reversal of steroid-resistant acute heart and liver transplant rejection in 1993.

HOW TO USE THIS MEDICATION: To decrease the incidence of first-dose reaction, before Orthoclone OKT3 is given, patients usually receive IV Solumedrol (prednisone), in addition to a histamine-blocking agent such as Benadryl and Tylenol. Orthoclone OKT3 is administered intravenously in a hospital over a 10- to 14-day period. Patients should be closely monitored during the first few doses of Orthoclone OKT3, and lab work performed prior to and during therapy. Lower doses or total withdrawn of other immunosuppressants should be employed during Orthoclone OKT3 therapy to avoid the potential for infections and malignancies.

POSSIBLE SIDE EFFECTS: *Common:* fever; chills; shortness of breath; nausea or vomiting; diarrhea; headache; hypertension; hypotension; shortness of breath; tremor; wheezing; chest pain; and tachycardia. *Less Common:* rash; and a spectrum of often serious, sometimes fatal, adverse events such as cardiac arrest, angina, heart failure, adult respiratory distress syndrome and pulmonary edema; central nervous system adverse events include seizures, brain dysfunction, acute aseptic meningitis, cerebral edema; anaphylaxis; increased risk for infection such as cytomegalovirus, herpes simplex, and fungal infections; and post-transplantation lymphoproliferative disorders (disease of the lymph nodes or lymphomas).

PRECAUTIONS:
- The combination of Orthoclone OKT3 and other immunosuppressants can increase the risk of infection and malignancies.
- Orthoclone OKT3 should only be administered when the patient has a clear chest X-ray and absence of fever.
- The use of Orthoclone OKT3 has been associated with serious, sometimes life-threatening reactions. It should be used with caution in patients with unstable angina, recent heart attack, heart disease, heart failure, uncontrolled hypertension, pulmonary edema, primary Epstein-Barr virus infection, COPD, and in those with a history of seizures or neuropathy.

For more information about Orthoclone OKT3, contact:
Ortho Biotech Inc.
Customer Service and Medical Information: 800-325-7504
700 Route 202 S., Raritan, NJ 08869-0670

ANTITHYMOCYTE IMMUNOGLOBULIN: Atgam

DESCRIPTION: Atgam is a horse anti-thymocyte serum. It is an effective immunosuppressant, which has been in clinical use since 1981. It is used primarily for the prevention and treatment of acute kidney transplant rejection and aplastic anemia. Atgam promotes the destruction of lymphocytes from circulation. The damaged cells are then cleared by the lymph system in the spleen, liver and lungs.

HOW TO USE THIS MEDICATION: Atgam is given intravenously and its dosage is determined according to body weight. It is administered in the hospital under close medical supervision. Some people may be allergic to Atgam, therefore, a test dose may be given. Before each dose, the patient is pretreated with an antihistamines such as Benadryl and Tylenol. For the treatment of acute rejection, Atgam is administered over a 10- to 14-day period.

POSSIBLE SIDE EFFECTS: *Serious:* shortness of breath, wheezing, chest pain or tightness, irregular heartbeats, dizziness or fainting, low blood pressure, spontaneous bruising, prolonged bleeding, nosebleeds and excessive rash on the chest and extremities. *Minor:* fever, chills, headache, night sweats, back pain, rash, diarrhea, nausea, pain at the infusion site and increased thirst.

PRECAUTIONS:
- Since Atgam is an immunosuppressant, your risk of infections is increased after treatment. Avoid crowded places and people who may have a cold, flu or bronchitis.
- Anaphylaxis is uncommon, but serious, and may occur at any time during therapy with Atgam.

For more information about Atgam, contact:
Pharmacia Corp.
Patient Information/Consumer Information: 888-691-6813
Patient Assistance Program: 800-242-7014
100 Rt. 206 North, Peapack, NJ 07976
Website: http://www.pnu.com

ANTI-THYMOCYTE IMMUNOGLOBULIN: Thymoglobulin
DESCRIPTION: Thymoglobulin is a polycolonal antibody used in treating episodes of acute rejection in kidney transplant recipients. The antibody neutralizes the action of the T lymphocyte, the primary cell responsible for mediating rejection. Thymoglobulin has been proven to be superior to Atgam in reversing acute rejection and preventing recurrent rejection in kidney transplant recipients. Studies in lung transplant recipients have not been conducted. The FDA approved Thymoglobulin in December 1998.

HOW TO USE THIS MEDICATION: Your transplant physician will administer this medication. He or she will determine the dose and length of treatment best suited for you. Side effects are usually manageable and reversible.

POSSIBLE SIDE EFFECTS: *Most Common:* fever, chills, headache, pain, opportunistic infection, decreased white-blood cells and blood platelets.

For more information on Thymoglobulin, contact:
SangStat Medical Corp.
Patient Information: 87-SANGSTAT (877-264-7828), Fax: 510-789-4400
Patient Assistance Program: 87-SANGSTAT (877-264-7828)
6300 Dumbarton Circle, Fremont, CA 94555
Website: http://www.sangstat.com

Prophylactic Medications:

These are medications that you will take to prevent and treat infections.

ACYCLOVIR: Zovirax, generic equivalent available
DESCRIPTION: Acyclovir is an antiviral drug that is used after solid organ transplantation to prevent and treat CMV (cytomegalovirus), herpes simplex infection (cold sores or genital herpes), chicken pox and *varicella zoster* (shingles) and Epstein-Barr virus (mononucleosis). This medication cannot give total protection against these viruses. Acyclovir is effective only against actively replicating viruses; it does not eliminate the latent herpes virus. The FDA approved IV acyclovir in 1982 and oral acyclovir in 1985. Acyclovir came off patent in 1997.

HOW TO USE THIS MEDICATION: Acyclovir is available in 200 mg, 400 mg or 800 mg capsules and in liquid form. Dosages can range from 200 mg to 3200 mg per day. It can be taken without regard to meals, but can be taken with food if it upsets your stomach. Acyclovir is poorly absorbed by the gastrointestinal tract and bioavailability is roughly 20%. To clear up your infection completely, continue taking this medicine for the full course of treatment even if you feel better in a few days. IF YOU MISS A DOSE OF THIS MEDICATION, take it as soon as possible. If it is almost time for your next dose, skip the missed dose and go back to your regular dosing schedule. Do NOT take two doses at once.

POSSIBLE SIDE EFFECTS: *Most Common:* nausea or vomiting, diarrhea and headache. *Less Common:* rash and itching.

CALL YOUR DOCTOR IF YOU EXPERIENCE: joint pain, persistent or severe headache, nausea, vomiting or diarrhea.

PRECAUTION:
- This medication will NOT keep you from spreading herpes to others. Therefore, it is best to avoid any sexual activity if either you or your partner has symptoms of herpes.

For more information about Zovirax, contact:
  Glaxo Wellcome Inc.
  Customer Response Center: 800-TALK-2 GW (800-825-5249)
  Patient Assistance Program: 800-TALK-2 GW (800-825-5249)
  P.O. Box 52185, Phoenix, AZ 85072-9711
  Website: http://www.glaxowellcome.com

ITRACONAZOLE: Sporanox
DESCRIPTION: Sporanox is an antifungal agent that is closely related to ketoconazole, but appears to have fewer adverse effects. It is given to help prevent various fungal infections, such as *Aspergillus* and *Histoplasmosis*.

HOW TO USE THIS MEDICATION: Sporanox comes in capsules of 100 mg. It is recommended that it be taken with food. IF YOU MISS A DOSE OF THIS MEDICATION, take it as soon as possible. If it is almost time for your next dose, skip the missed dose and go back to your regular schedule. DO NOT take two doses at once. To clear up the infection completely, continue taking this medicine for the full course of treatment even if you feel better. Since fungal infections clear slowly, you may have to take this medicine every day for several weeks or months. If you stop taking this medicine too soon, your symptoms may return.

POSSIBLE SIDE EFFECTS: *Most Common:* nausea or vomiting, headaches, abdominal pain, edema and skin rash. *Less Common:* fatigue, fever, hypertension, liver function abnormalities and diarrhea.

CALL YOUR DOCTOR IF YOU EXPERIENCE: unusual fatigue, yellowing of the skin or eyes, nausea or vomiting, loss of appetite, dark urine or pale stools.

PRECAUTIONS:
- Do not take Sporanox if you have had an allergic reaction to similar antifungals such as ketoconazole (Nizoral), miconazole (Monistat) and fluconazole (Diflucan).
- Sporanox should be used with caution in people with liver function abnormalities or in those who have experienced liver toxicity with other medications. Liver function monitoring should be performed periodically in all patients receiving continuous treatment for more than one month.
Drug Interactions:
- Sporanox may increase blood levels of cyclosporine, Prograf and Rapamune, therefore, it is important to make sure that your blood levels are monitored while taking this medication.
- Serious cardiovascular events may occur when Sporanox is administered along with the antihistamine astemizole (Hismanal), gastrointestinal agent cisapride (Propulsid), anti-psychotic agent pimozide (Orap) and anti-arrhythmic agent quinidine (Quinora).
- Sporanox may increase the effects of the anticoagulant warfarin (Coumadin), anticonvulsant carbamazepine (Tegretol) and calcium channel blockers verapamil and dihydropyridines, among others.
- Antacids can reduce the amount of Sporanox in your blood, possibly interfering with its effectiveness. Do NOT take this medication with antacids such as ranitidine (Zantac), famotidine (Pepcid), nizatidine (Axid) or within two hours of taking an antacid.

For more information about Sporanox, contact:
Janssen Pharmaceutica
Patient Information: 800-JANSSEN (800-652-6227)
Janssen Patient Assistance Program: 800-526-7736
4828 Parkway Plaza Blvd., Suite 220, Charlotte, NC 28217-1969
Website: http://www.janssen.com

CLOTRIMAZOLE: Mycelex
DESCRIPTION: Mycelex is used as a prophylactic antifungal agent. It offers protection against oral candidiasis or thrush. In addition, it is also marketed in a variety of preparations including vaginal suppositories and cream, topical lotion and lozenges. The FDA approved Mycelex in 1975.

HOW TO USE THIS MEDICATION: Oral lozenges are used for local prevention and treatment of oral candidiasis (thrush). After each meal, rinse mouth with water, then let one lozenge dissolve slowly in your mouth. DO NOT chew or swallow whole. IF YOU MISS A DOSE OF THIS

Too Good To Be True

In April 1994, after being misdiagnosed for three and a half years, I was diagnosed with bronchiol-alveolar cell carcinoma, and was told I had six months to a year to live. My wife, Dolores, immediately contacted UNOS and got a list of all the lung transplant centers in the United States. I discovered that most centers wouldn't transplant someone with my diagnosis. Eventually, my pulmonologist referred me to the University of Alabama. They had already done three transplants with the same diagnosis as mine. They agreed to an evaluation and, after all the tests, I was accepted into their program.

In August, my wife and I moved to Birmingham to wait. I had four false alarms, even going as far as the operating room. However, five and a half months later I received my double-lung transplant. I had an uncomplicated hospital stay and was released only nine and a half days later! The first day I got out, I walked a quarter of a mile! However, about two weeks after my surgery, I had to go back to the hospital to have some fluid drained from my chest. Luckily for me I was able to do this as an outpatient and was released the same day.

During the next few months I was extra careful and took all the precautions recommended to me. I had read up on the literature and knew what to expect and what could happen. I wore my mask in public, avoided crowded places, took my vitamins, exercised and stayed away from sick people. I was prepared.

After about six months post-transplant I felt like I was able to live a normal life again. At one year post-transplant I only needed to take eight pills a day; Neoral, Imuran and prednisone. That's it! I felt great. I had no side effects! No rejection! No complications at all! When I talked to other lung transplant recipients and heard about their problems, I started to fell guilty because I was doing so well. Even when I talked to people who were pre-transplant I tried to down play how well I was doing. I was so free of anything that I was afraid I would paint a false picture for them.

Maybe this was all too good to be true? It has now been over five years without any problems, although I always get a little worried when I go for my checkups. I don't fear rejection, but worry about the cancer returning. Each time I leave the hospital with a clean bill of health, I am very relieved. So every day I say my prayers and thank God that everything is okay.

– Sandy Naclerio, bilateral-lung transplant recipient,
Feb. 5, 1995

MEDICATION, take it as soon as possible. If it is almost time for your next dose, skip the missed dose and go back to your regular schedule. DO NOT take two doses at once. Do not eat or drink anything immediately after taking this medication.

POSSIBLE SIDE EFFECTS: *Very Rare:* nausea or vomiting.

For more information about Mycelex, contact:
Alza Pharmaceuticals Corp.
Patient Information: 800-634-8977
Alza Indigent Patient Assistance Program: 800-577-3788
c/o Alza Pharmaceuticals Corp., 1250 Bayhill Drive, Suite 300, San Bruno, CA 94066 *Website:* http://www.alza.com

CO-TRIMOXAZOLE: Bactrim, Septra, generic equivalent available
DESCRIPTION: Co-trimoxazole is an antibacterial agent with a combination of trimethoprim and sulfamethoxazole. Co-trimoxazole is used for the treatment of urinary tract infections and has been proved to be a versatile agent for the prevention and treatment of *Pneumocystis carinii* pneumonia in transplant recipients. The FDA approved co-trimoxazole in 1973.

HOW TO USE THIS MEDICATION: Co-trimoxazole tablets are available as a combination of 80 mg trimethoprim and 400 mg sulfamethoxazole or 160 mg trimethoprim and 800 mg sulfamethoxazole (DS or double strength). This medication is best taken with a full glass of water to prevent the formation of crystals in the urine. Drink several additional glasses of water daily unless otherwise directed by your physician. Drinking extra water will help to prevent unwanted side effects.

This medicine may be taken with food if it upsets your stomach. Dosage is usually one tablet three times a week. IF YOU MISS A DOSE OF THIS MEDICATION, take it as soon as possible. If it is almost time for your next dose, skip the missed dose and go back to your regular dosing schedule. Do NOT take two doses at once.

POSSIBLE SIDE EFFECTS: *Most Common:* stomach upset, nausea or vomiting, skin rash or hives and loss of appetite. *Less Common:* sensitivity to sunlight, diarrhea, dizziness and headache.

CALL YOUR DOCTOR IF YOU EXPERIENCE: skin rash or hives, swelling of the tongue, fever, sore throat, joint pain, cough, shortness of breath, vaginal irritation or discharge, paleness, unusual bruising or bleeding, or yellow discoloration of the skin or eyes.

PRECAUTIONS:
- Co-trimoxazole is contraindicated in patients with a known hypersensitivity to anti-infectives such as sulfonamide or trimethoprim.
- Co-trimoxazole is contraindicated in patients with liver damage and severe kidney insufficiency. However, co-trimoxazole can be given to patients with impaired kidney or liver function, but should be used with caution.
- For many months after you stop taking this medicine you may be more sensitive to sunlight or sunlamps, so take proper precautions.
Drug Interactions:
- For people who are allergic to sulfa drugs, there are alternative medications available such as dapsone.
- Co-trimoxazole may increase the effects of various agents including blood-thinning warfarin (Coumadin), anti-inflammatory methotrexate (Rheumatrex), anti-convulsant phenytoin (Dilantin) and oral anti-diabetes drugs.
- The trimethoprim in co-trimoxazole may increase kidney toxicity and reduce the effectiveness of cyclosporine.

For more information about Bactrim, contact:
Roche Pharmaceuticals
Patient Information: 800-526-6367
Medical Needs Program: 800-285-4484
340 Kingsland St., Nutley, NJ 07110-1199
Website: http://www.rocheusa.com

For more information about Septra, contact:
Monarch Pharmaceutical Corp.
Patient Information: 800-776-3637, Fax: 423-989-6279
Patient Support Program: 800-776-3637
355 Beecham St., Bristol, TN 37620
Website: http://www.monarchpharm.com

OFLOXACIN: Floxin
DESCRIPTION: Floxin is used to treat respiratory infections such as bronchitis and pneumonia. It is also used to treat mild to moderate urinary tract infections, sexually transmitted diseases, prostate infections, and skin infections. Floxin works against many organisms that traditional antibiotic treatments have trouble killing.

HOW TO USE THIS MEDICATION: Floxin is available in oral or intravenous form and for eye or ear administration. Tablets are available in 200 mg, 300 mg or 400 mg. When administered orally, drink a full glass of water with each dose. Drink several additional glasses of water daily, unless otherwise directed by your doctor. To clear up your infection completely, continue taking this medicine for the full course of treatment even if you begin to feel better in a few days. IF YOU MISS A DOSE OF THIS MEDICATION, take it as soon as possible. If it is almost time for your next dose, skip the missed dose and go back to your regular dosing schedule. Do NOT take two doses at once.

POSSIBLE SIDE EFFECTS: *Most Common:* nausea and insomnia. *Less Common:* vomiting, diarrhea, abdominal pain, dry mouth, headache, rash, fatigue, drowsiness, dizziness, fever, nervousness and decreased appetite. *Rare:* depression, hallucinations, tingling in the hands or feet, unusual sensitivity to the sun and high blood pressure.

CALL YOUR DOCTOR IF YOU EXPERIENCE: joint pain, swelling or rash, swelling of throat or tongue, difficulty breathing or itching and hives.

PRECAUTIONS:
- Do not take this medicine if you have had a severe allergic reaction to this or another antibiotic such as cibrofloxacin (Cipro).
- Floxin should be used with caution in patients with kidney impairment or with a history of colitis.
- This medicine may cause increased sensitivity to the sun. Avoid excessive exposure to the sun or sunlamps.
Drug Interactions:
- Do not take iron products or antacids containing aluminum, calcium or magnesium within two hours of taking this medicine.
- Do not take vitamins containing iron, calcium, magnesium or zinc within two hours of taking this medicine.

For more information about Floxin, contact:
Ortho-McNeil Pharmaceuticals
Medical Information: 800-682-6532
Patient Assistant Program: 800-797-7737
P.O. Box 938, Summerville, NJ 08876
Website: http://www.ortho-mcneil.com

CEFUROXIME AXETIL: Ceftin

DESCRIPTION: Ceftin is used to treat mild to moderate upper and lower respiratory tract infections. The FDA approved Ceftin in December 1987.

HOW TO USE THIS MEDICATION: Ceftin is available in 125 mg and 250 mg tablets. Continue taking this medicine for the full course of treatment even if you begin to feel better in a few days.

POSSIBLE SIDE EFFECTS: *Most Common:* diarrhea or loose stools, nausea or vomiting. *Less Common:* abdominal pain and cramps, indigestion, loss of appetite and changes in taste perception, headache, rash and itching, vaginitis, drug allergy and sleepiness.

CALL YOUR DOCTOR IF YOU EXPERIENCE: rash, fever, joint pains or diarrhea.

PRECAUTIONS:
- Ceftin should be used with caution in patients with gastrointestinal disease, especially colitis.
- As with other broad-spectrum antibiotics, prolonged administration of Ceftin may result in overgrowth of nonsusceptible microorganisms.

Drug Interactions:
- Ceftin should be used cautiously in patients with hypersensitivity to penicillins and any other antibiotics, and should not be taken with diuretics because these drugs are suspected to adversely affecting kidney function. In addition, drugs that reduce stomach acid may result in a lower bioavailability of Ceftin.

For more information about Ceftin, contact:
Glaxo Wellcome Inc.
Customer Response Center: 800-TALK-2 GW (800-825-5249)
Patient Assistance Program: 800-TALK-2 GW (800-825-5249)
P.O. Box 52185, Phoenix, AZ 85072-9711
Website: http://www.glaxowellcome.com

GANCICLOVIR: Cytovene

DESCRIPTION: Oral Cytovene is usually given after a course of IV ganciclovir in order to provide protection against cytomegalovirus (CMV) infection, especially for transplant recipients who are CMV negative and receive CMV positive donors. Its use in solid organ transplantation is relatively new, but so far it seems to be more effective than acyclovir in preventing CMV infections. The FDA approved Cytovene as an intravenous product in 1989, and the oral form was approved in 1994.

HOW TO USE THIS MEDICATION: Follow the directions for taking this medicine provided by your doctor. It is recommended that you take Cytovene with food to increase bioavailability and drink plenty of fluids. Cytovene comes in 250 mg and 500 mg capsules. Cytovene capsules should not be opened or crushed. IF YOU MISS A DOSE OF THIS MEDICATION, take it as soon as possible. IF YOU TAKE IT 3X A DAY and it is almost time for your next dose, take one dose now and another in six hours, and then continue with your regular schedule.

It is important to keep all of your doctor and laboratory appointments while taking this medication since it may lower your resistance to infection and reduce the number of blood cells needed for clotting. To prevent bleeding, avoid situations where bruising or injury may occur.

POSSIBLE SIDE EFFECTS: *Common:* headache, abdominal pain, lowered white-blood cell count, decreased platelet count, anemia, decreased kidney function, chest pain, joint pain, muscle weakness and edema.

CALL YOUR DOCTOR IF YOU EXPERIENCE: vomiting, fever, chills, cough, sore throat, unusual bleeding or bruising, rash or confusion.

PRECAUTIONS:
- Cytovene is contraindicated in patients with hypersensitivity to ganciclovir or acyclovir.
- Cytovene should be used with caution in patients with impaired kidney function.

Drug Interactions:
- Mixing Cytovene with other drugs that can be damaging to the kidneys, such as cyclosporine and amphotericin B, can increase the rate and extent of damage.

For more information contact about Cytovene, contact:
Roche Pharmaceuticals
Patient Information: 800-526-6367
Medical Needs Program: 800-285-4484
340 Kingsland St., Nutley, NJ 07110-1199
Website: http://www.rocheusa.com

FLUCONAZOLE: Diflucan
DESCRIPTION: Diflucan is an antifungal agent that is effective against a variety of fungal organisms, including *Cryptococcus* and *Candida*. It may also be used to prevent fungal infections in AIDS patients and following a bone marrow transplant. The FDA approved Diflucan in 1990.

HOW TO USE THIS MEDICATION: Diflucan may be taken orally or intravenously. Tablets are available in 50 mg, 100 mg, 150 mg or 200 mg. It may be taken without regard to food or meals. Follow the directions for using this medicine provided by your doctor. To clear up your infection completely, continue taking this medicine for the full course of treatment even if you feel better in a few days. Do not miss any doses. IF YOU MISS A DOSE OF THIS MEDICINE, take it as soon as possible. If it is almost time for your next dose, skip the missed dose and go back to your regular dosing schedule. Do NOT take two doses at once.

POSSIBLE SIDE EFFECTS: *Most Common:* nausea or vomiting, headache, skin rash, abdominal pain and diarrhea. *Less Common:* anaphylaxis and liver toxicity.

CALL YOUR DOCTOR IF YOU EXPERIENCE: skin rashes, darkening of urine, yellowing of the skin or eyes, loss of appetite or abdominal pain (especially on the right side).

Sink or Swim

Five years ago, I received a double-lung transplant at Shands Hospital in Florida. At the time, I had gotten approval from my HMO (Tufts) to "go out of region" for my transplant since I wasn't going to survive the long wait in Massachusetts. Luckily, all of my hospital bills were covered.

After my transplant, I decided to remain in Florida, and was notified by my HMO that my policy was going to be "terminated!" I remember how scared I was when I heard those words. I panicked. Right away, I began looking for a new job and found one at a large music distributor. They offered a policy (Aetna) that didn't have any waiting period or a pre-existing condition clause. Knowing my medical background, I knew I wouldn't have qualified for anything but a group policy.

At the same time, I was informed that I could convert my policy with Tufts to another policy with a different company (Allianz). This policy had similar benefits, but it was very expensive. Now, I had two policies; the one from my job was primary and the other policy was secondary. Unfortunately, after about five months on the job, I had to resign because of problems I was having with my transplant. I became eligible for short-term disability and was able to keep my health insurance.

Then the company I had worked for switched insurance carriers and I had to change to Cigna. Then I became eligible for Medicare. Once that happened I was forced to give up my policies with Allianz and Cigna. I was upset because Medicare didn't cover prescription drugs and those other policies did. After a month on regular Medicare, I switched to an HMO Medicare plan with Avmed through the Medicare+Choice plan. Because it was an HMO, they offered unlimited prescription drug coverage. This was to be my sixth health insurance company change in a year and a half!

Things were going great for a couple of years until I got a letter from Avmed. It started out by telling me how wonderful they were, etc., but the real zinger was they were reducing benefits. On Jan. 1, 2001, I was reduced to a $2,000-a-year limit on prescription drugs. Now that may sound like a lot to some folks, but for a transplant recipient it isn't. I gave them a call and told them about my need for these "life-sustaining drugs." Fortunately, Avmed realized that it was cheaper to give me the meds I needed instead of giving me another transplant. Now, my immunosuppressants are taken out of the medical portion of my insurance plan, rather than my annual limit on prescription drugs.

Medicare's contract with these HMOs is rewritten each year, and I'm scared to see what changes are in store for me next year. But, for now, I can afford my drugs and for that I am happy. I'll worry about tomorrow another day.

– Karen Couture, bilateral-lung transplant recipient,
Jan. 21, 1996

PRECAUTIONS:
- Maintain regular visits with your doctor in order to monitor your liver function.
- Diflucan should be used with caution in patients with pre-existing liver or kidney disease.

Drug Interactions:
- Diflucan may increase the amount of oral anti-diabetes drugs such as tolbutamide (Orinase), glyburide (Micronase) and glipizide (Glucotrol) in your blood causing low blood sugar.
- Diflucan may increase the amount of cyclosporine (Sandimmune,

Neoral), Prograf, phenytoin (Dilantin), warfarin (Coumadin), astemizole (Hismanal), hydrochlorothiazide and ritabutin.
- Diflucan may decrease the amount of cimetidine (Tagamet), rifampim (Rifadin) and theophylline.
- Do not take Diflucan if you are allergic to similar antifungals such as ketoconazole (Nizoral) and itraconazole (Sporanox).
- Do not take Diflucan with cisapride (Propulsid).

For more information about Diflucan, contact:
Pfizer Inc.
Patient Information: 800-682-6532
Pfizer Diflucan and Zithromax Program: 800-869-9979
P.O. Box 25457, Alexandria, VA 22313-5457
Website: http://www.pfizer.com

NYSTATIN: Mycostatin, Nilstat, generic equivalent available
DESCRIPTION: Nystatin is an antifungal agent that is effective against a wide variety of yeasts and yeast-like fungi, such as *Candida albicans.* It is used to treat a fungal infection of the mouth, called thrush (candidiasis).

HOW TO USE THIS MEDICATION: For oral administration, use nystatin as a swish-and-swallow solution or as lozenges. If your are using the swish and swallow, place half the dose in each side of the mouth. Swish the medicine around the entire oral cavity. Retain the dose in your mouth as long as possible before swallowing. Lozenges should be allowed to dissolve slowly in your mouth and should not chewed or swallowed. Do not eat or drink anything for 15 to 30 minutes after taking it, otherwise you will wash away its effect.
  To clear up your infection completely, continue taking this medicine for the full course of treatment even if you feel better in a few days. IF YOU MISS A DOSE OF THIS MEDICINE, take it as soon as possible. If it is almost time for your next dose, skip the missed dose and go back to your regular dosing schedule. Do NOT take two doses at once.

POSSIBLE SIDE EFFECTS: Nystatin is virtually nontoxic and is generally well tolerated by all age groups. Large doses may induce nausea or vomiting, diarrhea and abdominal pain.

PRECAUTIONS:
- Do not use this medication if you are allergic to nystatin.

For more information about Mycostatin, contact:
Apothecon (a division of Bristol-Myers Squibb)
Medical Information: 800-321-1335, Fax: 609-897-6968
Address: P.O. Box 4500, Princeton, NJ 08543-4500
Website: http://www.bms.com

For more information about Nilstat, contact:
Wyeth-Ayers Laboratories
Medical Affairs Drug Information: 800-934-5556
Professional Services/Indigent Patient Program: 800-395-9938
P.O. Box 8299, Philadelphia, PA 19101
Website: http://www.ahp.com/wyeth.htm

Gastrointestinal Drugs:

These medications are used to prevent and treat ulcers, heartburn, gastrointestinal reflux, and nausea or vomiting. They also act as an antacid. Most patients take one of these medications in the first weeks after transplantation to reduce stomach irritation and most patients continue to take them since prednisone causes increased acid in your stomach, which can lead to ulcer.

RANITIDINE (Zantac), **CISAPRIDE** (Propulsid), **FAMOTIDINE** (Pepcid), **METOCLOPRAMIDE** (Reglan)
HOW TO USE THIS MEDICATION: Use this medicine exactly as directed by your physician. IF YOU MISS A DOSE OF THIS MEDICINE, take it as soon as possible. If it is almost time for your next dose, skip the missed dose and go back to your regular dosing schedule. Do NOT take two doses at once. Additional antacids may be used with these medications, but check with your transplant coordinator first.

POSSIBLE SIDE EFFECTS: nausea or vomiting, constipation or diarrhea, headache, dizziness and drowsiness.

PRECAUTIONS:
Drug Interactions:
- Antacids have the ability to interfere with the action of antibiotics AND absorption of cyclosporine and Prograf. You should avoid taking antacids along with your antibiotics or immunosuppressants and do not take them less than two hours apart.
- Some antacid medications such as Reglan and Propulsid may cause drowsiness or dizziness. Do not drive or operate machinery while on these medications.

Diuretic Drugs:

A diuretic is a medication that helps your body rid itself of excess fluid, which may be caused by steroids. These medications will increase your secretion of urine. By increasing the amount of sodium and water that are removed from the body, this causes the patient to urinate more frequently.

This, in turn, decreases the amount of fluid (blood) your heart needs to pump and decreases blood pressure. You may have been taking one of these medications before your transplant. After your transplant, you may continue to take a diuretic.

FUROSEMIDE (Lasix), **BUMETANIDE** (Bumex), generics available
HOW TO USE THIS MEDICATION: Since these drugs act to increase urine flow, several common sense suggestions can make their use easier. The drug's effect may last from two to 12 hours, so plan your activities so that a bathroom is accessible. If an evening dose of a diuretic is required, take it in the early evening to prevent the inconvenience of excessive urination during sleep hours. Weigh yourself daily and keep a record. In general, large changes in body weight reflect fluid retention or fluid loss.

Follow the directions for using these medications provided by your doctor. IF YOU MISS A DOSE OF THIS MEDICINE, take it as soon as possible. If it is almost time for your next dose, skip the missed dose and go back to your regular dosing schedule. Do NOT take two doses at once.

Usually, after your transplant you will NOT need to take any potassium supplements with the diuretic even though you may have needed them before.

POSSIBLE SIDE EFFECTS: *Common:* light-headedness, fatigue, indigestion, diarrhea, skin rash and hives. *Less Common:* vomiting, yellowing of the skin and eyes, dermatitis and other skin reactions, and anemia.

PRECAUTIONS:
- It is important to have your blood pressure and blood electrolyte levels checked frequently when you are taking diuretics. Electrolytes are necessary for the body to work properly. Symptoms, such as dryness of the mouth, excessive thirst, muscle aches, nausea, headache, low blood pressure, and fatigue may indicate that electrolyte levels are abnormal.

Drug Interactions:
- Do not take any over-the-counter cough, cold, asthma or diet medications along with diuretics without asking your transplant coordinator first.
- Diuretics may change the sugar metabolism in your body; therefore, patients who are diabetic may need to have their medication adjusted.

Blood Pressure Lowering Medications:

There are many different types of medications available for the treatment of hypertension. Medications can lower blood pressure in many ways. Some dilate the blood vessels, others change the kidney's effect to control blood pressure, still others block part of the nervous system that increases blood pressure. Remember high blood pressure is very common when taking cyclosporine or Prograf and prednisone. The choice of blood pressure medication is determined by the patient's existing medical problems, such as diabetes, asthma or heart disease.

CALCIUM CHANNEL BLOCKERS (CCB) have been shown to block some of the effects of cyclosporine that may be responsible for causing high blood pressure. CCBs cause the blood vessels to expand in the kidney and throughout the rest of the body, which lowers blood pressure. CCBs also cause the removal of sodium from the body and works to slow the heart rate, which also aids in lowering blood pressure. Some common calcium channel blockers are diltiazem (Cardizem) and nifedipine (Procardia).

ANGIOTENSIN-CONVERTING ENZYME (ACE inhibitors) are another class of drugs used for the treatment of hypertension. These drugs work by inhibiting the effects of an enzyme in the body called angiotensin II, which causes constriction of blood vessels throughout the body. These drugs also help to protect the kidneys from progressive damage caused by hypertension or diabetes. Some common ACE inhibitors include enalapril (Vasotec), lisinopril (Prinivil) and quinapril (Accupril).

BETA-BLOCKERS work by blocking signals that activate muscles that constrict blood vessels, expand air passages and speed up the heart. The overall effect is a reduction in heart rate, which decreases blood pressure. Beta-blockers must be used with caution. Some common beta-blockers are atenolol (Tenormin), metoprolol (Lopressor) and propranolol (Inderal).

HOW TO USE THIS MEDICATION: Your physician will give you information on how to take this medication properly. IF YOU MISS A DOSE OF THIS MEDICINE, take it as soon as possible. If it is almost time for your next dose, skip the missed dose and go back to your regular dosing schedule. Do NOT take two doses at once. It is important that you check your blood pressure daily and take any anti-hypertensive medications exactly as prescribed.

POSSIBLE SIDE EFFECTS: headache, dizziness, fatigue, nausea, joint pains and rash.

CALL YOUR DOCTOR IF YOU EXPERIENCE: tender, bleeding or swollen gums, irregular heart beat, dizziness or swelling of the feet and hands.

PRECAUTIONS:
- Some of these medications can cause dizziness. Do not drive or operate machinery until you know how you react to this medication.

Antianxiety Medications:
These medications are used to help control anxiety in transplant patients, which is often caused by the side effects of prednisone and cyclosporine.

DIAZEPAM (Valium), **BUSPIRONE** (BuSpar), **LORAZEPAM** (Ativan), **ALPRAZOLAM** (Xanax), generic equivalents available
HOW TO USE THIS MEDICATION: Your physician will give you information on how to take these medications. IF YOU MISS A DOSE OF THIS MEDICINE and you take it regularly, take it as soon as possible. If it is almost time for your next dose, skip the missed dose and go back to your regular dosing schedule. Do NOT take two doses at once.

POSSIBLE SIDE EFFECTS: drowsiness, headache, weakness and lightheadedness.

PRECAUTIONS:
- Do not take these medications with alcohol, which can induce drowsiness.

Antidepressive Medications:
These medications are used to treat depression in transplant patients, which is very common in patients with chronic illness.

SERTRALINE HYDROCHLORIDE (Zoloft), **AMITRIPTYLINE** (Elavil), **FLUOXETINE HYDROCHLORIDE** (Prozac), generics available
HOW TO USE THIS MEDICATION: Your physician will give you information on how to take these medications. IF YOU MISS A DOSE OF THIS MEDICINE and you take it regularly, take it as soon as possible. If it is almost time for your next dose, skip the missed dose and go back to your regular dosing schedule. Do NOT take two doses at once. It may take several weeks before the full effect of these medications to be noticed.

POSSIBLE SIDE EFFECTS: drowsiness and dizziness.

PRECAUTIONS:
Drug Interactions:
- Do not take these medications with alcohol, which can induce drowsiness.
- Do not take any over-the-counter medications without talking to your transplant coordinator first.

Drug Interaction Dangers:

There is a real danger of drug interactions for transplant recipients who are on multiple drug therapies. Some of them can be potentially life-threatening. Always ask your doctor or pharmacist about interaction hazards whenever you begin a new medication, and before you take any over-the-counter medication.

The most likely encountered drug interactions occur between drugs that have similar effects, such as adding a depressant to ANOTHER depressant, or a stimulant to ANOTHER stimulant. Depressive agents include: alcohol, antianxiety agents, tranquilizers, anticonvulsants, antihistamines, certain high blood pressure drugs, muscle relaxants, narcotics and some pain relievers. Stimulants include: antidepressants, appetite suppressants, some asthma drugs, caffeine and nasal decongestants.

For more information, check out these resources:

Food and Drug Interactions (free brochure)
The National Consumers League
Phone: 202-835-3323, Fax: 202-835-0747, E-mail: info@nclnet.org
1701 K St., N.W., Suite 1201, Washington, DC 20006,
Website: http://www.nclnet.org/fooddruord.html

Deadly Drug Interactions: The People's Pharmacy Guide: How to Protect Yourself from Harmful Drug/Drug, Drug/Food, Drug/Vitamin Combinations is written by Joe and Teresa Graedon, authors of *The People's Pharmacy*. This book not only goes into great details about drug reactions but also contains information about what foods can cause deadly interactions. (St. Martin's Press, 1997, ISBN: 0312155107)

Alcohol and Transplant Medications:

Some of the medications often used by transplant patients are listed here, along with their potential interactions with alcohol. Always play it safe and check with your transplant team to learn exactly how your medications interact with alcohol. However, an occasional glass of wine or beer is usually not a problem.

ANTIANXIETY AGENTS (Valium, Ativan, Xanax): These drugs come with warning labels stating they should not be used with alcohol. They all depress the central nervous system, as does alcohol, and the combined effect can seriously slow down reaction times and impair judgment.

ANTIBIOTIC DRUGS: Alcohol doesn't appear to have specific effects on antibiotics, but the antibiotics are given for a reason. That reason itself may be cause enough for avoiding alcohol.

ANTIDEPRESSANT DRUGS: These drugs should not be used with alcohol because the combination greatly reduces motor skills and thinking processes. Alcohol itself is considered a depressant.

ANTI-FUNGAL MEDICATIONS: Ketoconazole (Nizoral) and metronidazole (Flagyl) both carry a risk. When these drugs are present, the body can't break down alcohol as it normally would.

AZATHIOPRINE (Imuran): When used in very small amounts, alcohol doesn't seem to have serious effects on this anti-rejection drug. However, immunosuppressive drugs can impair the liver, a problem linked with alcohol use and abuse.

BETA-BLOCKERS: Beta-blockers are used to treat high blood pressure. Alcohol does not seem to affect their actions, but always be careful when you are taking a number of other drugs as well.

CALCIUM CHANNEL BLOCKERS: These drugs, also used for high blood pressure, seem to slightly prolong and increase the effects of alcohol. When you have a calcium channel blockers in your system, you may react differently to alcohol than you did before.

CIMETIDINE (Tagamet): This drug is used to treat stomach ulcers. Alcohol doesn't have any special effect on it, but if you need it in the first place, you want to stay away from alcohol, which aggravates ulcers.

CYCLOSPORINE (Neoral/Sandimmune, etc.): Because alcohol can impair the liver's ability to use this drug, the levels of cyclosporine circulating in your blood may increase. Transplant patients should be extremely careful with alcohol and cyclosporine.

METOCLOPRAMIDE (Reglan): This drug is used to speed up the emptying of the stomach. Transplant patients sometimes take it for heartburn or to help move prednisone through the stomach quickly. If alcohol is present, it may be absorbed quickly and cause changes much sooner than normally expected.

NITRATES, NITROGLYCERIN: These medications decrease blood pressure by widening blood vessels. Alcohol also dilates blood vessels, so the effect is increased.

RANITIDINE (Zantac):This drug is used to treat gastrointestinal ulcers. Alcohol can only make a burning stomach burn more intensely.

WARFARIN (Coumadin): This is an anticoagulant used to prevent the blood from clotting too quickly. Small amounts of alcohol don't seem to interfere with its action. However, warfarin can markedly affect cyclosporine and Prograf levels.

Buying Prescription Drugs:

The cost of immunosuppressive drugs can be staggering. But, the costs can vary from one pharmacy to another. Even if you think you don't have to worry about the cost because your insurance is paying the bill, be careful. Many, if not most, health insurance policies now have a lifetime or annual cap and you don't ever want to reach that limit if you can avoid it.

Today it pays to be informed. Here are some things to think about when selecting a pharmacy in addition to cost:

- Will the pharmacy complete insurance claim forms and wait for reimbursement or will you have to pay up-front?
- Does the pharmacy routinely stock immunosuppressive drugs? If not, how much notice do they require?
- Does the pharmacy deliver free of charge?
- How long is the turnaround time from when the pharmacy receives the prescription to when you receive the medication?

FINDING THE BEST PRICE FOR PRESCRIPTION DRUGS: To find the best price for prescription drugs you should compare prices from a variety of different pharmacies. Don't forget to check your local pharmacy, in addition to the big chains. However, some of the lowest prices for prescription drugs are at "membership" organizations. Remember that the savings on an order of immunosuppressive drugs will often cover the annual membership fee. Likewise, membership in any organization with a prescription drug plan is well worth investigating.

Unfortunately, the only way to get the price for a drug BEFORE getting the prescription filled is to ask for the "self-pay" price. This is the price you would pay if you paid for it without insurance. Keep in mind that the price your insurance company pays will be less than the self-pay price.

Another way to cut your pharmacy bill includes telling your doctor you want to lower your medication costs, if possible. They may be able to use more generic drugs or use lower-costing brand-name drugs.

DRUG SUBSTITUTION: Most pharmacists offer generic substitutes for brand-name drugs that cost less. A generic drug must be the "therapeutic equivalent" of the brand-named drug and contain the identical amount of active medicine. However, generic drugs can be made with different dyes, flavoring, preservatives and fillers – the nonactive ingredients. Most of the time, these drugs are the same as the brand-names. However, sometimes

One Month's Supply of Prescription Drugs

Self-Pay or Cash Price (as of January 1, 2001)

Medication & Dosage	Statlanders	Chronimed	Wal-Mart	Walgreen's	Costco
Sandimmune/175mg/2x day	755.93	642.80	739.69	763.78	653.08
or Neoral/175mg/2x day	679.60	577.37	658.89	683.78	587.58
or Gengraf/175mg/2xday	612.31	519.69	568.70	603.78	419.58
or Prograf/2mg/2x day	381.67	324.57	347.97	374.39	329.69
Azathioprine/125mg/1x day	106.23	88.48	57.54	85.09	51.39
or CellCept/1gram/2x day	598.60	520.78	593.68	625.29	540.59
Prednisone/7.5mg/1x day	7.75	4.95	10.46	7.99	8.09
Axid/150mg/2x day	123.30	111.37	124.54	126.99	113.39
SMZ-TMP/M, W, F/1x day	4.95	5.42	11.84	10.79	6.99
Mycelex/10mg/2x day	78.72	64.90	79.46	84.59	84.29

there may be differences in the way they are absorbed in your body. This is especially important in the case of your immunosuppressive medications. To avoid problems, make sure your pharmacist doesn't switch any of your immunosuppressive drugs without informing you or your transplant physician. If you are taking a brand-name drug and want to continue to receive it, ask your physician to specify "brand medically necessary" on your prescription. Do not switch between different brands of any of your immunosuppressive medications.

PRESCRIPTION DRUG ASSISTANCE PROGRAMS: Most people don't realize that just about all pharmaceutical companies have a "Patient Assistance Program," which provides medications to people who cannot afford them. Your physician must apply to these programs on your behalf, but you can call and obtain the applications and information yourself. Most programs require that patients meet certain income requirements. Amounts and eligibility vary greatly from program to program.

There are approximately 55 drug manufacturers that offer some type of assistance to needy patients. The Cost Containment Research Institute has published a 32-page booklet entitled *Free and Low Cost Prescription Drugs*. To receive a copy, contact:

The Cost Containment Research Institute
Capital Hill, 611 Pennsylvania Ave. S.E., Suite 1010, Washington, DC 20003 Phone: 202-637-0038
Website: http://www.institute-dc.org

As a last resort, if you cannot afford your prescription medication, ask your doctor for some drug samples to help keep you going until you find a more permanent solution.

TAKE PRECAUTIONS:

"I refuse to give up, I refuse to feel sorry for myself, and I intend to live each day to the fullest of my ability."
– Linda Cornell

When Eating:

Stay away from salad bars and buffet tables since these foods are often left out for long periods of time. Serving spoons may be contaminated from all the people using them. Order well-cooked meats and eggs to avoid the chance of getting *Salmonella*. Never eat raw oysters or seafood, which can contain potentially lethal bacteria.

With Alcoholic Beverages:

If drinking alcohol is important to you, weigh the risks first. A little usually won't hurt, but, along with moderation, caution is the key. When you are taking a number of medications, as most transplant recipients are, and using alcohol the potential for drug interactions are great. These drugs not only interact with each other, but when alcohol is present the effects can be hard to predict. For example, the liver metabolizes azathioprine, and, when used in combination with alcohol, can cause liver damage as well as liver failure. If you must drink, don't do it when you need to take your drugs.

With Grapefruit Juice
and Cyclosporine or Prograf:

Grapefruit juice contains certain flavonoids, which can block an important enzyme in the liver responsible for gradually deactivating some drugs. Without the enzyme, drug levels can climb dangerously high. This has implications for transplant recipients who are on cyclosporine or Prograf and who also ingest grapefruit juice. This interaction cannot be predicted and can result in less-than-consistent blood levels; use with caution. You should not attempt to adjust your cyclosporine levels by drinking grapefruit juice on your own since a standard dose of grapefruit juice doesn't exist.

With Unpasteurized Juices,
Milk and Milk Products:

Some 98% of all juices, milk and milk products on the market are pasteurized. However, unpasteurized juices, particularly fresh-squeezed varieties, can be a threat to people with suppressed immune systems. Such was the case with bacteria-laden apple juice that caused one death and widespread illness in 1996. Keep in mind that fresh apple cider is unpasteurized. However, there's a way you can avoid getting ill by killing off any bacteria present by bringing the cider to a slow boil for one minute.

With Drinking Water:

Cryptosporidium is a naturally occurring microscopic organism found in the feces of humans, livestock and other animals. Individuals can be infected through contaminated drinking water or food or by contact with infected people or animals. When healthy adults ingest a number of parasites, they can cause flu-like symptoms (diarrhea, nausea, cramping, low-grade fever and vomiting) that usually last up to two weeks. However, *Cryptosporidium* can be a serious complication for individuals with weakened immune systems, infants and the elderly. In severe cases, the disease, called cryptosporidiosis, can develop into a prolonged, life-threatening cholera-like illness.

Cryptosporidium is prevalent in surface waters, such as rivers, streams, lakes and reservoirs. Recent studies show it is present in 65% to 97% of surface waters tested throughout the United States. Ground water sources are typically free from *Cryptosporidium* because of the natural filtration in the soil and rock. However, ground water under the direct influence of surface water is susceptible to contamination.

A waterborne outbreak poses the biggest concern because of its potential to infect many thousands of people, e.g., the 1993 Milwaukee outbreak that caused 403,000 cases of cryptosporidiosis, and more than 100 people died of contaminated tap water. *Cryptosporidium* is highly resistant to chemical disinfectants used in the treatment of drinking water. Therefore, physical removal of the parasite from water is an important component of the drinking water treatment process. If *Cryptosporidium* is detected in any public drinking supply, the results must be reported to Department of Environmental Protection (DEP). Currently, the Health Department tracks reported cases of cryptosporidiosis to determine any area wide trends that may implicate water treatment failure.

If there is a reported outbreak of *Cryptosporidium* in your area, safe drinking water sources include tap water that has been at a full and rolling boil for a minimum of one minute. Bottled water is also a safe bet providing it comes from protected underground sources, such as springs and wells. In addition, bottled water that has been subjected to distillation, reverse osmosis, and/or one-micron absolute filtration is free from *Cryptosporidium*. The International Bottled Water Association can tell you which companies use a process that guarantees removal of the parasite.

International Bottled Water Association
Information Hotline: 800-WATER-11 (800-928-3711)
1700 Diagonal Road, Suite 650, Alexandria, VA 22314
Website: http://www.bottledwater.org

Another option is to buy a water filter certified by the National Sanitation Foundation (NSF) International, a product testing organization. The filter should be marked "NSF Standard 53 for cyst reduction." *Cryptosporidium* parasites measure about four to six microns in diameter. For a list of tested and certified manufacturers, contact the NSF International.

National Sanitation Foundation
Phone: 800-NSF-MARK (800-673-6275) or 734-769-8010
P.O. Box 130140, Ann Arbor, MI 48113-0140
Website: http://www.nsf.org

Remember, do not to contaminate safe drinking water with ice cubes made from tap water that was not boiled. Don't drink juices made from concentrate or fountain sodas. Be careful not to swallow water while brushing your teeth. For more information on *Cryptosporidium*, contact your state's DEP, Health Department office or the Division of Parasitic Diseases of the Centers for Disease Control and Prevention.

Division of Parasitic Diseases
Phone: 770-488-7760
Centers for Disease Control and Prevention
MS F22, 4770 Buford Highway, N.E., Atlanta, GA 30341
Website: http://www.cdc.gov/ncidod/dpd/aboutdpd

When Swimming:

The water in oceans, rivers, lakes, pools, hot tubs and water parks can become contaminated by untreated storm drain water, sewage and leaking diapers, which pose an increased risk of developing a variety of respiratory and gastrointestinal infections. Standard chlorination and filtering does not kill the parasite, *Cryptosporidium*. If you swim, avoid immersing your head underwater or swallowing any water. Children should be required to wear special "leak-proof" rubber pants while swimming.

With Smoking:

You must not smoke. Smoking causes damage to the lungs, making it easier for you to develop a lung infection. You should stay away from smoke-filled areas as much as possible. If family members smoke, they must smoke outside of your home.

> *"One should never give the impression that one gets through this on their own. Not me. Thank God for friends and family, of course, but kitties help a lot too."*
> *– Deborah Drier*

With Pets:

Opinions on whether or not you can own a pet vary from transplant center to transplant center. Immunosuppressed patients may wish to keep their pets or adopt a new one. You should discuss the risks and benefits of pet ownership with your transplant doctor and veterinarian so that logical decisions concerning ownership and management can be made. Sociologists and psychologists agree that the unconditional companionship and emotional support that pets can provide are especially important for the infirmed and elderly. However, pets can be a source of infection, so you need to exercise caution. Nonetheless, the risk of acquiring a disease from direct contact with a personally owned, healthy, INDOOR pet is very small.

All new or existing pets should be screened for animal diseases. The most common agents that infect immunosuppressed patients include *T. gondii*, *Giardia spp.*, *Cryptosporidium parvum*, *Salmonella spp.*, *Campylobacter jejuni* and *Bartonella henselae*.

DOGS AND CATS should be routinely dewormed with drugs that kill heartworms, hookworms, roundworms and tapeworms. Flea control should be instituted. A physical examination should be performed yearly, and fecal examination should be performed twice yearly or more if you own an outside pet. Be aware of any clinical signs of disease associated with the gastrointestinal tract, eyes, respiratory tract, urinary system or skin, and seek evaluation and treatment as needed. If your pet has diarrhea or shows signs sickness, you should avoid contact with it and seek medical care.

Stay away from dog and cat feces. In the case of cat feces, they should be removed daily, preferably by someone other than the transplant patient. For individuals who live alone, an automatic cat litter box can solve the problem. (Littermaid makes a good one.) Always were a mask and gloves to prevent infection. Cat feces can carry *Toxoplasma gondii*, a parasitic organism that can be potentially fatal in immunosuppressed patients. Cats get the parasite from hunting mice, birds or other wild animals, so keep your cat indoors. And since cats often defecate outdoors, wear gloves when working in the garden and wash your hands well afterward.

In addition to direct contact, transmission of animal-to-human diseases can take place via mosquitoes, fleas, instruments, contaminated water and food. Inhalation and ingestion are also common, but injuries through bites and scratches can be just as risky. A scratch from your cat may cause cat scratch fever, which is a benign bacterial infection. If you've been experiencing a low-grade fever, fatigue, headaches and swollen lymph nodes, see your transplant physician immediately. Cat scratch fever can be fatal. If caught early and treated with antibiotics, infected individuals will almost always recover. Avoid activities that may result in cat scratches or bites. You may want to have your cat's claws surgically removed or use a low-tech alternative, called Soft Paws, through which your veterinarian glues a soft plastic covering over the nails, somewhat like acrylic nails.

Don't let your dog or cat lick your hands or face. After handling or petting animals be sure to wash your hands thoroughly. Be wary of stray animals and pets owned by other people.

BIRDS: Immunosuppressed owners of pet birds have been told they should avoid ownership due to concerns about *Cryptococcus neoformans* and *Mycobacterum avium*. *C. neoformans* are frequently isolated from soil and droppings of wild birds, especially pigeons, but it is rare in pet birds' droppings. Transplant recipients should avoid places where pigeon droppings are abundant. *M. avium*, which can cause avian tuberculosis, rarely develops in pet birds, although the infection may be more common in gray-cheeked parakeets and Amazon parrots. Persons with impaired immune systems should avoid contact with pet birds with *M. avium* infections and avoid handling any wild birds because they are more likely than pet birds to shed *Salmonella* and *Campylobacter spp*.

Transplant recipients should avoid all contact with bird droppings. The possibility of inhaling the dried fecal material is too great. Get someone to clean the cage for you or, if you must do it, wear a mask and gloves and immediately wash afterwards To reduce the risk of acquiring *Salmonella* and *Campylobacter spp.*, owners should feed their birds a high-quality diet, avoiding old seed that may have been contaminated during storage.

FISH: Fish can carry many parasites. If you must have them, have someone else clean their tank. A small number of *Mycobacterium marinum* infections have been reported among immunosuppressed persons. All of these cases occurred when the person was cleaning the tank.

OTHER ANIMALS: Transplant recipients should not own reptiles, since they are likely carriers and shedders of *Salmonella*. People who already keep reptiles as pets should:
- Always wash hands thoroughly after handling a reptile or reptile cage.
- Do not allow reptiles in the kitchen or other food preparation areas.
- Do not wash reptiles, their cages or their dishes in the kitchen sink. If the bathtub is used for that purpose, clean and disinfect it thoroughly.
- Do not let reptiles roam about the home.
- Remove the reptile from the home before a new child arrives.
- Keep reptiles away from children younger than 5 years of age and individuals with poorly functioning immune systems.

Small rodents, such as hamsters, gerbils, rats and mice, can also transmit *Salmonella*, *Campylobacter*, *Cryptosporidium* and *Giardia* infections. They can also affect your resistance to some immunosuppressive drugs, such as Orthoclone OKT3, so stay away from them.

Transplant recipients should avoid contact with farm animals, especially animals with diarrhea. They can carry several infectious agents, including *Cryptosporidium spp.* and *B. bronchiseptica*. Also, it may be a good idea to stay away from the circus or zoo, since the dried fecal material from these animals creates dust, which is not good for anyone. Horse, cat and dog shows present the same problem. Keeping horses can be hazardous to transplant recipients because of the microorganisms that can live in their feed. If you must keep horses, have someone else feed and clean their stalls.

When Gardening:

Gardening should be done with extreme caution, if at all. *Aspergillus fumigatus* is a fungus that lives in soil, decaying leaves and grass. When the soil is stirred up, it can be inhaled, which can lead to a condition called farmer's lung. It can be fatal to immunosuppressed patients if not treated early. Symptoms are flu-like and tend to appear in those prone to allergies. In general, patients are discouraged from gardening, but, if you must, wear a mask and gloves. This fungus also exists around any construction site where the soil is disturbed. It can also exist in ventilation and air conditioning systems that have been inactive for a long time. You should leave the house for a while the first time the air conditioner is turned on for the season; the same is true for your automobile.

When Traveling:

Travel to interesting areas of the world can be an enjoyable experience. However, travel plans should be tempered by good sense. In general, you can safely travel in North America, Europe, Japan and Australia. Any other possibilities should be discussed on an individual basis with your transplant coordinator. You should always get the recommended shots for the area you intend to travel, but check with your transplant coordinator first. Be careful to drink only bottled water and avoid drinks with ice cubes and salads.

If you decide to travel, NEVER pack your medications in your suitcase, keep them with you at all times. Your flight could get delayed or your luggage could get lost. It is a good idea to carry extra medications, and bring a copy of your prescriptions with you in case you run out. It is best to keep them in their original containers, so you don't have any trouble with Customs. Complete any routine checkups or blood work prior to your departure. Pack any relevant medical records, including a list of daily medications, allergies and vaccinations, and the names and phone numbers of your transplant center. You may also want to purchase travel insurance in the event that you might need to cancel or change your travel plans.

When flying, take along a mask in case someone seated close to you has a cold, and wear it at all times. Most major airlines mix fresh air with re-circulated air. The re-circulated air is run through filters to remove bacteria, pollen, dust and mold, but viruses that cause colds, flu, chicken pox and some other diseases are so small that sometimes filters can't capture them. Carry bottled water to keep yourself hydrated. It's also a good idea to check to see if your health insurance will cover you for medical emergencies outside of the United States before you travel. Always check with your transplant coordinator prior to leaving for the name and location of a transplant facility where you will be traveling.

For more information about traveling after your transplant, contact the National Kidney Foundation at 800-622-9010 to order their "Travel Tips" brochure.

With Vaccinations:

Vaccinations without the live virus (tetanus, diphtheria, H. influenza B and hepatitis B) can be safely given to transplant patients, and there is no restriction on being around people who have received them.

Other vaccines with live viruses, such as the conventional oral polio vaccination or the varicella virus (chicken pox) vaccination, should NOT be given to transplant patients since they could get the disease. Transplant recipients should not handle the feces or diapers or washcloths that have been used to cleanse the anal area of someone who received the polio vaccination for one month, since it is excreted in an active form in the feces of the person vaccinated. There is an alternative vaccine that is available for polio, called IPV (inactivated polio vaccine). This fits in the dead virus category and is safe for transplant patients to take, and vaccinated persons pose no threat to transplant patients, but check with your physician.

Other vaccines with live virus include measles, mumps and rubella (MMR). The Centers for Disease Control (CDC) does NOT recommend that these be given to transplant recipients since they could get the disease.

However, since the vaccine is not excreted in feces, it is not a problem handling the wastes of someone who has been vaccinated.

Some centers recommend an annual flu shot for patients, while others do not. Note that these are good for handling the flu but will not prevent the common cold. Your center may also recommend a tetanus shot every 10 years. Currently, there is no CDC recommendation for the varicella zoster vaccine (chicken pox). The FDA has a general caution against using the vaccine in immunosuppressed patients since it contains the live virus.

Transplanted children will need to continue their immunizations six months after surgery. The schedule they will follow is different from the one a child without a transplant would follow. Contact your transplant coordinator for information about immunizations for your child.

With Antibiotics:

Never take clarithromycin (Biaxin) or anything resembling erythromycin. It has been known to drive up the absorption level of cyclosporine and Prograf. Always check with your transplant coordinator or doctor whenever a nontransplant physician prescribes an antibiotic.

With Over-the-Counter Medications:

Do NOT take aspirin or any other nonsteroidal anti-inflammatory drugs, such as Advil, ibuprofen, Nuprin or Excedrin IB. These medications are often a problem for patients on cyclosporine and can reduce kidney function and even result in kidney failure. Patients need to take any over-the-counter medications with caution, especially ibuprofen which is available in many different drugs, including sinus medications and cold remedies. Also, aspirin is very irritating to the stomach and can cause bleeding ulcers. Use acetaminophen (Tylenol) only. Read labels carefully and always call your transplant coordinator before taking any over-the-counter medications.

PERSONAL CARE:

"Seems like I have something else to look forward to post-transplant; not going bald."
– JoAnn Davies

Skin Care:

In general, you will not need any special skin care unless you have problems with acne or dry skin. You may use any type of soap.

BRUISING: Extended prednisone use can cause the skin and its blood vessels to thin. To reduce the damage to your skin, be careful not to bump into any hard surface. Bruising can also be avoided by carefully monitoring your platelet count to make sure it isn't too low. Azathioprine, CellCept and Rapamune can decrease the platelet count in the blood. Platelets are a component of the blood that allow the blood vessels to clot.

If you do bang yourself, you may want to put some arnica gel on them to help heal them more quickly. If bruises become unsightly, you may want to consider using makeup to cover them up.

CUTS AND SCRATCHES: Long-term prednisone use can lead to impaired wound healing. In the case of cuts and scratches, keep the area clean and dry by washing with soap and water. You may want to clean with hydrogen peroxide, if desired, and apply an antibiotic ointment to prevent infection. For large cuts, dog bites or areas of skin that appear infected (redness, swelling, pus, increased tenderness), always call your transplant coordinator for information about proper treatment.

DRY SKIN: Use a mild soap for bathing and lotion if you have problems with dry skin. Keri lotion or Moisturel are some good over-the-counter lotions. Ammonium lactate (Lac-Hydrin), which requires a prescription medication, can be ordered if severe dry skin persists.

OILY SKIN OR ACNE: Acne is related to the testosterone-like effects of prednisone. You may have acne on your face, chest, shoulders or back. The primary measures used to control acne are aimed at removing the excess oil and preventing formation of whiteheads and blackheads.

Wash the areas thoroughly three times a day, scrubbing gently with a soapy washcloth to remove the oils, dead skin and bacteria. Use a soap that removes oil, but does not dry the skin (Basis). Do not use a soap that moisturizes (i.e., Dove, Caress) or harsh antibacterial soaps (i.e., Dial).

Benzoyl peroxide 5% to 10% cream or lotion, which can be purchased over-the-counter, is helpful in drying acne. It is extremely important to keep your hands away from your face, and don't pick or touch acne. Also, cleaners or gels containing salicylic acid – an ingredient that cleans pores – will help prevent acne before it starts. When acne is present, it is best not to use cosmetics. If acne persists, you may want to see a dermatologist.

SKIN INFECTIONS AND LESIONS: Any area of skin that is changing or that does not heal should be pointed out to the transplant nurse and/or dermatologist. Warts may be particularly difficult to treat after transplant since they are caused by a viral infection.

SUN EXPOSURE: Prednisone, antibiotics and some of the other medications after lung transplantation may make your skin more sensitive to the sun. You will probably burn and tan easier and faster than you did before your transplant. If you have blond or red hair and a fair complexion, you have an even greater chance of getting severe sunburn.

Transplant recipients have an increased chance of developing skin and lip cancers. These cancers are 10 times more common in transplant patients than in the general population. These cancers occur more often if you live in an area that has numerous sunny days or in an area of high elevation, and in people whose jobs require them to work in the sun.

The ultraviolet (UV) portion of sunlight is an invisible form of radiation that causes skin cancer by penetrating and changing skin cells. There are two types of UV rays: UVA, which damages the deeper layers of the skin, and UVB, which damages the top layer. Ultraviolet rays are present even on cloudy days and in shady areas. Wear broad-rimmed hats, long sleeves, gloves and slacks, and use sunscreen lotion on any exposed areas of skin. Avoid the midday sun, since ultraviolet rays are the strongest then. If you must be outside, plan to be outside in the early morning or late afternoon, when there are fewer ultraviolet rays. The window glass in cars cannot stop most harmful ultraviolet rays.

Lotions containing a sunscreen with a SPF of 30 or higher are best. Also, look for a sunscreen that blocks both types of ultraviolet light. No lotion protects completely, however, and all of them wash off quickly. Swim in the late afternoon rather than at midday, and reapply sunscreen after swimming. A daily application of a moisturizer that contains a sunscreen is advised. For those with oily skin, there are oil-free lotions available.

You should have an annual skin checkup to look for the presence of any unusual moles that may signal the beginning of skin cancer. *(Refer back to page 95 for more information about skin cancer.)*

Hair Care:

Prednisone will probably affect the condition of your hair. It is recommended that you wait until your prednisone dose is less than 20 mg per day before you have a permanent or color your hair. However, tints, dyes, bleaches and permanent wave lotions may cause your hair to break, so you might want to avoid them. Tell your hairdresser that you are on prednisone, and use a conditioner on your hair regularly.

INCREASED HAIR GROWTH: Excessive hair growth is a fairly common side effect of cyclosporine. This problem is especially annoying to women and children, particularly when facial hair increases.

You may bleach dark hair with a hair bleaching cream or lotion, such as Nair, Neet or Surgicream, but be sure to test an area of skin according to directions on the bottle. This cream causes severe irritation to the eyes and mucous membranes (even to lips), so apply it carefully.

You may want to trim excess hair with a pair of round-tipped scissors, but do not shave it. After your prednisone dose is less than 20 mg per day, you may use electrolysis for permanent hair removal; just make sure the machine is sterilized before each use. Waxing for eyebrows or bikini line is all right as long as you go to a salon to have it done. In addition, you may want to try the prescription drug, Vaniqa, which is used like a moisturizer, but contact your transplant coordinator first.

HAIR THINNING: Prograf can cause hair loss by weakening hair strands, which increase the hair's tendency to break off at the roots. Azathioprine has also been associated with hair loss. This problem usually begins after initiation of therapy, but hair fallout usually levels off. To minimize damage to your hair, make sure you use a good conditioner and a hard rubber or wide-toothed comb. Never brush your hair when dry; instead, comb it while it is still wet. Avoid treatments that can damage your hair, such as perms, dyes, tints and bleaches. You may want to cut your hair shorter, which will minimize the appearance of thin hair. Most hairdressers can put you in contact with a wig maker if the problem becomes severe.

Eye Care:

It is common to have focusing problems in the first few months after your transplant. Check with the transplant nurse or physician first if you feel you need to see an optometrist. It is recommended that you get a yearly eye exam because, over time, the medications can affect your eyes.

Dental Care:

It is a good idea to wait six months after your transplant to schedule your first dental visit; then schedule regular visits every three to six months. You may require prophylactic antibiotic therapy before any dental cleaning or work since your mouth is a warm, moist area in which bacteria can grow. Your prednisone dose should be as low as possible when dental work is done to reduce the possibility of infection, bleeding and increase the healing process.

Practicing good dental hygiene includes keeping your teeth, tongue and palate clean, in addition to flossing, which should be done regularly to help prevent yeast infections and tender, swollen gums. Overgrowth of the gums is a side effect of cyclosporine and appears to be exacerbated by poor oral hygiene. You can use a solution of hydrogen peroxide and water (do not swallow this) or mouthwash to clean your tongue and palate. Also, switch to an electric toothbrush to help reduce plaque and swollen gums.

Humidifiers:

During winter months it is recommended that a humidifier be used daily at your home. Cooler weather tends to dry the air, which ultimately dries the mucous membranes. Your mucous membranes are part of your protection against infection. Clean the humidifier every other day and use distilled water or a demineralizing filter when filling. Change the filter weekly.

HEALTHY EATING FOR TRANSPLANT RECIPIENTS:

"They increased my prednisone to 30 mg. Everyone say a prayer for me to stay away from food."
– Mary Ann Kluk

Immediately after transplantation, your nutritional needs increase due to the stress of surgery and the side effects of some medications. For this reason, you may need to make adjustments in your diet. For example, a common side effect of prednisone is an increased appetite and cravings for salts or sweets that can result in weight gain. Even though the diet after transplantation is often less restrictive than before surgery, a healthy eating plan can make the difference to your health and the health of your organ transplant. The following recommendations comply with the American Heart Association, the American Dietetic Association and the American Diabetes Association guidelines.

Adequate Nutrition:

A balanced diet is important after surgery to replace lost vitamins and minerals and provide enough protein and calories to promote healing. Those who have lost weight or had a poor appetite before surgery should concentrate on improving their bodies' nutrient stores. General guidelines for adequate nutrition include:
- Eat enough servings from each of the four basic food groups to ensure a well-balanced diet
- Eat two servings from the meat/protein food group for adults, teenagers and children
- Eat four servings from the breads/cereals food group for adults, four to six servings for teenagers and four servings for children.
- Eat two servings from the milk/dairy food group for adults, four servings for teenagers and three servings for children
- Eat four to six servings from the vegetables/fruit food group for adults and teenagers, and four servings for children.

General Guidelines for a Healthy Diet:

A registered dietician is available to you as part of the transplant team. He or she can help you plan your diet to meet your specific needs and tastes. A few simple changes in your eating habits can make a difference in your long-term health and the health of your transplant. This is a healthy way to eat for your whole family, so there's no need for separate meals.

MEAT AND PROTEIN FOODS: Choose fresh fish, chicken and turkey without skin; ground turkey; lean, well-trimmed beef, veal, lamb, pork; meatless protein such as dried beans, lentils, peas, tofu; egg whites or cholesterol-free egg powder; water-packed tuna; and low-fat, low sodium frozen dinners. Limit or avoid intake of fried chicken, duck; fatty cuts of meat; bacon, sausage, lunch meats, hot dogs; liver and organ meats; cured and smoked meats; fried fish; egg yolks (limit three per week); canned meats and fish; and regular frozen dinners.

BREADS AND CEREALS: Choose plain breads, English muffins, bagels; plain pasta and rice; hot or cold cereals with no or minimal added fat, sugar or salt. Low-fat, low-salt snack foods such as unsalted pretzels, air-popped popcorn, rice cakes, melba toast; low-fat, low-salt baked goods such as angel food cake, graham crackers, fruit cookies, gingersnaps and fortune cookies. Limit or avoid intake of: high-fat, high-sugar baked goods, such as Danish pastry, croissants, etc.; granolas with coconut or coconut added; salted chips, cheeses or butter crackers; and seasoned pasta and rice mixes.

MILK, CHEESE AND DAIRY PRODUCTS: Choose skim or 1% milk, evaporated skim milk or nonfat dry milk powder; low-fat or nonfat yogurt; and low-fat, low-salt cheeses. Limit or avoid intake of any milk containing more than 1% fat; cream, half-and-half, nondairy creamers; whipped cream; and whole-milk yogurt, sour cream and cheese.

FRUITS AND VEGETABLES: Choose all fresh and sundried fruits; all fruit juices (preferably unsweetened); raw or frozen vegetables prepared without fat or salt; homemade or low sodium canned soups, bouillon and broths; and low-sodium vegetable juices. Limit or avoid intake of coconut and coconut meat or juice; deep-fried or canned vegetables; vegetables with cream, cheese or butter sauces; packaged sauces and casseroles; regular soups, bouillon and broths; and pickles and olives.

FATS: Choose unsalted margarine made with liquid safflower, corn or sunflower oil; vegetable oils; low-fat diet salad dressings made without saturated oils; reduced-calorie mayonnaise or regular mayonnaise limited to one tablespoon. Cook with oils that are low in unsaturated fats, such as olive oil or canola oil. Limit or avoid intake of butter or margarine made with partially hydrogenated oil; foods containing salt pork, lard, meat fat, hydrogenated or partially hydrogenated solid vegetable shortening; products made with coconut or palm oil; regular salad dressings and those made with sour cream or cheese; salted nut snacks and peanut butter.

SWEETS: Choose fruit ices, gelatin, sherbets, low-fat frozen yogurt, ice milk; and desserts prepared with low-fat ingredients and little salt. Limit or avoid intake of ice cream, chocolate, doughnuts, pastries, cake, cookies and pies unless prepared to be low-fat and low-salt.

Stomach Upset:

Since transplant recipients are on a large number of medications, these drugs often cause stomach upset. Medications are available that can help. In addition, to help prevent problems, it is a good idea to avoid acidic foods like tomatoes and citrus; spices that can irritate your stomach, such as pepper, garlic, gloves, chili powder, nutmeg and mustard seed; alcohol, chocolate, peppermint and nicotine, which can cause the muscle between the stomach and the esophagus to relax and allow food to pass back up into the esophagus.

It is also a good idea to avoid lying down within two to three hours after eating; chew foods thoroughly and eat more slowly, so the stomach has less work to do; eat six small meals instead of three large ones; drink six to eight glasses of water each day. Also, eat a variety of foods in moderation, gradually increase your fiber intake and decrease the amount of fat in your diet. Some foods, such as grapes, bananas, broccoli and cauliflower, can cause gas, but instead of eliminating them from you diet, eat smaller amounts and enjoy them with other foods. Avoid swallowing air as you eat, don't talk with your mouth full and use a straw to sip drinks.

If you make these changes and you still have digestive problems after three to four weeks, see your doctor. He or she may be able to prescribe something or otherwise get to the root of the problem.

Weight Control:

Weight gain after transplantation is commonly due to steroid treatments, which can greatly increase your appetite. You can successfully control your weight by limiting the amount of high-calorie foods you eat and gradually increasing your physical activity to burn them off. Weight control should be considered a life-long endeavor.

If you are not sure your weight is healthy, ask your doctor. He or she can determine if your weight is a good one depending on your body build, how much of your body weight is fat, where your excess weight is located, your family history of medical problems, and personal history of any weight-related health problems, such as hypertension.

A responsible and safe weight-loss program should include the following: The diet should be safe. It should include all the recommended daily allowances for vitamins, minerals and protein. The weight-loss diet should be low in calories (energy) only, not in essential foodstuff. The weight-loss program should be directed toward a slow, steady weight loss. Expect to lose only about a pound a week after the first week or two. With many calorie-restricted diets there is an initial, rapid weight loss during the first few weeks, but this loss is largely due to fluid.

Avoid yo-yo dieting (losing and gaining weight over and over), which can permanently slow down your metabolism and increase the fat stores in your body, making it even more difficult to lose weight. Eat regularly; skipping meals may increase your appetite further or slow down your metabolism. Include exercise in your program. Regular exercise helps you lose pounds and controls weight, in addition to indirectly helping to reduce your blood pressure and reduce your risk for many other diseases.

Post-transplant patients, as well as those who suffer from high blood pressure, should avoid over-the-counter diet pills. These drugs contain ephedrine, which can increase blood pressure. Ephedrine, also called ephdra or ma huang, is in herbal formulations as well and should be avoided. Supplements that are designed to reduce weight through simple

What is Your Metabolic Rate?

Your metabolic rate is simply the number of calories your body needs to function, e.g., to breathe, to beat your heart, etc. How do you figure out yours?

Using a calculator, follow this formula, known as the Harris-Benedict formula, to get a general idea of your metabolic rate:

655 + (4.36 x body weight in pounds) + (4.32 x height in inches) - (4.7 x age in years).

The resulting number is how many calories it takes to support your metabolism at rest.

calorie restriction (e.g., Slim Fast, etc.) are typically safe if used in moderation and according to manufacturer guidelines. These products do not attempt to alter the metabolism or interfere with absorption of nutrients.

To lose weight and keep it off, limit your intake of fats, such as butter, gravy, cream, oil, mayonnaise, salad dressing and fried foods, as well as high-sugar sweets, such as candy, cookies, cakes and regular sodas. Try fruits or popsicles for dessert; limit foods that contain brown sugar, raw sugar, glucose, sucrose, dextrose, honey, syrup, molasses and fruit juice concentrate. Limit portions; no second helpings, select only one entree. Add a salad or vegetable if you are hungry; eat slowly and eat a variety of foods; drink plenty of water and low-calorie beverages. Limit high-calorie beverages between meals (soda, Kool-Aid and sweetened juices). Often people confuse feeling hungry with being thirsty, so drink lots of water.

Trim all visible fat from meat, including skin from poultry; steam or stir-fry vegetables in monounsaturated canola or olive oils; avoid frying meats, instead roast, bake or broil them. Avoid using whole eggs in recipes. Instead, use two egg whites for one egg or use 1/4 cup of egg substitute for one egg; use apple sauce in baked goods instead of oil or butter. One cup applesauce equals one cup oil or butter; replace low-fat for whole versions of yogurt, ice cream, sour cream, cheese and milk.

Limit fat intake to 30% or less of calories per day. Fat contains approximately nine calories per gram, which is why high-fat foods are also high-calorie foods. By contrast, protein and carbohydrates supply only four calories per gram. To calculate the percentage of calories from fat, multiply the number of grams of fat by nine, then divide by the number of calories per portion. Limit alcohol intake to no more than two ounces of liquor, eight ounces of wine or 24 ounces of beer a day if male, and 1.5 ounces of liquor, five ounces of wine or 12 ounces of beer a day if female.

HOW YOUR METABOLISM AFFECTS YOUR WEIGHT: Many people believe that weight gain is a result of a slow metabolism. But, in fact, it is rare that you find someone with a true medical problem related to his or her weight gain, such as a thyroid disorder that can slow metabolism. Many people have different rates of metabolism due to family history or other causes. However, the differences aren't significant enough to really affect our lives. It is true that men have a higher metabolic rate than women. Also, when people age, their metabolism slows down.

Certain foods increase your metabolic rate. Lean proteins and carbohydrates are harder to digest than foods high in fat. Therefore, just the act of digesting proteins and carbohydrates burns more calories than fat. For example, eating 100 calories of protein takes your body 25 calories to break down, whereas eating 100 calories of fat only takes your body 10 calories to break down, leaving you with more calories to burn off or store as fat.

Regular exercise can boost metabolism by allowing your muscles to do more work, and muscle burns more calories than fat because muscle tissue requires constant repair and replacement. Adding as much activity to your daily life as possible adds to the daily amount of calories you burn and helps to increase your metabolism.

Also, stop dieting and start eating. A caloric restriction of more than 500 calories a day can trigger your body to go into conservation mode, therefore slowing your metabolism to prevent starvation. Even moderate dietary restrictions can slow your metabolism. The best advice is to eat three square meals a day or six smaller meals a day and don't skip meals.

Preventing High Blood Pressure and Fluid Retention:

High blood pressure and fluid retention often occur as side effects of the medications taken after transplantation. Managing hypertension in transplant patients first involves weight control, exercise, stopping smoking, limiting alcohol intake and reducing the amount of sodium, saturated fat and cholesterol in your diet. The likelihood of developing high blood pressure while taking prednisone depends on the dose and duration of treatment. Cyclosporine and Prograf can also cause high blood pressure. The combination of prednisone and cyclosporine or Prograf makes it even more likely to develop high blood pressure. The first step in treatment is to restrict dietary salt. Sometimes this is all that is needed.

Sodium is a mineral that is essential for many normal body functions as it acts with water to maintain fluid balance and helps regulate blood pressure. It also helps to regulate the amount of fluid found between and inside cells, coordinate muscle contractions, expedite nerve impulses and help maintain the acid-base balance (pH) of your blood. However, your body requires much less sodium than the average American consumes. A mild

---

THE VOICE OF EXPERIENCE

A Moveable Feast!

All my life I have loved to cook and to eat. When I was home, I would eat a healthy diet, but when I went out, I would go wild. Whatever I wanted, regardless of calories or fat, I had. So, you can imagine how devastated I was when I lost my appetite, especially since eating had been one of the few enjoyable things I was able to do shortly before my transplant. But, about two weeks before "the call" came, just the taste and smell of food would make me gag. No matter what my friends brought me to eat or drink (and, boy, did they try!) everything turned my stomach even though I was hungry! Popsicles turned out to be the only food I could get down, but they were in no way satisfying!

Then, on May 8, I got "the call." After some initial complications and a longer-than-anticipated stay in the ICU, I came home three weeks later with a new, healthy lung. It was then that my appetite returned with a vengeance! Much to my delight EVERYTHING tasted positively delicious! I spent ALL of my waking hours eating. My friends were stunned to see how much I could consume. Only a month before they were almost to the point of force-feeding me, but now I could handle Vietnamese food, popcorn, Goobers and Dairy Queen all in one night. (Well, if you're going to do something, you may as well go all out, right?)

Anyway, after about a month of this, food and drink began to taste bad again. It tasted as though it had been seasoned with metal pipe shavings, if you can imagine such a thing. To avoid dehydration I had to force myself to drink by holding my nose and gulping it down. Then, thankfully, my doctor decided to change my Imuran to CellCept, and, miraculously, my appetite returned and has stayed with me ever since. Now going out to eat is once again the thrill that it used to be, and experimenting with recipes from various cooking magazines is a weekend pastime. Sure, I have gained a few pounds, but that's OK. Since I have a chubby face from the prednisone, I may as well have a little extra fat on my body as well!

– Lolly Gilmore, single-lung transplant recipient,
May 8, 1999

sodium (salt) restriction is recommended (2,400 mg or 2.4 grams of sodium per day). This is equivalent to roughly one teaspoon of table salt. People with hypertension who are also sodium sensitive may require even smaller sodium intakes (usually about 2,000 mg daily).

To reduce the amount of sodium in your diet, use herbs and spices to flavor foods. Eat fresh, unprocessed foods whenever possible, and shop carefully by checking the list of ingredients on the label. All ingredients are placed in order of the highest percentage of content first. Many of the so-called "healthy choices" are not as low-salt or low-sodium as they claim. When buying frozen vegetables, most of the greens have been blanched in boiling, salt water to help preserve them. Rinse before cooking.

Avoid table salt and salt substitutes, which still may contain a small amount of sodium; foods with visible salt, such as potato chips and crackers; salted, smoked, cured, pickled or canned meat, poultry or fish, such as cold cuts, sausage, bacon, hot dogs, anchovies, sardines, ham, regular canned tuna and salmon, and breaded fish. Avoid regular cheese and cheese spreads, pickles, vinegar, regular peanut butter and canned soups, which are high in salt. Look out for foods that contain sodium chloride, acetate, ascorbate, benzoate, bicarbonate, citrate, fumarate, glutamate (including monsodium glutamate or MSG), nitrate, nitrite and oleate. If you cook with wine, don't use cooking wines, which are loaded with salt; use real wines. Leave out salt in cooking and baking wherever possible. Use no-sodium baking soda and baking powder; and read the labels of over-the-counter medications, since both may contain significant amounts of sodium.

Preventing High Cholesterol:

After transplantation, many people tend to have high blood cholesterol levels partially due to their medications. Avoiding excessive dietary cholesterol, saturated fat intake and weight gain can help control blood cholesterol levels. After your transplant, your blood cholesterol level should be measured frequently. The ideal goal is less than 200 mg/dl. A cholesterol level of 130 mg/dl to 159 mg/dl is borderline high. A level of 160 mg/dl and above may be considered too high and may warrant attention.

Cholesterol is a fat-like substance that the body needs to function properly. Our bodies produce cholesterol in the liver, and we also get cholesterol from the animal products we eat. Vegetable products do not contain cholesterol. High-density lipoproteins (HDLs) carry the cholesterol from the arteries to the colon, where it is eliminated through waste. Low-density lipoproteins (LDLs) carry cholesterol to body tissues where it is deposited. LDLs are sticky and can attach themselves to the walls of the blood vessels, producing a build-up of plaque over the years. This accumulation makes the path for blood flow smaller and smaller. When the pathway becomes blocked, we experience a stroke or a heart attack. The low-density lipoproteins (LDLs) are the type of cholesterol we need to watch out for.

Making specific changes in the amount and type of food eaten can reduce cholesterol levels. Dietary changes include decreasing the total amount of fat, saturated fat and cholesterol. Increasing the consumption of fiber in the form of fresh fruits and vegetables, whole grains, beans and nuts is recommended. If you are overweight, weight loss is also encouraged. Experts recommend eating no more than 300 mg of cholesterol a day.

Saturated fats are found in animal, dairy and some plant products.

These fats become hard at room temperature. They include coconut oil, palm oil and cocoa butter. They tend to raise blood cholesterol levels. Polyunsaturated fats are found in plant products and become liquid at room temperature. Oils such as safflower, sunflower, corn and soybean are high in polyunsaturated fat. These fats tend to lower blood cholesterol. Monounsaturated fats, such as olive oil, canola oil and peanut oil, may also lower cholesterol levels.

To reduce your cholesterol, avoid foods that contain palm oil, coconut oil, lard, hydrogenated or partially hydrogenated vegetable shortening, butter, cream and cocoa butter; avoid gravy and cream sauces. Use broth to moisten meat; limit egg yolks to three to four per week (including foods containing eggs); and use soft margarine in limited amounts instead of butter. Choose foods such as seafood and poultry more often than beef, lamb, pork or cheese. Avoid organ meats and fatty meats such as cold cuts, sausage, bacon and fried foods. Choose 1% low-fat or skim milk and low-fat cheese. Begin an exercise program and don't smoke.

Eating a high-fiber diet will also help lower your cholesterol. Most Americans consume inadequate amounts of fiber. Experts recommend between 20 to 35 grams of fiber a day as a healthy guideline. There are two types of fiber, insoluble and soluble. Insoluble fiber includes foods like wheat bran, whole grain breads, bran cereals, vegetables (especially root vegetables). They help prevent constipation and provide a feeling of fullness, and can also prevent colon cancer. Soluble fiber includes foods like oat bran, oatmeal, citrus fruit, apples, strawberries, beans and barley.

Preventing High Blood Sugar:

Normally when we eat, our blood sugar rises as carbohydrates are absorbed in the gut. The body responds by secreting insulin. However, immediately after your transplant, high doses of steroid medications are given which can affect the way your body uses sugar. When this process goes awry, it results in higher-than-normal blood sugar. This problem (insulin resistance) is what causes "adult-onset" diabetes.

In order to prevent high blood sugar (hyperglycemia), a diet low in sweets is recommended. This diet will help keep your blood sugar normal and help prevent unwanted weight gain. If high blood sugar becomes a long-term problem, your doctor may order a diabetic diet for you.

To reduce the amount of sugar in your diet, avoid candy, cookies, pie, cake and ice cream; sugar-sweetened beverages, soda, lemonade, iced tea and Kool-Aid; sugar and honey; sugar-coated cereal; canned fruit in syrup; fruit yogurt made with sugar; syrup, jelly and jam.

Preventing Osteoporosis:

Steroids may cause bones to lose calcium, particularly if dietary calcium intake is inadequate. Osteoporosis is a common consequence of long-term steroid use. Dairy products are the main sources of calcium and should be included in the diet to help keep bones strong.

Your daily calcium needs change as you age. From birth to six months old, you need 400 mg per day. From six months to 1 year old, you need 600 mg. From 1 year to 5 years old, you need 800 mg. From age six to 10 you need 800 mg to 1,200 mg. From 11 to 24 years old, you need 1,200 mg to 1,500 mg. Pregnant or lactating women need 2,000 mg. Women ages 25 to 50 need 1,000 mg. Men ages 25 to 65 need 1,000 mg. Post-menopausal women need 1,500 mg if they are not taking estrogen and 1,000 mg if they are. Women and men over 65 need 1,500mg.

For transplant recipients, it is generally recommended that you need 1,500 mg per day through your diet and/or supplements. In addition, you need to take 400 IU to 800 IU of vitamin D supplements, which help the body absorb calcium. However, 30 to 60 minutes of sunshine weekly will provide enough vitamin D.

Not all calcium supplements are readily absorbable. The type most easily used by the body contain calcium carbonate. Newer products contain calcium with citrate and malate, which are acids that help the body absorb calcium. Check the label and dissolve a tablet in four ounces of white wine vinegar and stir. If it dissolves in a half hour, it's fine; if not, switch brands. Beware of dolomite and bone meal sources of calcium since some brands may be contaminated with lead.

To increase the amount of calcium in your diet, choose at least two servings of low-fat dairy products each day, such as two eight-ounce glasses of 1% low-fat or skim milk. An eight-ounce glass of milk contains 300 mg of calcium. Salt and excess protein and phosphorus (contained in meat) increase the loss of calcium. Don't drink caffeine, which causes calcium to be secreted into the urine. Avoid alcohol; as much as two drinks per day have been shown to keep the body from properly absorbing calcium and other minerals. Don't smoke since smoking interferes with estrogen activity, including estrogen replacement therapy, and can cause menopause to arrive at least five years earlier than normal. Additionally, studies indicate that cadmium, a heavy metal found in cigarette smoke, can cause extensive bone loss. Exercise to work your bones and build bone mass. Regular weight-bearing activity is vital to preventing bone loss.

Lowering Your Potassium Levels:

Potassium is a substance your body uses to control nerve and muscle function, including that of the heart. Depending on the amount of potassium in your body, you may need to monitor your intake. In addition, cyclosporine may increase in the level of potassium in your body. The following foods are high in potassium and may need to be avoided after transplantation: avocado; molasses; flounder and halibut; tomato juice; lima beans, black-eyed peas, kidney beans, lentils, split peas and pinto beans; potatoes and sweet potatoes; winter squash; yams; bran cereal; beet greens; bananas; mushrooms; sardines; honey-dew melon; plantains; prune juice; spinach; tomatoes; artichokes; nuts; skim milk and whole milk; dried apricots and cucumbers.

Food Safety:

When you are immunosuppressed, you are at a greater risk of obtaining food-borne illnesses. Learning to prepare and store foods properly can greatly reduce your chance of illness. In recent years, the Center for Disease Control and Prevention (CDC) reported finding *E. coli* bacteria in lettuce and undercooked beef. The *Cryptosporidium* parasite was found in raspberries. *Salmonella* was found in undercooked poultry, red meat, eggs and raw seafood. In addition, the CDC detected *E. coli* in watermelon, cantaloupe, alfalfa sprouts and tomatoes. *C. Jejuni* bacteria can be found in undercooked poultry and raw mushrooms. The following tips will help improve the safety of the foods you eat.

WHEN FOOD SHOPPING:
- Be alert for signs of spoilage. Don't buy fruits or vegetables that have soft spots or bruises.
- Never use food from cans that are bent, creased, rusting, bulging or leaking or that spurt liquid when opened. Don't taste. These spoilage signs may mean the deadly botulism organism is present.
- Read the label for the "sell by" date and the "use by" date. Do not purchase or eat foods whose date has expired or will expire in the next two days.
- Don't buy cracked eggs since they can harbor disease-carrying organisms.
- Take groceries directly home, especially during the summer months.

KEEP A CLEAN KITCHEN:
- Clean work surfaces often and remove all food particles. Sanitize cutting boards after each use with a bleach and water solution and let them air-dry. Also, clean sinks, counters, kitchen tables with a bleach solution or with antimicrobial soaps or sprays. The recipe for a homemade bleach solution is to mix one part bleach to nine parts water.
- Towels, dishcloths and sponges can harbor bacteria, so change them often. Toss sponges and scrub brushes into the dishwasher each night or boil them with a small amount of bleach if you don't own a dishwasher. Throw away any sponges, towels or dishcloths that have an odor. This may be a sign of bacterial growth.
- Wipe up spills in the refrigerator right away and keep shelves, sides and doors sanitized.
- Don't let dishes soak in the sink. The mixture of food, warm water and soap provides the perfect condition for bacterial growth.

PROPER FOOD HANDLING:
- Wash your hands in warm, soapy water before and after every step in the food preparation process, especially after preparing meat or poultry.
- If you have a cut or open sore on your hand, use plastic gloves or a plastic sealing bandage. Wounds are easy entry points to the body for bacteria.
- Be sure to wash all fresh fruits and vegetables with water and lemon juice using a vegetable brush, and peel before eating.
- Thaw meat, poultry or fish in the refrigerator, never on the counter. Bacteria thrive in food at room temperatures.
- Use one cutting board for raw meat and poultry and another one for chopping food that won't be cooked. Plastic boards that can be tossed in the dishwasher after each use are best. If you use a wooden cutting board, be sure to wash and scrub it after each use with soap and hot water, then sanitize with a bleach solution or antimicrobial spray.
- Beware of cross-contamination. Don't carry cooked meat to the table in the same dish you used to carry the raw meat to the grill.
- Avoid raw or under-cooked meat, poultry or seafood. Cook beef and lamb to at least 160° F; pork and poultry to 170° F.
- Cook eggs thoroughly until both the yolk and white are firm, not runny. Consider using pasteurized eggs instead of shell eggs whenever possible.
- Avoid sushi, raw oysters or any raw seafood. The bacteria *Vibrio,* which can be fatal, may be present.
- Avoid raw eggs (cookie or cake dough, eggnog, shakes and Caesar salad dressing) in any form.
- Stuff chicken or turkey just before roasting. This keeps the bacteria in raw

poultry from invading the starchy stuffing. Once cooked, poultry and stuffing should be stored separately in the refrigerator.
- Don't use old vegetables and fruits since they can harbor *Cryptococcus*. Avoid eating cauliflower with black spots on it.
- Wash the tops of canned goods before opening. Almost everything you buy in a supermarket was stored at one time or another in a warehouse, which may have been infested with rodents.
- Always add spices during cooking rather than at the end. Spices can harbor bacteria known as *Bacillus cereus*, which needs to be destroyed by heating thoroughly.
- Reheat leftovers on the stove or in the oven. Heating them in a microwave requires stirring or rotating to avoid cold spots, which can contain bacteria.

PROPER FOOD STORAGE:
- Keep cold foods colder than 40° F. Keep hot foods hotter than 145° F.
- Keep food out of the temperature danger zone: 40 to 145° F. Foods left out for more than two hours, even in heated serving units, invite bacteria to grow. Keep refrigerator temperatures below 40° F.
- Put raw seafood, poultry and meat in plastic bags so their drippings can't contaminate other foods.
- Keep eggs in their original carton and keep them in the main section of the refrigerator. Don't put them in the egg section of the door because the temperature there is higher.
- Keep your cupboards clean, dry, dark and cool. The ideal temperature is 50 and 70° F. Temperatures over 100° F are harmful to canned foods.
- Organize your cupboards with older cans up front for earlier use. Generally, canned goods keep for at least one year.
- Don't use frozen leftovers more than two weeks old.

VITAMINS AND MINERALS:

"I believe in vitamins very highly and I use quite a few. But, you must research, research and research some more."
– Karen Fitchett

The American Dietetic Association believes a healthy diet is the best source of vitamins. No one who is healthy and eats an adequate variety of foods should need vitamin pills. If your diet lacks variety, the first step should be to improve food choices. Food provides many other healthful compounds in addition to vitamins. However, when specific health problems or unusual dietary habits make it difficult to meet vitamin requirements through food, a vitamin supplement may be needed for good health. Before taking any vitamins, speak to a registered dietitian or transplant physician first. They are trained to help decide if extra vitamins could be helpful or harmful to your health, and if they may interact with any prescription medicine you are on.

Vitamins contribute to good health by regulating metabolism and assisting the biochemical processes that release energy from digested food. They are considered micronutrients because the body needs them in relatively small amounts compared with other nutrients, such as carbohydrates, proteins, fats and water. Of the major vitamins, some are water-soluble and some are oil-soluble. Water-soluble vitamins must be taken into the body daily as they cannot be stored and are excreted within one to four days. These include vitamin C and the B-complex vitamins. Oil-soluble vitamins can be stored for longer periods of time in the body's fatty tissue and the liver. These include vitamins A, D, E and K.

Over-the-counter vitamins come in various forms, combinations and amounts. In most cases, it is a matter of personal preference as to how they are taken. The amount you take should be based upon your own requirements. If there is no single supplement that provides you with what you are looking for, consider taking a combination of different supplements. Just be careful that you tabulate the total quantity so you aren't taking more than you should. Since sunlight may decrease the potency of most vitamins, make sure that you store them in a dark place or in a cool, dark container.

Minerals, like vitamins, function as coenzymes, enabling the body to quickly and accurately perform its activities. They are needed for the proper composition of body fluids, formation of blood and bones and the maintenance of healthy nerve function. Minerals are naturally occurring elements found in the earth. Minerals belong to two groups: macro (bulk) and micro (trace) minerals. Bulk minerals include calcium, magnesium, sodium, potassium and phosphorus. These are needed in larger amounts than the trace minerals. Although only minute quantities of trace minerals are needed, they are important for good health. Trace minerals include zinc, iron, copper, chromium, selenium and iodine. Because minerals are stored primarily in the body's bone and muscle tissue, it is possible to overdose on minerals if an extremely large dose is taken. However, toxic amounts will accumulate only if massive amounts are taken for a long period of time. Bulk and trace minerals are often found in vitamin supplements and multivitamin formulas.

Most vitamins and minerals are marketed as food supplements, not as drugs; therefore they aren't regulated, nor do they have the approval of the Food and Drug Administration. Many researchers have noted the need for controlled clinical trials to determine their safety and effectiveness. Many of the immuno-enhancers available, such as CoQ10 (Coenzyme Q) and the antioxidants, haven't been studied in transplant patients. So, it is unknown whether these substances are safe, and it is possible that they might antagonize the effects of immunosuppression.

Many recipients are encouraged by their transplant team to take multiple or specific vitamins and mineral supplements. All programs, however, agree that patients on prednisone need calcium in their diet and/or mineral supplements. The following are some of the frequently recommended vitamins and minerals for transplant recipients.

MULTIVITAMIN: A multivitamin is good for general replacement of essential vitamins for people with a very low calorie intake (fewer than 1,000 calories per day), poor appetite or intestinal absorption problems, and for those with limited variety in their diets or recovering from surgery.

Dosage is one tablet per day.

PRECAUTIONS:
- Multivitamins are generally safe as long as you don't take too much. Tabulate all of the vitamins you are taking to make sure you aren't getting too much, especially the nonsoluble vitamins, such as vitamins A, D, E and K.

CALCIUM SUPPLEMENTS: Calcium is one of the main building blocks of bones, teeth and muscles. A calcium supplement with vitamin D acts to replenish the calcium lost from your bones as a result of the action of prednisone. Vitamin D helps the body absorb calcium from the stomach.

The recommended dosage is 500 mg 3x day. Calcium is more effective when taken in smaller doses spread throughout the day and before bedtime. When taken at night, it also promotes a sound sleep. Make sure your brand of calcium will dissolve readily. *(See page 156 for instructions.)*

POSSIBLE SIDE EFFECTS: If taken in excess, calcium supplements can cause kidney damage. Also, too much calcium may interfere with the absorption of other nutrients, like iron.

MAGNESIUM SUPPLEMENTS: Your body needs magnesium to carry out many of its daily functions. A low level can cause muscle weakness, sleepiness and problems with your heartbeat. Also, a deficiency interferes with the transmission of nerve and muscle impulses. Medicines like cyclosporine and Prograf can cause your magnesium level to go down.

The recommend dose is 400 mg per day.

POSSIBLE SIDE EFFECTS: diarrhea.

PRECAUTIONS:
- Cirpo (an antibiotic) can affect the absorption of magnesium, so it should be taken two hours before magnesium.

ALTERNATIVE OR COMPLIMENTARY MEDICINE:

"Patients should avail themselves of everything and anything to help with the side effects as long as they get the go ahead from their transplant team."

Today nearly 40% of all Americans utilize some form of alternative medicine, according to a survey published in the *Journal of the American Medical Association*. This overwhelming consumer demand has accelerated the integration of alternative or complimentary medicine with mainstream or conventional medicine. The majority of alternative therapies, unlike mainstream medical practices, are not backed by scientific research that measures safety and effectiveness.

Issues that you should consider when deciding on an alternative therapy include: safety and effectiveness, expertise and training, adherence to state or local regulatory agencies and costs. Unfortunately, most insurance companies don't provide benefits for these types of medical treatments. Discuss all issues concerning treatments and therapies with your transplant physician BEFORE you give them a try. For more information about alternative medicine, contact:

The Office of Alternative Medicine (OAM)
Phone: 888-644-6226 or 888-644-6226 (TTY)
OAM Clearinghouse, The National Institutes of Health
P.O. Box 8218, Silver Springs, MD 20919
Website: http://www.altmed.od.nih.gov

Acupuncture:

Originating in China more than 2,000 years ago, acupuncture is based on points along the body that connect with 12 main and eight secondary pathways, called meridians. Chinese practitioners believe these meridians conduct energy or Qi between the surface of the body and internal organs. Qi regulates spiritual, emotional, mental and physical balance.

The opposing forces of yin and yang influence Qi. When yin and yang are balanced, they work together with the natural flow of Qi to help the body achieve and maintain health. Acupuncture is believed to balance yin and yang, unblock the flow of energy and restore health to body and mind.

During your first office visit, the practitioner may ask about your health condition, lifestyle and behavior. The actual treatment involves the insertion of hair-thin needles into specific points, which may involve heat, pressure or electromagnetic energy to stimulate points on the body.

According to a National Institutes of Health panel, clinical studies have shown that acupuncture is an effective treatment for nausea caused by surgical anesthesia and cancer chemotherapy, as well as for dental pain experienced after surgery. The panel also found that acupuncture is useful by itself or combined with conventional therapies to treat addiction, headaches, menstrual cramps, tennis elbow, fibromyalgia, osteoarthiritis, lower back pain, carpal tunnel syndrome and asthma and assist in stroke rehabilitation and surgery-related pain.

About 30 states have established training standards for certification, and an estimated one-third of certified acupuncturists in the United States are medical doctors. Generally, treatment may take place over a few days or several weeks. The cost per treatment typically ranges between $30 to $100, but it may be more. Sessions last approximately 50 minutes. An estimated 70% to 80% of the nation's insurers cover some acupuncture treatments. To find an acupuncturist in your area, contact:

The National Acupuncture and Oriental Medicine Alliance
Phone: 253-851-6896, Fax: 253-851-6883
14637 Starr Road, S.E., Olalla, WA 98359
Website: http://www.naoma.org

Aromatherapy:

Aromatherapy dates back thousands of years and uses essential oils extracted from flowers, leaves, stalks, fruits and roots for therapeutic purposes. The smell of essential oils stimulates the release of neurotransmitters in your brain. These brain chemicals can have affects that are calming, sedating, stimulating or euphoric. The oils are administered by several methods of inhalation: placing drops of oil on a handkerchief or in steaming hot water or using a diffuser – a device that spreads the vapors throughout a room – and by soaking in therapeutic baths.

Some of the conditions that may benefit from aromatherapy include: anxiety, asthma, colds, depression, fatigue, headache, indigestion, insomnia and nausea. You can conduct your own aromatherapy, but caution is advised. Essential oils are very potent due to their high concentrations. It is recommended that you read an aromatherapy resource book, take a course, or visit a qualified aromatherpist before experimenting on your own.

Currently, no licensing or accrediting boards exist for the practice of aromatherapy in the United States. Individual sessions cost $40 to $60 and can last approximately 60 minutes. To find a therapist in your area, contact:

The National Association for Holistic Aromatherapy
Phone: 888-ASK-NAHA (888-275-6242) or 314-963-2071,
Fax: 314-963-4454, E-mail: info@naha.org
P.O. Box 17622, Boulder, CO 80308
Website: http://www.naha.org

Biofeedback:

Biofeedback uses a simple electronic monitoring device, connected by electrodes to the skin's surface, to collect information on vital body functions, such as heart rate, blood pressure, brain wave activity and skin temperature, which is converted into a series of sounds or images. A practitioner assesses the feedback and teaches the client how to alter or slow down the signals through the use of relaxation and visualization.

Biofeedback may be appropriate for treatment of any physical or emotional illness that could benefit from improved relaxation skills, such as anxiety, headaches, migraines, high blood pressure, pain and stress-related disorders. Cost per session can range anywhere from $50 to $150 and last approximately 50 minutes. Currently, there is no state licensing for biofeedback practitioners. To find a practitioner in your area, contact:

The Biofeedback Certification Institute of America
Phone: 303-420-2902, Fax: 303-422-8894,
E-mail: bcia@resourcenter.com
10200 W. 44th Ave., Suite 310, Wheat Ridge, CO 80033
Website: http://www.bcia.org

Chiropractic Medicine:

Chiropractic is based on the belief that a strong, agile and aligned spine is the key to good health. Trauma or poor posture can result in spinal misalignment (called subluxation) that puts pressure on the spinal cord, leading to illness and diminished or painful movement. With the backbone in its proper position, the nervous system is free to send out the necessary signals for the body to function normally.

A chiropractor identifies and corrects the misalignments through spinal manipulation and adjustment. He or she may also integrate massage therapy techniques to alleviate tension and/or spasm, and/or may use heat, cold or ultrasound for muscle relaxation. In addition, chiropractors may offer exercises to support the benefits gained from manipulation and to help prevent future problems.

Chiropractic may be an appropriate form of treatment for shoulder, back, joint, knee and neck pain, disc problems, headaches, whiplash and sports injuries. During your first visit, in addition to obtaining a complete medical history, the practitioner will perform an examination and possibly x-ray your spine. Your chiropractor should be able to discuss the anticipated number of treatments necessary for your diagnosis, which can range from two to 15 visits depending on the severity of your condition. The initial visit can cost $50 to $100 and lasts approximately 30 to 60 minutes. Follow-up visits cost $20 to $50 and last approximately 10 to 20 minutes.

All states require chiropractors to be licensed, graduate from an accredited college of chiropractic medicine and pass the National Board of Chiropractic examination, as well as a state board exam. To find a chiropractor in your area, contact:

Herbal Medicine:

Herbs and plants have a long history of treating symptoms and promoting health. Herbal medicine uses the roots, stems, leaves and flowers of plants for medicinal purposes. The U.S. Food and Drug Administration (FDA) has approved approximately 200 plant products for sale to the public as dietary supplements. The FDA does not subject dietary supplements to an extensive pre-market approval process as it does with new drugs, but the agency can remove a supplement from the market if it is determined to be unsafe. In addition, herbal products have less stringent manufacturing guidelines than medications and can be sold in the United States even if there is no proof that they are safe or effective.

Combining herbs with immunosuppressant drugs may actually counteract their effect. For example, studies have found that St. John's Wort (used as an antidepressant) may reduce the effectiveness of cyclosporine. Any product that claims to stimulate or enhance the immune system should be avoided by transplant recipients. These include echinacea, goldenseal, cat's claw and pau d'arco. In addition, some herbal products claim to detoxify the liver or kidney, such as milk thistle and burdock, but it is unknown if they are safe. In addition, the following herbs are known to be toxic or associated with illness and should be avoided: chaparral, comfrey, ephedra (ma huang), germander and magnolia-stephania preparation.

Always consult your transplant physician before taking any herbal or homeopathic supplement or remedy. Keep in mind that herbs are nature's medicines, meaning they have the ability to cause pharmacological actions and responses just as synthetic medications can. If you must take herbs, use only single-item products. If you experience a side effect, it will be that much easier to pinpoint the source. Immediately report any noticeable changes in your health to your transplant coordinator.

Purchase products from a quality manufacturer and look for products that include the name and address of the manufacturer, expiration date, dosage suggestions, milligrams (mg) or percentage strength of the active ingredients in each dose, and a list of all other ingredients. Also, do not exceed the dosage or duration of therapy suggested on the label and look for products that guarantee standardization of active ingredients. If you decide to consult with an herbalist, make sure you see a reputable therapist experienced in their use.

Currently, no licensing or accrediting boards exist for the practice of herbal medicine in the United States. Various holistic professionals – naturopaths and practitioners of traditional Chinese medicine – use herbal remedies as part of their healing treatment. The initial session can cost from $15 to $60 and last 30 to 60 minutes. Follow-up visits are less expensive and usually last only 10 to 15 minutes. To find an herbalist, contact:

Hypnotherapy:

Hypnotherapy is a technique whereby the therapist guides the client into a trancelike state called hypnosis. This state is induced by verbal suggestions, relaxation techniques and by having the patient observe a continuously moving object. In a hypnotic state, the client becomes relaxed, capable of intense concentration and open to suggestions for change. It is recognized as an effective technique for medical and psychological treatments.

When you are in a state of hypnosis, the practitioner will guide you toward changing habits, beliefs or behavior. No one can be forced into a hypnotic state against his or her will. Once in that state, you will be fully aware, can speak and be able to stop the session if you feel uncomfortable. The motivation to participate in treatment and the hope that treatment will be effective are essential factors in benefiting from hypnosis.

Hypnotherapy may be appropriate for the treatment of addictions (including smoking), anxiety, behavioral problems, weight problems, fears and phobias, hypertension, insomnia and stress-related disorders.

Practitioners certified in hypnotherapy have completed a training program approved by the American Board of Hypnotherapy or have passed an examination approved by the same board. It is recommended that you find a practitioner who is also a licensed psychiatrist, psychologist or social worker. Sessions cost approximately $40 to $150 and can last 30 to 50 minutes. To find a hypnotherapist in your area, contact:

The American Board of Hypnotherapy
Phone: 800-872-9996 or 714-261-6400, Fax: 714-251-4632,
E-mail: aih@ix.netcom.com
16842 Von Karman Ave., Suite 475, Irvine, CA 92714
Website: http://www.hypnosis.com/abh/abh.html

Homeopathy:

Homeopathy believes symptoms are the body's attempt to heal itself. Homeopathic remedies, prepared from plant, animal or mineral substances, encourage symptoms to run their course instead of suppressing them. Homeopathy believes effective medicine should trigger symptoms that are similar to the illness itself, thus activating and strengthening the body's immune system.

A homeopathic medicine, containing an extremely small amount of the substance that naturally produces symptoms similar to the illness, is administered. This concept is based on the "Law of Similars," which states that a substance taken in large amounts by a healthy person can cause illness or symptoms. But, if taken in minuscule amounts by a sick person, the same substance would benefit the body through the acceleration of healing. These remedies are nontoxic and free of side effects. The necessary strength and dosage amount is specific to each person.

Homeopathic medicine may be appropriate for treating acute infection, allergies, asthma, infectious diseases, substance abuse, among others. Some practitioners are medical doctors with a diploma in homeopathy credential (D.Ht.) or doctors of osteopathy (D.O.). They must pass a written and practical competency exam. Other practitioners are certified in classical homeopathy and must have 500 hours of training, plus one to two years of experience before they are permitted to take the exam.

The initial visit, which includes a full medical history and examination, can cost approximately $100 to $130 and last 60 minutes. Follow-up visits to evaluate your response to the treatment can cost on average $50 and last 20 to 30 minutes. To locate a practitioner in your area, contact:

The National Center for Homeopathy
Phone: 703-548-7790, E-mail: info@homeopathic.org
801 N. Fairfax St., Suite 306, Alexandria, VA 22314
Website: info@homeopathic.org

Massage:

Massage is the practice of kneading or manipulating muscle and other soft tissue with the intent of improving health and wellbeing. It dates back to ancient Chinese, Greek and Roman cultures. Today, massage therapy consists of numerous techniques, such as Swedish massage, sports massage, trigger point, Rolfing, reflexology, etc. Massage is believed to help improve circulation, balance and coordination, posture, flexibility, relaxation and elimination of muscle waste, as well as eliminate and prevent muscle adhesions.

Massage may be appropriate for treating anxiety, arthritis, back pain, bronchitis, circulation problems, constipation, headaches, labor and delivery pain, muscle spasms, muscle pain and soreness, muscle tension, neck pain, sciatica, shoulder pain, recurring injury and stress-related disorders. However, if you suffer from any of the following conditions, massage may not be appropriate: acute infectious diseases, aneurysm, bruises, cancer, fever, hematoma (broken blood vessels), hernia, high blood pressure, inflammation due to tissue damage or from bacteria, osteoporosis, phlebitis (inflammation of a vein), skin conditions and varicose veins.

The credentials of massage therapists vary from state to state, with some states requiring schooling in a program accredited by the American Massage Therapy Association, along with licensing. It is recommended that you seek a practitioner who, in addition to completing program requirements, has passed the National Certification Examination for Therapeutic Massage and Bodywork. Treatments typically last from 30 to 60 minutes and can cost $50 to $60 per hour, or $30 to $40 per half hour. To locate a practitioner, contact:

The American Massage Therapy Association
Phone: 847-864-0123, Fax: 847-864-1178
820 Davis St., Suite 100, Evanston, IL 60201
Website: http://www.amtamassage.org

Naturopathy:

Naturopathy is not a single medical theory, but a combination of healing approaches drawn from various parts of the world, such as acupuncture, nutrition, counseling, exercise, herbal medicine, homeopathy, osteopathy and tradition Chinese medicines, among others. Naturopaths teach their clients lifestyle changes and make recommendations on diet, exercise and eating habits to encourage self-responsibility for health. Gaining the health benefits of naturopathic care requires the individual to make a commitment to changing dietary and lifestyle habits.

Naturopaths obtain a Doctor of Naturopathic Medicine (N.D.) degree from a four-year, graduate-level, naturopathic medical college. The first two years of schooling are similar to that of traditional medical school, while the last two years focus on naturopathic approaches with an emphasis on nutrition. Some states regulate the practice of naturopathy; in those states, candidates must also pass a state or national board examination.

Initial visits to a naturopathic physician can cost $80 to $100 and last 60 to 90 minutes. Follow-up visits cost $55 to $90 and last 30 to 60 minutes. To locate a naturopath in your area, contact:

The American Association of Naturopathic Physicians
Phone: 206-298-0126, Fax: 206-298-0129,
E-mail: hulinc@mindspring.com
601 Valley St., Suite 105, Seattle, WA 98102
Website: http://www.naturopathic.org

EXERCISE:

"Last year, I never thought I'd be alive at this time, much less fly across the country and go bicycling, golfing and play tennis with my husband."
– Carol Lewis White

Exercise was an important part of your life while you waited for your new organ, as this helped to maintain your level of function during the wait. After transplantation, exercise will help you return to a normal, functional lifestyle and will help you make the most out of your new life!

For the first few weeks after your transplant, it is common to fatigue easily. Because of the many years of decreased activity, it will take several weeks or months of a consistent exercise program for your muscles to "catch up" with your improved lung function.

Most transplant centers incorporate some type of physical rehabilitation program into their postoperative regimen. However, exercise for the transplant recipient should be considered a life-long pursuit that is never-ending. Exercise helps to maintain weight, reduce the loss of calcium from bones, increase muscle strength and improve the proportion of muscle to body fat stores, in addition to working your heart and lungs.

The same golden rules of exercise that you practiced before your transplant apply here as well. Start slowly, be sure to warm up and cool down, to listen to your body and breathe. To maximize the use of your new lungs and improve your function, your exercise program should consist of endurance exercises and flexibility and strengthening exercises. However, BEFORE STARTING ANY EXERCISE PROGRAM, CONTACT YOUR TRANSPLANT PHYSICIAN, who can advise you on an exercise program that is right for you. *(Turn to pages 266 and 270, and copy the worksheets provided to help you keep track of your progress.)*

Endurance Exercises:

Endurance exercises uses large muscle groups in a rhythmic manner that can be sustained for increasing periods of time. These exercises improve the ability of your heart and lungs to supply oxygen and nutrients to the rest of your body. The exercise must be strenuous enough to condition your cardiopulmonary system, but not so vigorous as to damage your muscles, joints and bones. You may participate in any form of noncontact sport or activity, such as walking, cycling, swimming and low-impact aerobics.

The intensity of the exercise is measured by your perceived rate of exertion. Since it may take four to six months to return to cycling or

Taking Flight

As long as I can remember I have always wanted to run. When I was little, I was fast. I could do the 100m pretty well. But unfortunately that didn't last as my lung disease progressed. My first recollection of feeling different from others was in the fifth grade. It was gym day and time for long-distance running. I remember sitting on the side of the curb as I watched everyone else run over the hill. I will never forget that feeling of being left behind.

Maybe that's why I have always had a burning desire to run. Silently I hoped that one day I would know what it would feel like to take flight as I had seen them do. It wasn't until my doctor told me I could have a lung transplant that I believed someday that it would come true.

On Oct. 27, 1994, I received my transplant. The first few months exercising were fairly difficult. It was a new thing for me to have my legs tire before my lungs. I started slowly, and, after six months, I started to jog slowly on the treadmill. It was a beautiful spring day in May when I decided it was time to go farther. I was a little scared and a lot nervous but felt an inner need to lace up and step outside. My heart was beating loud and fast, but my Nikes seemed to move on their own. Within moments, I was running along the same street I had watched so many run on before. I started to smile and take deep breaths. I felt like I was flying that day, and nothing since has ever compared. I ran and I was alive. It was amazing.

Then in 1998, I attended the U.S. Transplant Games. I took great pride in a couple things during those three days. One was that I, a double-lung transplant recipient, won a race running! It was the 100 m run and I ran the hardest I ever had in my life. I won my heat and went on to take the silver medal overall. The medal was nice, but the smile on my dad's face was worth much more.

It seems like a dream sometimes when I think of how my life has changed. I still have a very strong commitment to exercise because I will never forget where I came from. I believe exercise played a large role in saving my life, and it continues to play a large role in maintaining my good health. And, I still run. As far and as much as I can.

– Dottie Lessard, bilateral-lung transplant recipient,
Oct. 27, 1994

---

swimming, most patients start with walking or exercising on the treadmill. Recent studies suggest that a leisurely walk, three to five times a week, may offer benefits comparable to those derived from more intense exercise.

Flexibility Exercises:

Flexibility in the chest is often a problem for patients after their lung transplant. This is a result of cutting muscles, fascia (tissue covering, supporting and separating muscles) and skin during surgery. In the beginning, your body stretches the skin in order to heal the incision. As time goes on this will lessen, but you may experience tightness around your rib cage, hunched shoulders, a limited range of motion and poor posture. Doing daily stretches will help to increase your range of motion and flexibility in your chest.

Many people think they don't have enough time to stretch, yet will go ahead and watch several hours of television at night. If you can set aside just 10 to 15 minutes every day for stretching, you will be increasing your range of motion, helping your muscles relax and creating healthy scar tissue all at the same time. In order to avoid straining yourself, you should warm up your muscles first before stretching. Do some light warm up exercises or stretch right after you get out of a hot shower when your muscles are warm. When stretching, hold each movement for only one to two seconds. Do not bounce; just let the muscles slowly elongate. Also, on the first stretch, don't challenge yourself too much, just go through the motion. Once you've done a few, then you can go for a more challenging stretch. Repeat each stretch approximately six or seven times.

Here are a few stretches to start out with. Remember to start slowly and do not strain. Stretching should not cause any pain or require a lot of effort on your part. You will increase your flexibility a little bit more each day, so be patient. The following stretches are for your chest and torso:

1) Raise your arm out to your side, up over your head and stretch; alternate each arm. If you want a more challenging stretch, you can lean over to the side at the waist.
2) Raise your arm up in front of you and stretch; alternate each arm; then do both arms.
3) Place both hands behind your head and bend over at the waist. Twist at your trunk and point your elbow toward the ceiling.
4) Stand with feet about shoulder width apart; clasp your hands behind your back; pull hands downward toward the floor. Alternate with raising your hands up behind your back.

Strengthening Exercises:

Strengthening exercise, or resistance training, is very desirable after your transplant. Resistance training is important because it helps strengthen your bones and muscles, which may be weakened due to the effects of prednisone and cyclosporine. The most popular type of resistance training is weight-lifting. To work best, you should try to incorporate one exercise for each of the major muscle groups (chest, back, shoulders, abdomen, arms, thighs and legs). You should begin working with a personal trainer who can get you started and teach you the safe way to use the various equipment. The main principles of weight-lifting include:

1) Begin with a weight you can comfortably lift 10 to 12 times. If you can't reach 12, then you are lifting too much.
2) Stay in control; raise the weight slowly up and down.
3) Remember to breathe during the effort, and avoid holding your breath. Most lifters exhale with each lift and inhale on their way down.
4) Slowly work up to three sets of repetitions. You should start to fatigue by the end of the third set.
5) If you can do 12 repetitions in three sets without a lot of strain, then increase the weight at your next workout.
6) Lift two to three times a week, but make sure you get a full day's rest in between sessions.

If you develop discomfort in your muscles or joints, reduce your exercise intensity for a few days and contact your physical therapist.

MENTAL HEALTH ISSUES:

"Transplant doesn't just give you a new set of breathers, it gives you a second chance to do things differently the second time around."
– Gail Brower

The time following your transplant can often be a very difficult adjustment period. It is common for people to experience mood changes, in part due to the medications, effects of major surgery and all the stresses that have occurred recently. Some may even experience brief periods of depression and/or irritability or short temperedness. It should be noted that elevated levels of anxiety and depression are a normal reaction to acute stress associated with a medical crisis. However, if periods of anxiety and/or depression are prolonged and are significantly interfering with your quality of life, contact your transplant coordinator, social worker or doctor. Support groups can provide valuable help for many transplant patients, while some may benefit from a referral for counseling in their community.

It is not uncommon for children to have difficulties adjusting to life after their transplant. They may have been away from school and other children for quite a while. The child may find him or herself looking different from his or her peers, with increased hair growth and moon face. For families who experience difficulties with their child, it is recommended that they participate in family therapy sessions with a trained child-life counselor, psychologist or psychiatrist.

Anxiety/Panic Disorders:
Anxiety disorders are distinguished by certain characteristics including worrying constantly and fears of the unknown. They can be triggered by the stress of a job loss or divorce, or may be caused by physical conditions, such as hyperthyroidism, or by medications. In more severe cases, the patient may become preoccupied with catastrophic thoughts and visions, so much so that it can become extremely impairing.

The effects of anxiety are felt in varying degrees from person to person but are common in transplant recipients. In severe cases of anxiety, a person may experience panic attacks, which are intermittent, brief episodes of heart palpitations, chest pain, dizziness, shortness of breath, sweating, shaking, feelings of choking, hot or cold flashes, faintness, nausea and fear of losing control. Steps you can take to minimize the symptoms of anxiety include:
- Cut back on caffeine
- Exercise
- Practice relaxation and deep-breathing exercises
- Keep a journal to help track anxiety triggers
- Schedule less in your life.

If these measures don't work, seek help from your transplant physician, who may prescribe medication or counseling. Most patients get relief from drug therapy within three to four weeks.

Depression:
Depression is an often-misused term to describe feeling down, blue, angry, sad or just plain unhappy. True depression – also called clinical depression – is a collection of symptoms that last some time and interfere with your ability to function in many areas of life.

Depression can be caused by a combination of factors, such as extreme stress, an under-active thyroid (hypothyroidism) and some medications. Steroids, such as prednisone, can trigger chemical changes that lead to depression in some transplant patients. The first step in treating depression is recognizing the problem. Symptoms of depression include:
- Loss of interest in things you used to enjoy
- Feeling sad, blue or down in the dumps
- Extreme tiredness or low energy
- Restlessness or inability to sit still
- Insomnia or sleeping too much
- An increase or decrease in appetite or weight
- Feelings of worthlessness or guilt
- Thoughts of death or suicide
- Problems concentrating, remembering or making decisions
- Headaches, backaches, upset stomach and digestive problems, sexual problems, anxiety, worry, pessimism or hopelessness.

Fortunately depression is very treatable and usually involves taking an antidepressant medication. Common ones include fluoxetine (Prozac), sertraline (Zoloft), paroxetine (Paxil) and amitriptyline (Elavil). See your transplant physician for help. A clinical psychologist or therapist may also be recommended. If you have depression, it is important to know it's not your fault and is not a sign of weakness, laziness or poor willpower.

SEXUALITY AND RELATIONSHIPS:

"In the beginning, my husband was a little overprotective of me. He acted funny, like he was unsure what he should be doing. But, as I progressed, he got better."
– Carol Lewis White

Some couples feel that they need to protect the newly transplanted organ and are fearful that sexual activity will be too stressful. This is not so. Kissing, intimacy and sexual activity are safe. However, be careful to avoid strain across your incision for at least four to six weeks after surgery and make sure your partner doesn't have any open sores on his or her mouth or genitals. During the early months, your sexual interest and functioning may not be consistent. If you have concerns about either, discuss these with a member of your transplant team.

Safe Sex:
Because the medications that you will be taking after transplantation put you at a higher risk for sexually transmitted diseases, it is strongly recommended that you use condoms, but only for those who are NOT in a stable, monogamous relationship. These diseases behave aggressively in transplant recipients due to their low immunity.

Pregnancy:
Obviously, birth control is necessary unless pregnancy is desired. However, if you want to get pregnant, you should weigh the risks carefully and speak to your transplant physician before becoming pregnant. There have been a number of reports of successful pregnancy following transplantation. However, most of this experience has been in kidney and heart transplant patients. It is important to realize that there is very little information

Picking up the Pieces

Tornadoes can be mysterious things; you never know when they might hit. When they do, they scatter everything and you are left to pick up the pieces. My tornado hit when I was hospitalized while waiting for a heart and lung transplant. Pieces of my life were scattered and shredded, and for a while it seemed impossible to pick up the pieces. I lost most of my friends while I was hospitalized. My boyfriend left me during the waiting period saying he couldn't handle the hospital and sickness. I also had to leave school in the middle of the semester and contend with the fact that I did not complete my freshman year.

On Dec. 23, 1997, I received my transplant. I had a rough time after surgery. I didn't know where I was, nor, who I was. I had problems remembering things. After I got my transplant I was forced to reckon with and fix the turmoil left behind. This included learning to trust again. I am lucky I found someone who saw me through the transplant. We fell in love and I agreed to marry him.

Through the whole ordeal, there was no question that I would be going back to school. Moving back was interesting; my mother cried her eyes out. She was terrified for me and never expected me to pack up and leave on my own two feet. While back at school, I became vice president of Harley Hall, and got elected as vice president of the overall Board of Residence Halls. I also handled all the programming for a conference held at the college in addition to my five classes, homework and lab work. So it pushed my stress level up pretty high. When it got too stressful for me, I learned to just take a week off. I would hibernate in my room and do schoolwork. That kept me sane, kept me from getting behind and kept me from getting sick.

Now, the sky has cleared. Some storm clouds still linger from my tornado, but none of them can do any damage. The sun is shining and I see a rainbow on the horizon.

– Sara Marie Henke, heart and right-lung transplant recipient,
Dec. 23, 1997

---

available on lung transplantation and pregnancy. In addition, a consensus within the medical community regarding the safety of pregnancy after lung or heart-lung transplantation just doesn't exist. The long-term effects of pregnancy on lung function are not clear. Each center has its own opinion on whether it is considered safe.

However, all pregnancies in transplant recipients are considered high-risk. In general, transplant recipients are asked to wait three to four years after transplantation before becoming pregnant to assess their risk for developing obliterative bronchiolitis syndrome. They should have good, stable transplant function. Any medical conditions, such as diabetes and hypertension, should be well-controlled, and immunosuppression should be at maintenance levels. However, counseling needs to address the possibility of unfavorable outcomes.

Some of the more common problems associated with pregnancy and transplant recipients include hypertension and premature births. The general opinion within the medical community on breast-feeding has been that female transplant recipients should not breast-feed because the medications can be present in breast milk.

Since 1991, Thomas Jefferson University Hospital has been operating the National Transplantation Pregnancy Registry to study the effect that pregnancy has on the health of the mother, her transplanted organ and her baby. The registry contains information on more than 2,000 pregnancies, including information on pregnancies fathered by transplant recipients.

Currently, the registry has information regarding 12 pregnancies in lung transplant recipients and five pregnancies in heart-lung transplant recipients. Due to the small number of patients, it is difficult to formulate any conclusions or recommendations about the safety of pregnancy in lung transplant recipients. For more information, contact:

> **The National Transplantation Pregnancy Registry**
> Phone: 877-955-6877 or 215-955-2840, Fax: 215-923-1420
> Thomas Jefferson University Hospital, Department of Surgery,
> Transplant Program, 605 College Building, 1025 Walnut St.,
> Philadelphia, PA 19107

Relationships:

Being in a relationship with a transplant patient, or anyone with a chronic illness, can be a tremendous stressor even when things are going well medically. Most likely, the fears are not one of being with someone "abnormal." Rather it's probably a fear of going through the struggle again. Recipients need to recognize that partners and caregivers have emotional needs, and the intensity of this experience may create a whole array of acute stress reactions, including anger, isolation, withdrawal, depression, etc. If this becomes an issue, family counseling is advised.

EMPLOYMENT:

"You must give up the life that you planned in order to live the life that awaits you."
– Karen Fitchett

One of the goals of transplantation is to return people to a productive, active lifestyle. For some, that may mean continuing their education or raising their children. For others, that may mean looking forward to returning to school, taking on a new job or resuming previous employment.

Going Back to School:

Returning to school can be something to look forward to. However, schools can be a haven for a variety of illnesses that can be passed on to others. Lung transplant recipients are especially vulnerable to respiratory infections. Therefore, it is advisable to notify your classmates that your immune system is compromised. Ask them to let you know when they are sick so you can take the necessary precautions. You can stay relatively safe around people with colds as long as you wear a mask, wash your hands and keep them away from your face.

For children, most parents wonder when their child will be ready to return to school. Be sure to check with your transplant physician before they return to the classroom. You may want to meet with your child's teacher, school nurse, guidance counselor/social worker and principal to explain the situation. Also, make arrangements for your transplant coordinator to speak directly with the school staff, so they will have a clear idea about what your child is able to do and cannot do. Remember to give the school nurse your daytime phone number and your transplant physician's number. Your child can participate in gym activities as long as there are no contact sports involved. Otherwise, students are encouraged to participate in school activities.

Getting Back to Work:

Before getting back to work, you should ask your doctor if he or she thinks you are well enough. Ask for any precautions that you might have to take to protect yourself against health risks specific to your anticipated work setting and job duties. Most patients who are able to return to work return to a job they once held before. However, some transplant recipients may find that going back to their previous job may be potentially harmful to their health and that they need to be retrained. According to Paris et al, in a study of 99 lung transplant recipients, return-to-work rates were somewhat disappointing. Only 22% were employed after undergoing lung transplantation, 38% were unemployed but medically able to work, while 29% were disabled and 10% had retired.

THE VOICE OF EXPERIENCE

Life Promoted Here

In 1997, I was diagnosed with a rare lung cancer, called bronchiol-alveolar carcinoma. I was 30 years old at the time and working as a lobbyist at a women's public policy organization in Washington, D.C. After trying many different treatment options, including chemotherapy, I discovered an experimental lung transplant program for individuals with this type of cancer at the University of Alabama in Birmingham. In February 1998, I was placed on the transplant waiting list, and my job gave me a leave of absence while I moved to Birmingham to wait.

On Oct. 11, 1998, the call came. The surgery went smoothly, and I was released from the hospital 10 days later. Recovery, however, was difficult. The first two months I struggled with the surgical pain and CMV. At the two-month mark, however, I returned to the temporary job I had in Birmingham. I only worked four hours a day, but it helped me to regain my strength and gave me a focus as I recovered from surgery.

In December, my doctors said I could go home to Washington, D. C. I returned to my lobbyist position on Jan. 7, 1999. It was quite a celebration with my co-workers, who had been a faithful support team and "prayer warriors" throughout my illness. For a while, my transplant story attracted a lot of attention, but the novelty has worn off a little. I like to think of my lung transplant as a unique part of my story rather than my sole identity.

By February, I had the strength to work a full week. My employers have continued to give me flexibility through the ups and downs. I have had a few bouts with rejection, as well as CMV. A laptop-computer, pager and cell phone help keep me accessible when I am out of the office.

I feel better then ever, and am glad to be back in the job I enjoy so much. The stability of my employment has helped keep some sense of "normality" to my life as I cope with my never-ending medical needs. I was recently promoted to the position of Director of Legislative and Legal Affairs, and I see that as a wonderful vote of confidence in my abilities.

– Andrea Aulbert, bilateral-lung transplant recipient,
Oct. 11, 1998

If you are doing well following your operation, you may be able to resume your former job on a part-time basis in three to six months with a minimal amount of restrictions. However, the first year after your transplant will be filled with many clinic visits, blood tests, physical therapy, etc., and it may be difficult to incorporate this schedule with your old job.

Transplant recipients who have been out of the work force for long periods of time tend to have the greatest difficulty in returning to work. Some of the barriers to finding new employment after transplantation include: hiring discrimination on the basis of medical history, restrictive cost or unavailability of health insurance, poor local or regional economic conditions, limited education or work skills, changes in priorities for recipients who value leisure activities over work, and the perception by the patient that these obstacles are insurmountable.

When looking for a new job, you may want to start working as a volunteer first to see if it is a suitable job for you. If so, then gradually progress to part-time, then a full-time job. However, before going back to work, make sure you understand the effects that this will have on your health insurance and any other benefits you might be receiving. Always remember to refer to the Americans with Disabilities Act's guidelines regarding when to disclose a disability to a potential employer.

Finding an employer offering good health insurance benefits can be a challenge. Often large companies will be a more likely source of coverage, since insurers of large companies are better able to absorb the costs. According to the Health Insurance Portability and Accountability Act (HIPAAA), employees with a disability must be offered the same insurance benefits provided other employees. Exclusion periods for pre-existing conditions must be reduced or eliminated for new employees who previously had group health insurance coverage, including Medicare and Medicaid, providing there was no break in coverage lasting more than 63 days.

Employment and its Effect on Social Security/Medicare/Medicaid:

If you've been on Social Security and decide to go back to work, you will need to notify the Social Security Administration and tell them of your intentions. Fortunately, Social Security has a work incentive program to protect you as you try working again. You will begin a "trial work period," during which time you will receive your full disability benefits in addition to any earnings on the job. If you earn more than $530 (adjusted annually) in any one month, it is considered a "trial work month." You may work up to nine trial months (not necessarily consecutive) over a five-year period and earn as much as you can, without affecting your benefits.

After your trial work period ends, Social Security will evaluate your work. Generally, if your earnings average $740 per month (adjusted annually) or less, your benefits will continue. If you earn more than $740 per month on average, your benefits will end after a three-month grace period. Any work expenses related to your disability will be considered when your earnings are calculated. If you become unable to work due to your medical condition within five years after your benefits have stopped, your benefits can be reinstated with no waiting period.

Changes in the Medicare law will extend Medicare coverage for many working people with disabilities who are under the age of 65. These changes will allow a working person, as long as he or she still has a disabling condition, to get Medicare coverage for four and one-half years longer than under current law. This means you will keep your premium-free Medicare hospital insurance (Part A) coverage for at least seven years and nine months after the end of your trial work period. You will still have to pay a premium to get Medicare Part B coverage.

This law, called the Ticket to Work and Work Incentives Improvement Act (HR 1180), also allows individual states to permit an employed individual with a disability to buy into Medicaid, even though the individual is no longer eligible for Social Security or SSI benefits because his or her medical condition has improved. These changes went into effect Oct. 1, 2000.

Social Security has several booklets available to help explain the impact returning to work has on your benefits:

Working While Disabled: How Social Security Can Help (Publication No. 05-10095)

Work Incentives for People with Disabilities (Publication No. 64-030)

To receive a copy of these free booklets, contact the Social Security Administration at 800-772-1213. For more information, check out their website at: http://www.ssa.gov

The Americans with Disabilities Act:

The Americans with Disabilities Act of 1990 (ADA) was designed to protect the employment rights of disabled people. Employers are required to make reasonable accommodations as needed for disabled workers. Reasonable accommodations include, but are not limited to, improved access to work facilities, restructuring of job duties and schedules, reassignment to other positions, purchasing new equipment or modifying existing ones, and modifying job examinations, training materials or policies. If an employer can prove that an accommodation would pose an undue hardship to the business (too difficult or too expensive to provide) the employer may not have to provide it.

Whether or not you inform a potential employer about your disability is your decision. According to the Americans with Disabilities Act, an employer cannot ask you if you have a disability, only if you can perform the tasks required to do the job. An employer also cannot ask you if you are on medication, have ever been hospitalized or how many times you were absent due to illness. If your disability is invisible and you do not need an accommodation, you probably should not disclose. However, if you plan to ask for a job accommodation, e.g., a change in job duties, you will need to make your disability known at the time of the interview. If you do choose to disclose your disability, you may want to indicate how you have been able to overcome obstacles in the past. Be positive and focus on what you can do, not on what you can't do.

The Americans with Disabilities Act (ADA) prohibits discrimination on the basis of disability in five different areas:
1) Employment, including: job hiring, firing, promotion, pay and other job-related issues
2) State and local government activities, including: public education, courts, voting, town meetings, etc.
3) Public transportation, including: subways, commuter rails, Amtrak (the

Air Carrier Access Act prohibits discrimination by air carriers against individuals with a physical or mental impairment)

4) Public accommodations, including: restaurants, retail stores, hotels, movie theatres, private schools, recreational facilities, etc.

5) Telecommunications, including: telephone and television access for people with hearing and speech disabilities.

To be protected by the ADA, you must have a disability as defined by the ADA. The ADA defines disability as a physical or mental impairment that substantially limits one or more of the major life activities, such as breathing, walking, sleeping, working, self-care, etc. The ADA does not specifically name all of the impairments that are covered. For more information about the law, you can call the Department of Justice's ADA Information Line: 800-514-0301 or 800-514-0383 for TDD, or check out their website at: http://www.ufdoj.gov/crt/ada/adahom1.htm

Vocational Rehabilitation:

If you are unable to return to your former job or don't have a job to return to, you will need to find out what kinds of work are suited to your particular personality, strengths and abilities. One of the most overlooked resource for people returning to work is a vocational rehabilitation program. These state and federally-funded programs offer services, at no cost, to disabled people entering a new field of work. These services can range from counselors who can help develop a career plan, to tuition for job training or college courses. The process goes something this:

1) You must attend an orientation meeting.

2) A counselor is assigned to your case.

3) Your counselor decides if you are eligible for their services. Basically, if you have a medical condition and want to work, you will qualify.

4) A determination is made about what kinds of services are needed, such as retraining or going back to school.

5) A plan is written and agreed to.

6) The plan is put into action. A case is considered successfully closed after the client has worked for 90 days.

Not only can rehabilitation or training programs help you get a new job, but your disability benefits will be protected while you have an active case. To find the state agency nearest you or contact your local Department of Labor and Employment. If you are a veteran with a service-related disability, the Veterans Administration may provide help.

DONOR ISSUES:

Some centers have a policy of not telling the patient anything about their donor, while other centers provide some basic information such as sex, age and cause of death. Curiosity about the donor is natural. Some people may dream about their donor. Some recipients worry that they may take on the emotional, psychological or physical characteristics of the donor, but this will not happen. Recipients may develop personality changes and strong food cravings, but these are often a result of the medications.

Each transplant program establishes its own guidelines for recipient-donor communications, and, while some strongly encourage it, others don't think it's a good idea. Some recipients wish to know who their donor was, while some do not. Others may wish to meet the family of the donor. However, the majority of transplant centers wish to protect both the donor family and the recipient and will maintain confidentiality for both parties. Many donor families have a strong desire to hear something from the recipient acknowledging the value of the gift they gave to the recipient.

Writing to Your Donor Family:

If you wish, you can write an anonymous letter to your donor family and give it to the transplant coordinator or send it the organ procurement organization (OPO) that was involved in your transplant. Personal cards and letters from recipients can give donor families great comfort as they mourn the loss of a loved one. Don't let the passage of time stop you from offering this way of thanking your donor family. The following are some guidelines and suggestions to help you get started:

- Include a few words on how the transplant has changed your life. What kinds of things can you do now that you couldn't do before?
- Describe your transplant experience. Include a brief description of your illness and what the wait was like for you and your family.
- Talk about yourself (first name only). What are your hobbies or occupation? Do you have a spouse, children? Are you writing as the parent of a child who received a transplant?
- Describe some special events that you would not have experienced without a transplant. Did you get married? Have you become a parent or grandparent? Did you celebrate a special birthday?

There are a few things you should keep in mind when you write to your donor family. Be sensitive; the family has lost a loved one and they are grieving, so be sure to extend your sympathy along with your gratitude. Transplant professionals also recommend that you be sensitive about religious comments since you don't know the religious background of the donor family. Remember you are the positive aspect of all this and cannot cause them anymore pain than which they already feel by communicating with them. It has been demonstrated that families find great solace in being given the chance to enhance the lives of others through organ donation.

Finally, keep your letter anonymous. Confidentiality is required. Sign your first name only and omit your address, phone number and any other identifying information. Once you've written your letter, put it in an unsealed envelope. Then, on a separate piece of paper, write your full name, phone number and the date of your transplant. Send both items to your transplant coordinator or OPO. They will review your card or letter to ensure that you kept yourself anonymous and will then notify the donor family that it has received a letter for them. Some may not be ready to receive such mail, in which case the OPO will hold it for them. Others may be eager, not only to receive it, but to write a response. The majority will fall somewhere in between. Whatever happens with your letter, you will never regret writing it. If you aren't sure what to say, just keep it simple, keep it sincere and get it done. Your donor family deserves it.

In some circumstances, if both parties are mutually agreeable, transplant recipients can meet their donor family. Usually this is only done after a minimum of one year has passed since the transplant.

FUTURE TRENDS:

"The greatest thing to happen to transplantation would be no more list, after that, no more rejection drugs or at least ones that are much more user-friendly."
– Karen Fitchett

Successful lung transplantation has been performed in this country for more than 15 years. It has allowed for the treatment of many end-stage lung diseases that otherwise would have been fatal. Survival rates have improved substantially as experience with this procedure has increased. However, several problems still remain. While early survival rates are good, long-term survival of lung transplant recipients has been stagnant for the past seven years. Other problems include the scarcity of donor lungs, harsh therapeutic regimens, and the constant threat of infection and rejection.

Enhancing the survival for transplant recipients is the focus of much research. Some of the ways scientists are trying to improve survival rates include: improving preservation of the lungs, developing safer immunosuppressive drugs, and developing a better understanding, detection and treatment of chronic rejection.

Experimental Drugs:

Medicines used today to prevent organ transplant rejection are expensive and dangerous. They suppress all immune responses, thereby exposing the recipient to infection and cancer. However, new medicines are currently being developed that will prevent and treat graft rejection without the need for global immunosuppression. The majority of these new drugs are antibodies. There are both humanized and animal-derived antibodies. To create them, scientists induce the growth of a tumor in a host. Within a few weeks, the tumor causes an accumulation of fluid. This fluid is removed, processed and packaged. How these antibodies work is not completely understood, but the majority of these new drugs are designed to block the body's ability to signal something foreign is dangerous to the body.

ANTI-CD11A: XOMA Ltd. is collaborating with Genentech Inc. to develop this humanized monoclonal antibody (Mab). Anti-CD11 binds to the CD11a component on T cells. It selectively inhibits T cell migration, adhesion and activity without depleting T cell numbers or suppressing the entire immune response. Phase I/II clinical trials of Anti-CD11a in kidney transplant recipients began in March 2000. For more information, contact:

XOMA Ltd.
Phone: 510-644-1170
2910 7th St., Suite 100, Berkeley, CA 94710
Website: http://www.xoma

BT1-322 (Anti-CD2): is a mouse-derived monoclonal antibody. Phase I and II clinical trials have demonstrated that adding BT1-322 to commonly used immunosuppressive therapy reduced the incidence of rejection in liver transplant recipients by 70%. For more information, contact:

BioTransplant Inc.
Phone: 617-241-8780
Charlestown Navy Yard, Building 75, 3rd Ave., Charlestown, MA 02129
Website: http://www.biotransplant.com

CD40L: A group of doctors at the University of Wisconsin, the Naval Medical Research Institute and Biogen Inc. have explored the use of a monoclonal antibody specific for CD40L. In 1996, they used rhesus monkeys with kidney transplants that were treated for 28 days with CD40L-specific monoclonal antibody 5C8. This agent prevents T cells from signaling each other, otherwise known as co-stimulation. 5C8 was shown to prevent and reverse acute rejection, thereby prolonging kidney allograft acceptance. The monkeys were treated for six months with 5C8.

Subsequently, the monkeys did not reject their kidneys, which where still functioning normally for over 16 months despite the fact that they had been given no immunosuppression after the initial course of treatment. The animals also appeared to have normal immune systems. This treatment puts medicine one step closer to being able to offer transplants without the inherent risks of current treatments.

In 1999, researchers from the National Institutes of Allergy and Infectious Diseases in collaboration with Biogen began phase I/II clinical trials on the use of CD40L mAb to prevent rejection in kidney recipeints. Although this agent yielded promising results in pre-clinical trials, adverse events have temporarily halted patient enrollment. However, clinical samples obtained from the trials have proved valuable in studying the interaction between CD40L and rejection. For more information, contact:

Biogen Inc.
Phone: 617-679-2000
14 Cambridge Center, Cambridge, MA 02142
Website: http://www.biogen.com

ERL080: is a novel formulation of MPA, the active part of CellCept and offers the potential to reduce upper gastrointestinal side effects often associated with that drug and still retain the same efficacy. This product is currently in Phase III clinical trials. For more information, contact:

Novartis Pharmaceuticals
Phone: 800-742-2422
59 Route 10, East Hanover, NJ 07936
Website: http://www.pharma.us.novartis.com

EVEROLIMUS (formerly known as SDZ-RAD): Certican is a derivative of rapamycin and has potent immunosuppressant and anti-proliferative

WHAT ARE CLINICAL TRIALS?

A clinical trial is a research study to answer questions about a new drug or treatment's safety and effectiveness. Once researchers testing new drugs or treatments in the laboratory get promising results, they begin planning clinical trials. These are only tested on people after laboratory and animal studies are done. Clinical trials of experimental drugs proceed through four phases:

Phase I Study: In this phase researchers investigate a new drug or treatment in a small group of 20 to 80 healthy volunteers. This phase takes several months to evaluate its safety, determine a safe dosage range, and identify side effects. 70% of experimental drugs pass this initial phase of testing.

Phase II Study: In this phase, the study drug or treatment is given to a larger group of 100 to 300 people to further evaluate its safety and effectiveness and can take several months to a couple of years. The majority of phase II studies are randomized; meaning a group of patients receives the experimental drug, while the other or "control" group receives a standard treatment or placebo. Sometimes, neither patients, nor researchers, know who is getting the experimental drug; these types of studies are called "blinded." Only one-third of new drugs complete phase I and phase II studies.

Phase III Study: During this phase, the study drug or treatment is given to a very large group of 1,000 to 3,000 people to confirm its effectiveness, monitor side effects, compare it to other treatments, and collect information that will allow the drug or treatment to be used safely. Most phase III studies are randomized and blinded trials and typically last several years. Once this phase is completed, the pharmaceutical company requests for FDA approval to begin marketing the drug. The majority of drugs that enter this phase successfully complete testing.

Late Phase III/Phase IV Studies: Late phase III/phase IV studies are done after the drug or treatment has been marketed. Pharmaceutical companies will usually compare their drug with other drugs already on the market or monitor the drug's long-term effectiveness and impact on a particular population.

properties. It has an action distinct from cyclosporine and Prograf, as it inhibits growth factor-dependant cell proliferation. Preclinical trials of everolimus proved that it is at least as efficient as sirolimus in preventing graft rejection. Everolimus is designed to be taken along with Neoral and may offer the potential to reduce the need for steroids.

Everolimus is currently being studied in the largest multi-center clinical trial of any transplant drug for ALL types of transplanted organs. It is currently in Phase III trials for the prevention and treatment of rejection in kidney, heart and liver recipients. It is also in Phase III trials for the prevention and treatment of rejection (obliterative bronchiolitis syndrome) in lung recipients. It is expected that everolimus will be available for kidney transplantation sometime in 2002. For more information, contact:

Novartis Pharmaceuticals
Phone: 800-742-2422
59 Route 10, East Hanover, NJ 07936
Website: http://www.pharma.us.novartis.com

FTY 720: displays a completely novel mechanism of action that has not been observed with any other immunosuppressant drug. This agent is designed to re-route lymphocytes into the lymph nodes before they reach the new organ, essentially tricking the body into not recognizing the transplanted organ as foreign, thereby potentially prolonging organ life without impairment of the immune response to systemic infection. When used in combination with cyclosporine and other existing therapies, this drug may allow for dose reduction of other agents to minimize side effects.

FTY 720 is in Phase II trials for the prevention of organ rejection in kidney transplantation. FTY 720 will be considered a primary drug for immune suppression. For more information, contact:

Novartis Pharmaceuticals
Phone: 800-742-2422
59 Route 10, East Hanover, NJ 07936
Website: http://www.pharma.us.novartis.com

ISATX247: is designed for the prevention of organ rejection after transplantation and for treatment of autoimmune diseases such as arthritis and psoriasis. In preclinical trials, ISAtx247 appears to be less toxic than cyclosporine. Phase IA trials have been completed and Phase IB trials are presently underway with an expected completion date of later this year. Phase II trials will commence in 2001 for kidney and liver transplantation. For more information, contact:

Isotechnika Inc.
Phone: 780-487-1600, E-mail: sgillis@isotechnika.com
17208 -108 Ave., Edmonton, Alberta, Canada T5S 1E8
Website: www.isotechnika.com

MEDI-507: is a humanized antibody directed against the CD2 T cell (humanized form of BTI-322). It is currently in Phase II clinical trials for the treatment of graft-vs.-host disease (GvHD) in bone marrow transplant recipients. GvHD is a common and often fatal outcome of bone marrow transplantation. GvHD occurs when donor cells attack the tissue of the recipient. For more information, contact:

MedImmune Inc.
Phone: 301-417-0770
35 W. Watkins Mill Road, Gaithersburgh, MD, 20878
Website: http://www.medimmune.com

New Technologies for Predicting, Diagnosing and Preventing Rejection:

HLA MATCHING/TISSUE TYPING: The obstacles to using HLA matching in lung transplantation are substantial. Currently, donor lungs and recipients are allocated according to blood type and size only. The lung's short ischemic time and the order in which organs are removed have prevented the use of HLA testing. Additionally, HLA matching would require the need for a large recipient pool in order to identify an appropriate recipient for allocation. Because most patients are in urgent need of a transplant, most transplant centers prefer to accept the first available organ rather than wait for a better match to come along. Using HLA matching could increase the waiting time to transplantation and mortality. However,

HLA typing could be useful AFTER transplantation to help guide the degree of immunosuppression and the need for surveillance bronchoscopies.

DIAGNOSTIC TECHNOLOGIES: Currently, graft rejection is diagnosed by the symptoms of organ failure and biopsy. New technologies for the detection of the immunological changes preceding rejection are being developed using magnetic resonance imaging (MRI) and radionuclide imaging, both noninvasive means of monitoring rejection. Others techniques include using biopsy, blood and urine samples to detect the markers that predict rejection prior to organ injury.

INDUCING IMMUNE TOLERANCE: Considered the ultimate approach to transplant rejection, inducing immune tolerance would involve retraining the body through brief treatment around the time of transplantation, so that the immune system would "tolerate" the grafted organ without the need for long-term immunosuppressant drug therapy.

Researchers at the University of Pittsburgh Medical Center (among others) are injecting bone marrow at the time of transplantation with hopes that this will enhance the cellular environment called "chimerism." Chimerism is defined as the coexistence of recipient and donor immune cells. The name comes from the chimera, a creature in ancient Greek mythology that was made up of parts from various animals. This concept grew from the observation by Dr. Thomas Starzl that some liver and kidney transplant patients, who have had stable graft function for many years, could be safely withdrawn from all immunosuppression. When Dr. Starzl studied the patients who seemed to be tolerant he found that donor cells were throughout the recipient's body. He termed this finding "microchimerism."

Research containing 26 lung transplant recipients reports simultaneous infusion of donor bone marrow at the time transplantation reduced the incidence of acute and chronic rejection. In patients who did not receive bone marrow the incidence of chronic rejection was 33%, compared to 5% in those patients who received the infusions. For more information, contact:

The Thomas E. Starzl Transplantation Institute
4th Floor Falk Medical Bldg., 3601 Fifth Ave., Pittsburgh, PA 15213
Phone: 877-640-ORGN (877-640-6746) or 412-648-3200
Website: http://www.sti.upmc.edu

Emerging Technologies:

XENOTRANSPLANTATION: The severe shortage of human organs for transplantation has renewed interest in the potential use of organs obtained from other species, called xenotransplantation. In the future, it may be possible to use animal-to-human transplants when no human organs are available. Research into using animals for transplant purposes is not new, but started as far back as the late 1960s. The use of pig heart valves is common today, but the pig cells are killed first.

The focus of the majority of research in this area has been on the development of transgenic pigs (pigs injected with human DNA). Research into using nonhuman primates has virtually stopped because of many complications encountered with their small size, slow breeding and the emotional attachment human beings have to them. Pigs, on the other hand, have a physiology quite similar to that of man and their organs are roughly the same size. In addition, pigs breed quickly, have large litters and are eaten by millions of people throughout the world. However, even with the transgenic organs, patients will still need to take special immunosuppressive drugs for the rest of their lives.

Currently, the FDA has approved clinical trails involving cellular and tissue xenotransplants, rather than whole vascularized organs. Researchers have successfully transplanted fetal pig cells into the brains of people with advanced Parkinson's Disease and strokes, and into animals for Huntington's disease, epilepsy and spinal cord repair. In addition, pig pancreatic islet cells secreting insulin have been transplanted into patients with diabetes.

In response to the many questions about safety, xenotransplantation has been banned by the United States and United Kingdom. However, the Food and Drug Administration has established an Advisory Panel on Xenotransplantation along with the National Institutes of Health and the Centers for Disease Control and Prevention to develop a patient registry that will monitor xenotransplant patients on a lifelong basis and keep donor tissues in archives for future reference.

Recently, scientists at BioTransplant Inc. have developed an inbred group of miniature pigs that do not pass on porcine endogenous retrovirus to human cells in the laboratory. BioTransplant believes the discovery of a noninfecting pig line could eliminate one of the biggest concerns about xenotransplantation, disease transmission. In addition, researchers at PPL Therapeutics Inc., the company that created "Dolly the sheep," have produced the first clones of an adult pig. These two developments brings researchers one step closer to making modified pigs whose organs and cells can be successfully transplanted into humans.

Nextran, a subsidiary of Baxter International Inc., concluded trials in late 1999 in which specially engineered pig livers were used as filters outside the body to perform human liver functions, called xenoperfusion. The next step is to ask the U.S. Food and Drug Administration for permission to perform trials where the organ is actually transplanted inside the body. Imutran, a British biotechnology company and a unit of Swiss pharmaceutical giant Novartis AG, is planning to perform the first transplants of animal organs into humans. These trials could begin in 2001.

STEM CELL TRANSPLANTATION: Stem cells have the potential to differentiate not only into blood cells, but also into many tissues. The primary source of stem cells in the body is bone marrow, but other sources may be obtained from peripheral-blood stem cells and umbilical cord blood. NIH-supported researchers have generated mature liver cells from stem cells in the bone marrow, and similar results have been seen for muscle cells, bone, cartilage, brain, and blood. Stem cell transplantation may be used to replace or assist failing organs and to treat neurological disorders.

TISSUE ENGINEERING: Advances in cell biology and stem cell transplantation has enabled scientists the ability to grow entire new organs from only a few cells in the laboratory. Ultimately, scientists will be able to actually grow new kidneys, hearts or any organ or tissue. The creation of man-made tissues or organs, known as neo-organs, has already been used to grow replacement livers and hearts in rats and dogs. Researchers at the Massachusetts Institute of Technology, Children's Hospital of Boston and Advanced Tissue Sciences Inc., a bioengineering company, are working together to develop the technology for use in humans.

The procedure utilizes a three-dimensional dissolvable polymer scaffold that is molded into the shape of the organ to be replaced. Cells are attached to the scaffold and as they grow, they fill in the framework. By the time cell growth is completed, the scaffold has dissolved and the old organ can be removed, if necessary. Scientists at Children's Hospital in Boston have successfully grown heart valves from cells using this new technique.

The creation of tissue for medical use is already in use to a limited extent in hospitals across the United States involving fabricated skin, cartilage, bone, ligament and tendon. Various human trials of tissue engineering are underway to test the ability of bone growth promoters to heal acute bone fractures. However, the development of large, complex organs such as livers, kidneys, hearts may be far off in the future. To date, only the factors responsible for bone and blood vessel growth have been characterized. To generate other organs, the specific molecules for their development must be identified and produced reliably.

GENETIC TRANSFER TECHNOLOGIES: With the completion of the rough draft of the entire set of human genes by the International Human Genome Project, scientists have identified anti-inflammatory genes, which raises the possibility of gene transfer to reduce the anti-graft immune response. This process involves treating an organ prior to transplantation to activate or dampen specific genes. The goal of this process is to modify the genes known to be involved in the very early stages of rejection, helping to quite the immune system within the organ itself and preventing some of the initial damage which occurs at the time of transplantation.

SUMMARY:

We are living in an exciting time for transplantation. Dedicated teams of doctors and researchers give HOPE to countless numbers of transplant patients. Although, lung transplantation has a way to go in matching the survival rates of other organs, extending life for people faced with life-threatening diseases, even if it is for a limited amount of time, is a major victory.

Transplantation, for some, can be perceived as a "mixed miracle." Your life is prolonged, but not necessarily problem-free. Problem-free living is a luxury few people experience, with or without a transplant. After the first year is over, life really does get back to some degree of normalcy, and many of those earlier restrictions you had to adhere to will be lifted.

Live life to the fullest; just use common sense. Remember you still have an immune system; the immunosuppressive drugs don't wipe it out completely. You received your transplant in order to live a better life, not to live in a "bubble." The challenge of being a transplant recipient is to learn to recognize issues as they arise, seek help when needed and, above all, enjoy the time transplantation has offered you.

BIBLIOGRAPHY:

American Academy of Pediatrics. "Guidelines for Health Supervision." *News and Comment*, May 1982.

Angulo, F., Glaser, C., Juranek, D., Lappin, M., and Regnery, R. "Caring for Pets of Immunocompromised Persons." *The Journal of the American Veterinary Medical Association* 1994; 205 (12): 1711 - 6.

Armenti, V., Coscia, L., McGrory, C., and Moritz, M. "Research Addresses Concerns About Pregnancy After Transplantation." Stadtlanders' *LifeTIMES* magazine 1998; (3): 28 - 30.

Armenti, V., Gertner, G., Eisenberg, J., McGrory C., and Moritz, M. "National Transplantation Pregnancy Registry: Outcomes of Pregnancies in Lung Recipients." *Transplant Proceedings* 1998; 30: 1528 - 30.

"Basiliximab Approved for Use in Renal Transplant Patients." *American Journal of Health System Pharmacy* 1998; 55: 1444 - 5.

Blankenberg, F., Robbins, R., Stoot, J., Vriens, P., Berry, G., Tait, J., and Strauss, H.W. "Radionuclide Imaging of Acute Lung Transplant Rejection with Annexin V." *Chest* 2000; 117: 834 - 40.

Briffa, N., and Morris, R. "New Immunosuppressive Regimens in Lung Transplantation." *The European Respiratory Journal* 1997; 10: 2630 - 7.

Chronimed Pharmacy. "Drug Identification Sheet." *Encore* magazine, Spring 1996, 28 - 9.

Church Ball, Joanne. "Getting Back to Work: A Guide for Transplant Recipients." Stadtlanders' *LifeTIMES* magazine 1998; (3): 18 - 9.

Clinical Nutrition Service, Clinical Center, National Institutes of Health. "Vitamins and Good Health," March 1997.

"Corticosteroids-Glucocorticoid Effects." *United States Pharmacopei Drug Information 1997, Vol. 3, Advice for Patients: Drug Information in Lay Language*, 583 - 8.

Credit, Larry P., Hartunian, Sharon G., and Nowak, Margaret J. *Your Guide to Complementary Medicine.* Avery Publishing Group, Garden City Park, New York 1998, ISBN: 0895298317.

Daar, A.S. "Animal-to-Human Organ Transplants – A Solution or a New Problem?" *Bulletin of the World Health Organization* 1999; 77 (1): 54 - 8.

Department of Dietetic, Massachusetts General Hospital. "Healthy Eating for Organ Transplant Recipients," fact sheet.

Donaldson, S., Nocotny, D., Paradoteski, L., and Arts, R. "Acute and Chronic Lung Allograft Rejection During Pregnancy." *Chest* 1996; 110: 293 - 6.

Eskinazi, Daniel P. "Factors that Shape Alternative Medicine." *Journal of the American Medical Association* 1998; 280 (18): 1621 - 3.

Harkness, Richard. "Drug Interaction Dangers." *Bottom Line Personal*, Oct. 30, 1992, 3.

Hausen, Bernard, and Morris, Randell E. "Review of Immunosuppression for Lung Transplantation." *Clinics in Chest Medicine* 1997; 18 (2): 353 - 66.

Horning, Neil R., Lynch, John P., Sundaresan, Sudhir R., Patterson, G. Alexander, and Trulock, Elbert P. "Tacrolimus Therapy for Persistent or Recurrent Acute Rejection After Lung Transplantation." *The Journal of Heart and Lung Transplantation* 1998; 17: 761 - 7.

Hwang, Mi Young. "Alternative Choices: What it Means to Use Nonconventional Medical Therapy." JAMA Patient Page, *Journal of the American Medical Association* 1998; 280 (18): 1640.

Kahan, Barry D., Rajagopalan, P.R., and Hall, Michael for the U.S. Simulect Renal Study Group. "Reduction of the Occurrence of Acute Cellular Rejection Among Renal Allograft Recipients Treated with Basiliximab, A Chimeric Anti-Interleukin-2 Receptor Monoclonal Antibody." *Transplantation* 1999; 67 (2): 276 - 84.

Keenan, R., Konishi, H., Kawai, A., Paradis, I., Nunley, D., Iacono, A., Hardesty, R., Weyant, R., and Griffith, B. "Clinical Trials of Tacrolimus Versus Cyclosporine in Lung Transplantation." *Annals of Thoracic Surgery* 1995; 60: 580 - 5.

Lappin, Michael R. "Pet Ownership in Immunosuppressed People." The North American Veterinary Conference, 1997 Proceedings, 297 - 300.

Lemke, Gina. "Solid Organ Transplantation Part II: Secondary Medications." TRIO'S *LifeLines* newsletter, Nov./Dec. 1996.

McCallum, Marlo. "A Toast to Your Health, Should it Involve Alcohol?" Chronimed Pharmacy's *Encore* magazine, Winter 1995, 12 - 3.

McGee, C., Fox, M. D., and Loyd, J.E. "The Feasibility of HLA Matching for Lung Transplantation." *Clinical Transplantation* 1996; 10: 564 - 7.

McGinn, Le, and Harker, Kelli. "Pediatric Lung Transplantation Program: Patient Handbook." Pediatric Lung Transplant Team, Children's Hospital at Shands, University of Florida, 1999.

Meyers, Bryan F., and Patterson, G. Alexander. "Lung Transplantation: Current Status and Future Prospects." *World Journal of Surgery* 1999; 23: 1156 - 1962.

Mooney, David J., and Mikos, Antonios G. "Growing New Organs." *Scientific American*, April 1999.

Nashan, B., Light, S., Hardie, I.R., Lin, A., and Johnson, J.R. for the Daclizumab Double Therapy Study Group. "Reduction of Acute Renal Allograft Rejection by Daclizumab." *Transplantation* 1999; 67 (1): 110 - 5.

National Center for Complimentary and Alternative Medicine Clearinghouse. "Acupuncture Information and Resources Package." Publication Z01- April 1999.

National Heart, Lung, and Blood Institute. "Heart and Heart-Lung Transplants," fact sheet, August 1997.

National Institute of Allergy and Infectious Diseases, National Institutes of Health. "Status of NIH-Sponsored Basic and Clinical Research on Transplantation," February 2000.

National Institutes of Diabetes and Digestive and Kidney Diseases. "Choosing a Safe and Successful Weight-Loss Program," NIH Publication No. 94-3700, December 1993.

National Kidney Foundation. "Drug Substitution in Transplantation: Recommendations to the Health Care Community, Executive Summary," 1998.

"New Fruit Juice Safety Regulations." TRIO's *Membership Update*, June 1998.

Nicoletti, Paul. "The Human-Animal Bond: Risks of Zoonoses." The North American Veterinary Conference 1997 Proceedings, 301 - 2.

Painter, Patricia. "Exercising After Transplant." The American Association of Kidney Patients' *Renalife* magazine, Vol. 8 (1): 11 - 3.

Paris, W., Diercks, M., Bright, J., Zamora, M., Kesten, S., Scavuzzo, M., and Paradis, I. "Return to Work After Lung Transplantation." *The Journal of Heart and Lung Transplantation* 1998; 17: 430 - 6.

Pham, S., Rao, A., Zeevi, A., McCurry, K., Keenan, R., Vega, J., Kormos, R., Hattler, B., Fung, J., and Starzl, T. Department of Surgery, Thomas E. Starzl Transplant Institute, University of Pittsburgh, Pa. "Effects of Donor Bone Marrow Infusion in Clinical Lung Transplantation." *Annals of Thoracic Surgery* 2000; 69 (2): 345 - 50.

Piascik, Peggy. "New Therapeutic Monoclonal Antibodies Target Kidney Transplant Rejection and Cancer." *Journal of the American Pharmaceutical Association* 1998; 38 (3): 379 - 80.

Pierre, Colleen. "Food Safety Goes Far Beyond 'Mad Cow' Scare." *The Sun-Sentinel,* April 25, 1996: 11.

Rager, Dennis, and Rager, Kris. "The ADA and Disclosure of Your Transplant." TRIO's *LifeLines* newsletter, July/August 1996: 7.

Regan, John. "Cryptosporidium and Drinking Water: What You Should Know." Gainesville Regional Utilities, Water and Wastewater Systems informational pamphlet, 1999.

SangStat Medical Corp. "Medication Noncompliance in Transplant Recipients: Incidence, Determinants, Consequences, and Solutions" brochure, 1998.

Silverman, Harold M. (Editor). *The Pill Book.* Bantam Books, 1996.

Smith, Ellen. "Water, Water, Everywhere: Can Your Drinking Water Hurt You?" Stadtlanders' *LifeTIMES* magazine 1996, (2): 26 - 7.

Social Security Administration. "What You Need to Know When You Get Disability Benefits," Publication No. 05-10153, June 1999.

Squires, Sally. "Tips to Keep Kitchen Bacteria in Check." *The Sun-Sentinel*, Dec. 21, 1995: 6.

Stadtlanders. "Is It Safe To Take Over-The-Counter Diet Pills To Lose Weight?" *LifeTIMES* magazine 1998; (3): 31.

Stankiewicz, Lynn, Midelfort, Judy, and Thompson, Sharen. "Going Home after Heart and Lung Transplantation." Society of Heart and Lung Transplant Social Workers pamphlet, 1991.

Strohecker, James. "Medicine for the 21st Century." *Utne Reader*, March/April 1999: 83 - 8.

TransCare Prescription Services. "Your Medications and More!" booklet, October 1996.

TRIO and the International Bottled Water Association. "What You Should Know About Your Drinking Water" flyer, June 1997.

TRIO New England. "Ouch! Cat Scratch Fever," *ORGANized* newsletter, December 1994.

University of Miami Donor Family Aftercare Program. "Writing to Donor Families: A Way to Say Thank You," brochure.

U.S. Department of Justice, Civil Rights Division. "A Guide to Disability Rights Laws." Disability Rights Section, 1996.

U.S. Food and Drug Administration. "Supplements Associated with Illnesses and Injuries." *FDA Consumer magazine*, Sept./Oct. 1998.

Warren, Jim. "New Tissue Replacement Technique Could Have Major Impact on Organ Shortage." *Transplant News Digest*, Transplant Chronicles; Vol. 6 (3): 12.

The Washington Post. "U.S. Warns of Tap Water Peril in Cases of Immune Weakness." *The Boston Globe*, June 16, 1995.

Weiss, Robin A. "Xenografts and Retroviruses." *Science*, Vol. 285, Aug. 20, 1999: 1221 - 2.

Whyte, R., Rossi, S., Mulligan, M., Florn, R., Baker, L., Gupta, S., Martinez, F., and Lynch III, J. "Mycophenolate Mofetil for Obliterative Bronchiolitis Syndrome After Lung Transplantation." *Annals of Thoracic Surgery* 1997; 64: 945 - 8.

Young, Stephanie. "How Metabolism Does – and Doesn't – Affect Your Weight." *Glamour*, April 1998, 84 - 6.

Glossary:

A

A1AT: Alpha-$_1$ antitrypsin deficiency emphysema.

Acute: Having rapid onset, severe symptoms and a short course.

Adult respiratory distress syndrome: A form of restrictive lung disease due to abnormal permeability of either the pulmonary capillaries or alveoli.

AIDS: Acquired immune deficiency syndrome.

Alveolar: Pertaining to the air cell of the lungs.

Alveolus (pl. alveoli): Air cell of the lungs.

Ambulatory: Able to walk; not confined to bed.

Anaphylaxis: A severe, potentially fatal allergic reaction.

Anastomosis: The surgical connection between two tubular structures.

Anemia: A symptom rather than a disease in itself, characterized by too few red blood cells in the bloodstream, resulting in insufficient oxygen to tissues and organs.

Anesthesia: Partial or complete loss of sensation with or without loss of consciousness as a result of administration of a drug, usually by injection or inhalation.

Aneurysm: Localized abnormal dilatation of a blood vessel, usually an artery, due to birth defect or weakness of the wall of the vessel.

Angina: Severe pain and constriction about the heart.

Antibody: A protein molecule produced by the body's immune system that help the white-blood cells fight foreign substances, such as bacteria, viruses or a transplanted organ.

Anticoagulant: An agent that prevents or delays coagulation of the blood.

Anticonvulsant: An agent that prevents or relieves convulsions.

Antigen: A substance that the body considers foreign, such as bacteria, viruses or a transplanted organ. When the body detects an antigen, it makes antibodies to fight it.

Antimicrobial: An agent that destroys or prevents the development of microorganisms.

Anti-rejection drugs: Medicines that help slow down your body's immune system. These drugs help to protect your new organ from being rejected.

Aplastic anemia: Anemia caused by deficient red cell production due to disorders of the bone marrow.

Arrhythmia: Irregularity or loss of rhythm, especially of the heartbeat.

Arterial septal defect: A hole in the wall that separates the upper chambers of the heart, which may require surgical repair.

Aseptic: Free from the presence of microorganisms.

Aspiration: The taking in of foreign matter into the lungs.

Atherosclerosis: Thickening, hardening and loss of elasticity of the walls of the arteries.

Atypical mycobacteria: A species of organisms belonging to the *Mycobacteriaceae* family that can cause tuberculosis.

Autoimmune disease: Disease in which antibodies are produced against the body's own normal tissue. This immune reaction is the basis of a variety of diseases including diabetes, rheumatoid arthritis and lupus, among others.

Autologous blood transfusion: Transfusion of blood that has been donated by the patient in advance of surgery.

B

B cell: A type of lymphocyte that arises in the bone marrow and spleen. They are present in the blood, lymph and connective tissue, and are important in producing circulating antibodies.

Bilateral: Pertaining to, affecting or relating to two sides.

Bioavailability: The rate and extent to which an active drug enters the general circulation.

Biopsy: The removal of a small piece of living tissue for examination under a microscope, usually performed to establish a diagnosis.

BiPAP (bi-level positive airway pressure): A device for noninvasive support of inspiration and expiration of air from the lungs.

Blood gas volumes: Represents the level of oxygen and carbon dioxide in the blood, in addition to the blood's pH or acidity or alkalinity.

Bone marrow: Soft tissue located in the cavities of bones. Bone marrow is the source of all blood cells.

BOOP (Bronchiolitis obliterans with organizing pneumonitis): BOOP is a condition characterized by pneumonia-like symptoms in conjunction with bronchiolitis obliterans. It involves the small airways and alveolar ducts and is associated with chronic inflammation in the surrounding alveoli. Clinically, most patients have a history of a slowly resolving viral pneumonia spanning weeks or a few months, a persistent, nonproductive cough, difficulty breathing and flu-like symptoms with fever, sore throat, discomfort and fatigue. Approximately half of all patients present with shortness of breath and two-thirds present with crackles during inspiration. Pulmonary function tests demonstrate a restrictive pattern with a reduction in diffusing capacity and gas exchange.

Bronchial: Pertaining to the bronchi or bronchioles.

Bronchiole: One of the smaller subdivision of the bronchial tubes.

Bronchiolitis obliterans: A condition described following inhalation of toxic fumes, as a consequence of respiratory infections, in association with connective tissue disorders and after bone marrow, lung or heart-lung transplantation. The lungs reveal fibrous scarring of the small airways as a result of damage to the bronchiolar cells, during the repair phase that leads to irreversible airflow obstruction. Wheezing, nonproductive cough and gradual onset of shortness of breath characterize this disorder.

Bronchitis: Inflammation of the mucous membrane of the bronchial tubes.

Bronchoalveolar lavage: Washing out the cavity of the bronchi and the alveoli.

Bronchodilator: A devise used to dispense medication by inhalation to open up the bronchial tubes.

Bronchoscopy: Examination of the bronchi through a bronchoscope.

Bronchostenosis: Constriction or narrowing of the bronchus.

Bronchus (pl. bronchi): One of the two main branches leading from the trachea to the lungs providing the passage way for air movement.

Bullous disease: The presence of small sacs or bubbles, which may be filled with fluid.

BUN: Blood, urea and nitrogen.

C
Cadaveric: Pertaining to a dead body.

Candidiasis: Infection of the skin or mucous membrane with any species of *Candida*, but chiefly *Candida albicans*. Usually localized in skin, nails, mouth, vagina, bronchi or lungs.

Cardiac: Pertaining to the heart.

Cardiac-assist devices (CADs): Technological devices that assist the heart in performing its functions.

Cardiopulmonary bypass: During a surgical procedure, a device used to take blood from the body, oxygenate it, then return it to the patient's circulation under pressure.

Cataract: A clouding of the lens of the eye, its capsule or both.

Catheter: A small, flexible plastic tube inserted into the body to administer or remove fluids.

Cerebral angiogram: A series of x-ray pictures taken in rapid sequence of the blood vessels of the brain following the injection of an opaque substance. This technique is used to define the size and shape of various veins and arteries.

Cerebrovascular: Pertaining to the blood vessels of the brain.

Chimerism: A state achieved over time where the cells of the donor organ are present in the body tissues and blood of recipients after organ transplantation.

Chromosome: A linear thread in the nucleus of a cell containing DNA, which transmits genetic information.

Chronic: Designates a symptom or disease showing little change or of slow progression; opposite of acute.

Chronic obstructive pulmonary disease (COPD): A group of diseases that all share one common feature, difficulty in expelling air from the lungs.

Cirrhosis: Chronic disease of the liver.

CMV (cytomegalovirus): A viral infection common in transplant recipients that can effect the lungs and other organs; also a member of the group of herpes virus.

Colitis: Inflammation of the colon.

Compliance: The degree to which a patient follows medical instructions and protocols.

Congenital: Present at birth.

Contraindication: Any symptom or circumstance indicating the inappropriateness of a form of treatment otherwise advisable.

Contusion: An injury in which the skin is not broken; a bruise.

Coronary arteries: Blood vessels that supply blood directly to the heart muscle.

Corticosteroids: A class of drugs that have anti-inflammatory properties and that slow down your body's immune system, simply called steroids.

CPAP (continuous positive air pressure): A device for noninvasive support of inspiration and expiration of air from the lungs.

Creatinine: A waste product made by the body that shows how well the kidneys are working.

Crossmatch: A blood test that tells if a donor's organ is a good match for your body. A negative crossmatch means that there is no reaction between the patient and the donor and a transplant can be performed.

Cushing's syndrome: A condition that can result from prolonged administration of steroids. Symptoms include protein loss, obesity, fatigue and weakness, osteoporosis, absence of menstruation, impotence, blood vessel fragility, edema, excess hair growth, diabetes and skin discoloration.

Cytokines: Chemicals that are involved in growth regulation.

Cytolytic: Pertaining to the destruction and dissolving of living cells.

Cytotoxic or killer T cells: A type of T cell that is formed after mature T cells interact with antigens present on foreign cells; these are the cells that cause graft rejection and kill foreign cells.

D

Dermatitis: Inflammation of the skin as evidenced by itching, redness and various skin lesions.

Diabetes: A disease in which the body does not make or properly use insulin, making it hard to break down sugar.

Dialysis: A method of removing waste products from the blood of patients whose kidneys cannot do this on their own.

Diastolic: Pertaining to that period of the heart cycle in which the muscle fibers are relaxed.

Disseminated: Scattered throughout an organ or body.

Diverticulitis: Inflammation of a sac in the intestinal tract, especially in the colon, causing stagnation of feces in the colon and pain.

Donor: Someone who furnishes blood, tissues or organs to be used in another person.

E

Edema: The buildup of excess water or other fluid in cells, tissues or cavities. Swollen ankles are a common sign of edema.

EEG (electroencephalogram): A recording made of the electrical activity in the brain.

Electrolyte: Ionized salts in blood, tissue fluid and cells including salts of sodium, potassium and chlorine.

Embolism: A sudden obstruction of a blood vessel by an abnormal particle (such as an air bubble) circulating in the blood.

En bloc: In surgery, to remove as a whole or as a clump.

Endogenous: Produced or arising from within a cell or organism.

End-stage organ failure: A condition that leads, ultimately, to functional failure of an organ. Some examples are emphysema (lungs), cardiomyopathy (heart) and polycystic kidney disease (kidneys).

Esophagus: A muscular tube that leads from the throat to the stomach.

Extracorporeal membrane oxygenator (ECMO): An external device that oxygenates blood delivered to it from the body and returns it to the patient.

Extubated: Removal of a tube, such as a breathing tube.

F

FDA (Food and Drug Administration): The governmental agency responsible for the regulation of food, medical devices and medicine.

Fibromyalgia: A condition that involves chronic muscle pains, trigger points, tender points and nonrestorative sleep.

Fibrosis: Abnormal formation of fibrous tissue.

G

Gastrointestinal: Pertaining to the stomach and the intestine.

Gastrointestinal reflux: A backward flow of fluids from the stomach.

Gene: The basic unit of heredity.

Generic drugs: Drugs not protected by a trademark. In the United States, generic drugs are required to meet the same bio-equivalency test as the original brand-name drug.

Genetic disease: A disease due to an abnormal condition of one or more genes. While most diseases have some genetic component, the term genetic disease is usually applied to those cases where one or two genes determine the disease, such as sickle cell anemia and cystic fibrosis.

Gingival hyperplasia: Overgrowth of the gums surrounding the teeth.

Glaucoma: Disease of the eye characterized by increase in pressure, which results in a decrease in size of the optic nerve and blindness.

Glucose: A type of sugar found in the body. Glucose levels are important for transplant patients to watch, especially if they have diabetes.

Graft: (n.) A transplanted organ, tissue or cells; (v.) to transplant.

Graft-vs.-host disease: A common and serious complication of bone marrow transplantation where there is an immunological attack by cells within the donated bone marrow that recognize the host cells as foreign and attack the patient's own tissue.

Gram stain: The staining of bacteria for identification.

H

Helper cells: A type of T cell that enhances the production of antibody-forming cells, cytotoxic T cells, and initiates many other immune responses.

Hematocrit: A test that measures the amount of red cells in the blood.

Hemodynamic: Pertaining to the forces involved in circulating blood through the body.

Hemorrhage: Abnormal internal or external discharge of blood.

Hepatitis: A disease that causes liver damage.

Herpes: A family of viruses that infect people. Herpes simplex causes lip and genital sores, while herpes zoster causes shingles.

Hirsutism: A condition characterized by excessive growth of hair or the presence of hair in unusual places.

Histocompatibility testing: A test to determine how closely the HLA antigens of the donor and recipient are matched and the likelihood that the recipient will reject the donor tissue. Commonly referred to as "tissue typing."

Histoplasmosis: A systemic, fungal, respiratory disease due to *Histoplasma capsulatum.*

HLA (human leukocyte antigens): A type of antigen that is present on the surfaces of virtually all cells, tissues and organs in the body, and normally serves to alert the immune system to the presence of infectious agents. These antigens are the major targets of the recipient's immune response after transplantation and are used to evaluate tissue compatibility for the possibility of transplantation.

HMO (Health Maintenance Organization): An alternative health care delivery system that arranges for the provision of medical services through selected doctors and hospitals. An HMO emphasizes preventive health care and early diagnosis as effective ways to maintain good health and avoid extensive treatment later.

Humanized: To endow with human characteristics or attributes.

Hyperglycemia: An increase of blood sugar, as in diabetes.

Hyperinflation: Excess of air in anything, especially the lungs.

Hypersensitivity: Abnormal sensitivity to a stimulus of any kind.

Hypertension: High blood pressure.

Hyper-thyroidism: Reaction to the secretion of too much thyroid hormone, which regulates metabolism.

Hypotension: Low blood pressure.

Hypo-thyroidism: Condition in which inadequate levels of thyroid hormone are circulating.

I

Immune response: The reaction of the immune system to foreign substances.

Immune system: The system that protects the body from invasion by foreign substances, such as bacteria, viruses and forms of cancer cells.

Immunity: The ability to resist a particular infectious disease.

Immunologic disease: A disease due to a dysfunction of the immune system.

Immunosuppressant: A drug that lowers the body's natural defenses.

Immunosuppression: Therapy, usually pharmaceutical, to reduce the magnitude of the immune response. Immunosuppression is the treatment for organ transplant rejection and autoimmune disease.

Implantation: Insertion of an organ into a new location.

Incentive spirometer: A device that uses visual and vocal stimuli to stimulate the patient to perform the breathing test using maximum effort.

Indication: A sign or circumstance that indicates the proper treatment of a disease.

Induction therapy: Early high-dose therapy to induce graft acceptance.

Infectious mononucleosis: An infection that primarily affects lymphoid tissue and is characterized by enlarged, often tender lymph nodes and spleen with a great increase of mononuclear leukocytes in the blood.

Inflammation: The way the body reacts to injury or "invasion," such as an infection. Signs of inflammation include: redness, heat, local swelling and pain.

Infusion: A liquid substance introduced into the body via a vein for therapeutic purposes.

Insulin: A protein that helps the body use glucose.

Interstitial: Pertaining to spaces within an organ or tissue.

Intra-aortic balloon pump: A devise used to decrease the work of the heart and increase blood flow to the coronary arteries.

Ischemic: Local and temporary deficiency of blood supply.

J

Jakob-Creutzfeldt disease: A progressive and inevitably fatal, slow virus disease of the central nervous system, characterized by progressive dementia and seizures that affects adults in midlife.

Jaundice: A condition in which the skin and eyes appear yellow because there is too much bilirubin (orange colored or yellowish pigment in bile) in the blood.

K

L

Latent: Lying hidden, quiet and not active.

Lesion: An area of altered or diseased tissue.

Living related donor: A living person donating an organ who is related by blood (not a spouse) to the person receiving the transplant.

Living-lobar lung donor: A living person who donates a part or lobe of their lung to the person receiving the transplant.

Lobe: A well-defined part of an organ. In the lungs, lobes include the superior and inferior lobes of the left lung and the superior, middle and inferior lobes of the right lung.

Lobectomy: Surgical removal of a lobe of any organ or gland.

Lung volume reduction surgery: A surgical procedure for patients with severe emphysema whereby the hyperinflated portion of the lung is removed so the patient's chest wall and diaphragm can return to normal positions, easing breathing.

Lupus: An autoimmune disease in which antibodies attack various types of connective tissue throughout the body.

Lymph: A fluid that carries lymphocytes, bathes the body tissues, and drains into the lymphatic vessels.

Lymphatic vessels: A network of channels, similar to the blood vessels, which transport lymph to the immune organs and into the bloodstream.

Lymphocyte: A type of white-blood cell.

Lymphokines: Powerful chemical substances secreted by lymphocytes. These molecules help and regulate the immune response.

Lymphoma: A general term for the growth of cancerous tissue in the lymphatic system.

Lymph nodes: A round body consisting of an accumulation of lymphatic tissue found at intervals along the course of lymphatic vessels.

M

Macrophage: A large and versatile immune cell that acts as a microbe-devouring cells, an antigen-presenting cell and an important source of immune secretions.

Major histocompatibility complex (MHC): A group of genes that controls several aspects of the immune response. MHC genes code for self markers on all body cells.

Malignant: Describing a tumor that is cancerous.

Mean: In statistics, a number derived by adding all the numbers or values in a given set and dividing that sum by the number of values; syn. average.

Median: In statistics, a number obtained by arranging the given series in order of magnitude and taking the middle number.

Meningitis: Inflammation of the membranes of the spinal cord or brain.

Metastasis: Movement of bacteria or body cells, especially cancer cells, from one part of the body to another.

Metastasize: To invade by metastasis.

Monoclonal antibody: An antibody arising from a single clone that is active against a single target antigen.

Monokines: Powerful chemical substances secreted by machrophages. These molecules help direct and regulate the immune response.

Mortality: The number of deaths in a given population.

Mucous: Pertaining to a sticky fluid secreted by the mucous membranes.

Myocardial infarction: A condition caused by obstruction of one or more of the coronary arteries; synonymous with heart attack.

Myofascial: Muscle and its fibrous membrane covering that supports and separates muscles.

N

Natural killer cells: Large cells that take on tumor cells and infected cells.

Neutrophil: A white blood cell that is an abundant and important phagocyte.

Nebulizer: An apparatus for producing a fine spray or mist.

Noncompliance: The failure of the patient to cooperate by carrying out the portion of the medical care plan under his or her control.

Non-heart beating donor: A category of patients in whom cardio-pulmonary resuscitation has failed or for whom life-support has been deemed futile and discontinued with the agreement of family members. The history of the non-heart beating donor goes back to 1951and was the original type of donor before the establishment of the concept of brain death.

O

Obliterative bronchiolitis syndrome: A term used to describe chronic rejection of transplanted lungs; the presence of inflammation of the walls and tissue of the bronchioles, with obliteration and scarring that results in fibrosis.

Obstructive lung disease: A group of diseases characterized by obstruction to airflow, as seen in patients with asthma, emphysema, cystic fibrosis and chronic rejection.

Ocular: Concerning the eye or vision.

OPO (Organ Procurement Organization): A nonprofit organization that works with hospitals to identify potential organ donors and procure medically suitable organs for transplantation.

OPTN (Organ Procurement and Transplantation Network): A governmental agency that oversees the national organ sharing policies.

Osteoarthiritis: Joint inflammation brought about by wear and tear causing cumulative damage to articular cartilage.

Osteoporosis: A term for describing any disease process that results in reduction in bone mass.

Oxygen saturation: Oxygen content of blood divided by oxygen capacity and expressed in volume percent.

P

Pancreatitis: Inflamed condition of the pancreas.

Panel reactive antibodies (PRA): A test to measure what percent of a serum sample reacts to a panel of known antigens.

Pasteurization: The process of heating a liquid at a moderate temperature for a definite period of time in order to destroy bacteria without changing the liquid's chemical composition.

Patency: The state of being freely open.

Pathogen: A microorganism or substance capable of producing a disease.

Perfusion: Passing of a fluid, such as blood, through spaces.

PFTs (Pulmonary function tests): A number of different tests used to determine the ability of the lungs to exchange oxygen and carbon dioxide.

Phagocyte: A large white-blood cells that contribute to the immune defenses by ingesting microbes, other cells and foreign particles.

Physiotherapy: Treatment with physical and mechanical means, such as massage or electricity.

Placebo: An inactive substance given to a group of patients as part of a clinical trial.

Platelet: A small blood cell needed to form normal blood clotting.

Pleura: The membrane that surrounds both lungs. It is moistened with a secretion to reduce friction during respiration.

Pleural: Pertaining to the pleura.

Pneumonia: Inflammation of the lungs caused primarily by bacteria, viruses and chemical irritants.

Pneumothorax: Collection of air or gas in the pleural cavity. The gas enters as the result of a perforation through the chest wall or pleura covering the lung. Also, known as a lung collapse.

Polycolonal antibodies: Antibodies produced by many clones which, together, react with one or more antigens.

Primary care physician: A family physician or general medical doctor you choose from an HMO's network of physicians who becomes your personal plan doctor and provides and coordinates all of your health care.

Prophylactic: Pertaining to any agent or regimen that contributes to the prevention of infection or disease.

Prophylaxis: Observance of rules necessary to prevent disease.

Psoriasis: A common, chronic disease of the skin consisting of red elevated areas on the skin frequently located on the scalp, knees and elbows.

Psychosis: A mental disorder of such magnitude that there is a personality disintegration and loss of contact with reality.

Q
QOD: Every other day.

R
Reimplantation response: Accumulation of fluids in the lungs due to left-sided failure of the heart, i.e. more blood is supplied to the pulmonary circulation than is removed; otherwise known as acute pulmonary edema.

Rejection: The degradation or destruction of transplanted material at the cellular level by the patient's own immune system. This immunological response, if not controlled, will eventually lead to organ failure.

Renal: Having to do with the kidneys.

Reperfusion: Returning nutrients and oxygen to an organ or tissue.

Replication: The process of duplication of genetic material.

Restrictive lung disease: A group of diseases characterized by reduction in lung volumes, while expiratory airflow is normal, as seen in patients with sarcoidosis or interstitial fibrosis.

Rheumatoid arthritis: An autoimmune disease in which the membranes lining the capsule of a joint, particularly in the hands and feet, are attacked by the immune system.

S

Sepsis: A pathological state, usually accompanied by fever, resulting from the presence of microorganisms or their poisonous products in the blood.

Serology: The scientific study of the watery portion of the blood after coagulation.

Serum: The watery portion of the blood after coagulation. Also, serum from an animal rendered immune against an organism to be injected into a patient with disease from the same pathogen.

Shingles: A herpes viral infection that usually affects a nerve causing pain in various areas of the body.

Shunt: An irregular passage or one artificially constructed to divert flow from one main route to another.

Spirometer: An apparatus that measures the air capacity of the lungs.

Spirometry: Measurement of the air capacity of the lungs.

Spleen: An elongated organ located in the abdomen, composed of spongelike tissue consisting of lymphatic tissue.

Sputum: Substance expelled by coughing or clearing the throat.

Stem cells: Cells from which all blood cells derive. The bone marrow is rich in stem cells.

Stent: Any material used to hold tissue in place or to provide support for surgical or pathological connection of two tubular structures.

Suppressor T cells: A type of T cell that suppresses production of antibody-forming cells and shuts down the immune response.

Systemic: Pertaining to the whole body rather than one of its parts.

Systolic: Pertaining to that part of the heart cycle in which the muscle fibers are contracted.

T

Tachycardia: Abnormally rapid heart rate; usually defined as a heart rate over 100 beats per minute.

Tachypnea: Abnormally rapid respiration.

T cells: Small white-blood cells that orchestrate and/or directly participate in the immune defenses. Also known as lymphocytes, they are processed in the thymus and secrete lymphokines. There are three different types of T cells: Helper T cells, cytotoxic or killer T cells and suppressor T cells.

Telemetry: The transmission of data electronically to a distant location.

Thoracic: Pertaining to the chest.

Thorax: That part of the body between the base of the neck above and the diaphragm below.

Thromboembolism: A blood clot that obstructs a blood vessel that has become detached from its site of formation.

Thrush: A fungal infection of the mouth that produces white spots on the tongue and throat; caused by *Candida albicans*.

Thymocyte: A cell in the thymus that migrated there from the bone marrow. As these cells develop they mature and some of these cells leave the thymus to become various types of T cells.

Thymus: A primary lymphoid organ, high in the chest, where T cells proliferate and mature.

Tissue typing: Techniques utilized to determine the compatibility of tissues to be used in grafts and transplants with the recipient's tissues and cells.

Tolerance: A state of immunologic nonresponsiveness to one or more foreign antigens.

Trachea: The main trunk by which air passes to and from the lungs.

Transplantation: To transfer tissue or an organ from one body to another.

U

Ulcerative colitis: Ulceration of the mucous membranes of the colon.

UNOS (United Network for Organ Sharing): A government-funded organization that links all organ procurement organizations and transplant centers, contracted by the federal government to insure that all organs are shared as fairly as possible.

V

Vaginitis: Inflammation of the vagina.

Vascular: Pertaining to or composed of blood vessels.

Vasodilators: A drug that dilates the blood vessels.

Vasopressors: Agents used to stimulate contraction of muscles of the capillaries and arteries.

Ventilation: The inspiration and expiration of air from the lungs.

Ventilator: A mechanical device for artificial respiration of the lungs.

Ventricular: Pertaining to either of two chambers of the heart that, when filled with blood, contract to propel it into the arteries.

Ventricular assist device: A device that replaces the pumping action of a diseased or nonfunctioning heart.

Ventricular septal defect: An opening in the wall that separates the lower chambers of the heart, which may undergo spontaneous closure in infancy, lead to heart failure, require surgical closure or be accompanied by pulmonary vascular disease; a congenital defect present at birth.

Vesicle: A small blister-like elevation on the skin containing fluid.

W

White-blood cells: Cells in the blood that fight infection and play a role in rejection.

X

Xenotransplantation: Transplantation between members of different species; for example, the transplantation of animal organs into humans.

Y

Z

Zoonotic: Pertaining to diseases transmitted from animals to man under natural conditions.

Zoonoses: A group of diseases capable of being transmitted from animals to humans.

Resources:

The following is a list of national organizations that provide resources to transplant patients, recipients and their families. Check your local library or Yellow Pages to find organizations that may be available in your area.

Organ Donation & Transplantation Organizations:

American Bone Marrow Donor Registry

Patient Search Information: 800-7-A-MATCH (800-726-2824) or 508-792-8969, E-mail: info@crir.org or http://www.crir.org
Donor Operations Center: 800-736-6283
The University of Massachusetts Medical Center, Dept. of Pediatrics, 55 Lake Ave., Worcester, MA 01655

The American Bone Marrow Donor Registry is composed of two distinct divisions, a Patient Advocacy Office and a Donor Operations Center. The Patient Advocacy Office coordinates the patient search process through the American Registry centralized file and through international donor sources, accessing a total of approximately 3 million donors. The Donor Services Division is responsible for donor education, recruitment, subsequent compatibility testing and advocacy.
Website: http://www.neosoft.com/~jakardna

Anatomic Gift Foundation Inc.

Phone: 800-300-LIFE (800-300-5433), Fax: 301-953-2570
13948 Baltimore Ave., Laurel, MD 20707

The Anatomic Gift Foundation is dedicated to the procurement, preparation and provision of nontransplantable human organs and tissues for medical science and education. Scientific applications include the study and treatment of HIV, hepatitis, cancer, diabetes and asthma.
Website: www.anatomicgift.com

COMET (The National Council on Minority Education in Transplantation)

Fax: 516-546-4253, E-mail: physicals1@aol.com
P.O. Box 7401, Freeport, NY 11520

COMET was formed to increase organ and tissue awareness and donation, with emphasis on minority involvement. It provides information and education about organ and tissue donation to the public, assists donor families and assists transplant candidates and recipients.
Website: http://transweb.org/comet/index.html

The Coalition on Donation

For brochures: 800-355-SHARE (800-355-74273)
For information: 804-330-8620, Fax: 804-323-7343,
E-mail: coalition@unos.org
1100 Boulders Parkway, Suite 500, Richmond, VA 23225-8770

The Coalition on Donation is made up of approximately 47 organizations and 48 local coalitions around the country dedicated to educating the public about organ and tissue donation. In partnership with the Advertising Council, the Coalition has developed a national public education campaign for organ and tissue donation employing multimedia strategies (e.g., TV, print, radio, etc.) on the local and national level.

Contact the coalition to receive a free copy of the "Share your life. Share your decision" brochure. The coalition also has available organ donation campaign kits, which include: audiocassette, VHS cassette, poster, magazine ad, newspaper ad and "What you can do" list, buttons, removable bumper stickers, Post-It Notes, window decals, T-shirts and baseball caps, all for sale. It also publishes a bimonthly newsletter called *neXus*.
Website: http://www.shareyourlife.org

Israel Penn Transplant Tumor Registry
Phone: 513-558-6006
University of Cincinnati, 231 Bethesda Ave., ML 0558, Cincinnati, OH 45267
Dr. Israel Penn began collecting data on transplant tumors in 1968. In the mid '70s, the Cincinnati Transplant Tumor Registry was formed. After his death, the registry was renamed the Israel Penn Transplant Tumor Registry. Currently, the registry contains records on more than 13,000 patients who have developed some type of cancer since transplantation.

James Redford Institute for Transplant Awareness
Phone: 310-441-4906, E-mail: jrifilms@aol.com
PMB 214, 10573 W. Pico Blvd., Los Angeles, CA 90064-2348
Facing the choice of liver transplantation or death, James Redford waited six months for the donor liver that ultimately saved his life. Following his surgery, Redford launched the James Redford Institute for Transplant Awareness (JRI), an organization devoted to educating the public about the importance of organ and tissue donation. The institute utilizes film and educational outreach programs to raise awareness and build public acceptance. It currently has two films available:
Flow is a 16-minute drama targeting teenagers, which can be used to teach the topic of organ and tissue donation. *Flow* and its educational kits are distributed by the Coalition on Donation (804-327-1438).
The Kindness of Strangers is a 104-minute documentary film, which examines the complex world of organ donation and transplantation. For domestic distribution and to rent the film or inquire about future video copies, contact: Direct Cinema Limited at 310-636-8200 or E-mail: dclvideo@aol.com. For international distribution, contact: Jane Balfour Films Limited (011-44-171-267-5392), E-mail: jbf@janebalfourfilms.co.uk
Website: http://www.jrifilms.org

The Living Bank
Phone: 800-528-2971, Fax: 713-961-0979, E-mail: info@livingbank.org
P.O. Box 6725, Houston, TX 77265-6725
The Living Bank is an international organization dedicated to the enhancement of organ and tissue donorship and transplantation. It provides a registry and referrals for those who want to donate tissues, bones or vital organs for transplantation or research. It also has a speakers bureau which provides general information about organ donation and transplantation. The Living Bank also has pins, decals, etc. for organ donor awareness and a newsletter called *The Bank Account*. *Website:* http://www.livingbank.org

Marie "Mitzi" Singel Foundation
Phone: 219-548-7021, E-mail: staff@mitzisingelfoundation.org
505 N. Washington St., Valparaiso, IN 46383
The Marie "Mitzi" Singel Foundation was established in 1997 to honor

the memory of Mitzi, a double-lung transplant recipient. The foundation has created and maintains an online educational system to ensure that all individuals associated with transplantation (especially lung transplantation) are connected through the most current technologies to optimize quality of life of transplant recipients. In addition, the foundation's "Patient to Patient Forum" was designed for transplant patients, their family members and friends to receive information about all phases of transplantation. *Website:* http://www.mitzisingelfoundation.org

National Kidney Foundation Inc.
Phone: 800-622-9010 or 212-889-2210 (in New York), Fax: 212-689-9261, E-mail: info@kidney.org
30 E. 33rd St., Suite 1100, New York, NY 10016

In addition to providing services to kidney patients, the National Kidney Foundation (NKF) promotes organ and tissue donation through their Transplant Athletics program. It helps coordinate the U.S. Transplant Games, held every other year and Team USA's delegation to the World Transplant Games and the World Winter Transplant Games, which are held in the years between the U.S. Games. Through the TransAction Council, it provides advice and assistance to transplant recipients through its educational symposia, publications and other support services. NKF also publishes *Transplant Chronicles*, a quarterly newsletter and provides advocacy and support through the National Donor Family Council. *Website:* http://www.kidney.org

National Marrow Donor Program
Phone: 800-MARROW-2 (800-627-7692), Fax: 612-627-8577, E-mail: webdata@nmdp.org
3433 Broadway St., N.E., Suite 500, Minneapolis, MN 55413

The National Marrow Donor Program (NMDP) facilitates unrelated donor stem cell transplants for patients with life-threatening blood diseases who do not have matching donors in their families. Currently, the NMDP facilitates more than 100 transplants each month. The NMDP provides a single point of access for all sources of blood stem cells used in transplantation, marrow, peripheral blood and umbilical cord blood. The Registry is able to search its own database and provide physicians with information on multiple stem cell sources for life-saving transplants. *Website:* http://www.marrow.org

National Minority Organ and Tissue Transplant Education Program
Phone: 800-393-2839 or 202-865-4888, Fax: 202-865-4880
Howard University Hospital, 2041 Georgia Ave., N.W., Suite 3100, Washington, DC 20060

The National Minority Organ and Tissue Transplant Education Program (MOTTEP) is a national education and awareness campaign that works to implement strategies to increase the percentage of organ and tissue donations in minority communities. It has some excellent educational materials, available in English and Spanish, such as pamphlets, research reports and videotapes. *Website:* http://www.nationalmottep.org

The National Transplant Pregnancy Registry
Phone: 877-955-6877 or 215-955-2840, Fax: 215-955-1420
Thomas Jefferson University Hospital, Department of Surgery, Transplant

Program, 605 College Building, 1025 Walnut St., Philadelphia, PA 19107

Thomas Jefferson University Transplant Program established the National Transplant Pregnancy Registry in 1991 to study the effect pregnancy has on the health of the mother, her transplanted organ and her baby. It also includes information on pregnancies fathered by transplant recipients.

Newlungs.com

Newlungs.com is an online guide to preparing for, obtaining, recovering from and living with a lung transplant. Written from a patient's point of view, it also offers a list of resources, major transplant centers and patient support sites. *Website:* http://www.newlungs.com

The Nicholas Green Foundation

Phone: 707-875-2263, Fax: 707-875-2653
P.O. Box 937, Bodega Bay, CA 94923

In 1994, seven-year-old Nicholas Green was murdered during a robbery while vacationing in Italy with his family. His parents, Reg and Maggie Green, made the decision to donate his organs, and later established the Nicholas Green Foundation to increase awareness worldwide of the importance of organ donation. The foundation has videos available: *The Nicholas Effect* and *Thank you, Nicholas.* To get a copy, contact: Corporate Productions, 4516 Mariota Ave., Toluca Lake, CA 91602 or call 818-760-2622 or fax 818-760-8619. (Now available in Spanish.) In addition, the foundation has created The Nicholas Green Scholarship Fund, which provides scholarships to outstanding college students who want to study abroad. For more information about the Scholarship Fund, contact Robert Powell at 617-624-7116. The Nicholas Green Foundation is also funding annual awards for an outstanding elementary school student in every state. For more information, contact Peter Rosenstein at 202-785-4268. *Website:* http://www.greenfoundation.com

The Pulmonary Retransplant Registry

Phone: 519-663-3159, Fax: 519-663-3858, E-mail: rjnovick@julian.uwo.ca
c/o Dr. Richard J. Novick, Multi-Organ Transplant Program
London Health Sciences Centre, University Campus, P.O. Box 5339,
339 Windermere Road, London, Ontario, Canada N6A 5A5

The Pulmonary Retransplant Registry, established in 1991, is a collaborative effort among worldwide centers performing lung retransplants. The registry includes data on 250 patients from 48 centers in North America, Europe and Australia.
Website: http://www.lhsc.on.ca/prr/index.htm

Second Wind Lung Transplant Association Inc.

Phone: 888-855-9463 or 727-442-0892 (in Clearwater),
Fax: 727-442-9762, E-mail: secondwind@netzero.net
300 S. Duncan Ave., Suite 227, Clearwater, FL 33755-6457

The Second Wind Lung Transplant Association publishes a membership directory of lung transplant patients and *AirWays*, a newsletter which comes out six times a year. The association also hosts an annual educational conference, provides support to patients and is working to establish chapters of Second Wind throughout the country.
Website: http://www.2ndwind.org

Transplant for Life
Phone: 818-783-LIFE (818-783-5433), Fax: 818-986-5576,
E-mail: unitedforlife@aol.com
20400 Ventura Blvd., Woodland Hills, CA 91364
    Transplant for Life was organized to build awareness in the interfaith community of the critical shortage of organs and about the importance and permissibility of organ and tissue donation. Originally built around the National Donor Sabbath Weekend, it has created the "Transplant for Life Guide," a five-step action plan that includes information and materials needed to educate members, such as scriptural references and donor cards. This plan is easily adapted to all major religions.
Website: http://www.transplantforlife.org

Transplanthealth
    Transplanthealth is a website put together by the Cincinnati Transplant Institute that provides comprehensive information before and after transplantation, including interactive tools, links and other helpful resources for transplant candidates, recipients, their families and caregivers.
Website: http://www.transplanthealth.com

Transplant Recipients International Organization (TRIO)
Phone: 800-TRIO-386 (800-874-6386) or 202-293-0980 (in DC),
Fax: 202-293-0973, E-mail: trio@primenet.com
1000 16th St., N.W., Suite 602, Washington, DC 20036-5705
    Through TRIO's national headquarters and a network of local chapters, TRIO serves its members in the areas of support, advocacy, awareness and education. TRIO has formed the TRIO Insurance Task Force, which can answer many of your insurance-related questions. TRIO has also established The Donor Family Task Force to provide support and bereavement groups to donor families. It has published the *TRIO Guide for Coping with Communication,* which gives advise about written communication between recipients and donor families. In addition, TRIO has a legislative fact sheet and a website called the "Legislative Action Center" where you can find current legislation pertaining to issues important to transplant recipients.
Website: http://congress.nw.dc.us/trorg
    TRIO has also established the "Lend A Helping Ear Program," which is a peer-support group of transplant volunteers who have donated their time to answer questions from transplant patients. TRIO also has green ribbon pins and stickers available for purchase. It also provides annual educational scholarships for transplant recipients and donor family members wishing to further their education. TRIO and United Airlines have developed a partnership to provide airplane tickets for transplant patients through United's "Charity Miles Program." TRIO publishes *LifeLines*, a bimonthly newsletter and, *Membership Update*, a monthly publication.
Website: http://www.primenet.com/~trio

Transplant Speakers International Inc.
Phone: 732-972-3765
P.O. Box 6395, Freehold, NJ 07728
    Transplant Speakers International (TSI) is an organization consisting solely of transplant recipients and organ and tissue donor families. Since its inception in July 1998, the organization has devoted itself to educating the public through live public speaking engagements

presented from a donor-recipient perspective. TSI also offers public speaking training seminars to donor families and transplant recipients who would like to become involved in educating the public. These seminars are offered free of charge. *Website:* http://www.transplant-speakers.org

Transplant World
Phone: 561-234-1736
664 Azalea Lane, Suite C, Vero Beach, FL 32963
Transplant World is a virtual community that enables transplant recipients to share their stories and tell the world that transplantation works. If you would like to share your story, E-mail it and any accompanying photos to Jennifer Benjamin at jben@transplantworld.org *Website:* http://www.transplantworld.org/index.html

TransWeb
Phone: 734-998-7314, Fax: 734-998-6710, E-mail: transweb@umich.edu
c/o The Northern Brewery, 1327 Jones, Suite 105, Ann Arbor, MI 48105
Transweb is an educational resource devoted to transplantation and organ donation. It is perhaps the largest transplant-related website on the World Wide Web. *Website:* http://www.transweb.org

United Network for Organ Sharing (UNOS)
Donation related information: 800-355-SHARE (800-355-74273)
Patient Inquiries: 888-TX-INFO-1 (888-894-6361)
Media Inquiries: 804-327-1432 or http://www.newsroom@unos.org
Ordering Information: 804-330-8541 or online
Research Inquiries: 804-330-8576, Fax: 804-323-3794 or online
1100 Boulders Parkway, Suite 500, P.O. Box 13770, Richmond, VA 23225-8770
UNOS is a private organization that manages the Organ Procurement and Transplantation Network (OPTN), under contract with the U.S. Department of Health and Human Services, to ensure equal access for all patients needing organs for transplantation. UNOS coordinates the logistics of matching the organs, collecting, analyzing and publishing transplant data, and educating health professionals about the donation process.

In addition, UNOS has created an area on its website for patients and their families who've just discovered they need a transplant in order for them to better understand the process and help them make the best choices in choosing a transplant center. The site, called "Transplant Living," (www.patients.unos.org), features "Transplant 101," a step-by-step guide through every stage of the organ transplant process. It also includes helpful information on financing transplants, local support groups, instructions on how to get on waiting lists, as well as past experiences from transplant recipients, professionals and family members of organ donors.

A special highlight of the website is the "Transplant Patient DataSource" (http://www.patients.unos.org/tpd). It is designed to provide the latest statistics on survival rates, the size of waiting lists and waiting times, and the current supply of donated organs, nationally, by state and by transplant center. Patients without Internet access can always call in requests for information. *Website:* http://www.unos.org

UNOS BOOKLETS/BROCHURES/BOOKS/MAGAZINE:
What Every Patient Needs to Know: This free booklet is designed to help

patients and their families through the organ transplant process. Incorporating material from UNOS' three earlier patient brochures ("What Every Patient Should Know," "Questions a Patient Should Ask" and "Financing Transplantation,") this booklet provides information about preparing for one's transplant, developing a financial strategy, the transplant itself and life after transplantation.

Donate Life[sm] organ and tissue donation brochure: This brochure dispels myths, answers commonly asked questions, reveals donation statistics, and includes a donor and family notification card.

UNOS Update Magazine: This free monthly periodical highlights newsworthy information about UNOS and donation and transplantation.

Transplantation Information Kit: Patients and members of the general public can receive a free patient information kit about a specific organ or a general information kit about organ transplantation. This information is mailed within 48 hours of request.

Understanding Brain Death Card: This resource provides an explanation to the patient's family on the definition and meaning of brain death, and is intended to complement the discussion by healthcare professionals.

Organ & Tissue Donation: A Reference Guide for Clergy (4th edition): This updated guide was created to provide clergy with state-of-the-art information in a readily accessible format and provide resources for OPO personnel involved in donor family discussions, education and hospital development. This notebook also features article reprints, abstracts and a bibliography.

UNOS Organ Procurement, Preservation and Distribution in Transplantation (2nd edition): Every donor hospital unit should have this comprehensive reference manual authored by national leaders. This book covers the entire donation process (evaluation through preservation, histocompatibility and legalities) and its coordination.

UNOS REPORTS AND STUDIES:

1997 Report of Center Specific Graft & Patient Survival Rates: These organ-specific volumes provide the number of transplants performed at each transplant program over a given time period plus the survival rate at each program. More current information can be found on the UNOS website, through the Transplant Patient DataSource.

1997 Report of the OPTN: Waiting List Activity and Donor Procurement: This report provides detailed data that reflect organ procurement practices of each UNOS region and OPO in the United States. More current information can be found on the UNOS website, through the Transplant Patient DataSource.

Statistical Annual Report: Data and analyses are provided in this annual report of the U.S. Scientific Registry for Organ Transplantation and the Organ Procurement and Transplantation Network. Includes information for the most recent 10-year period.

UNOS AUDIO/VISUALS:

OPTN/UNOS Slide Presentation: This set of slides presents an overview of organ donation and transplantation for the general public and professional audiences. This resource, in a Powerpoint formate, can be downloaded from www.unos.org->resources->product catalog.

Brain Death Video: This video educates health professionals on the diagnosis of brain death.

The Wendy Marx Foundation for Organ Donor Awareness
Phone: 202-546-7270, E-mail: WEMarx@aol.com
322 S. Caroline Ave., S.E., Suite 201, Washington, DC 20003
   The Wendy Marx Foundation for Organ Donor Awareness has provided funding for a medical fellowship for doctors who want to learn more about organ donation and transplantation. It also supports the U.S. Transplant Games and has developed the U.S. Sports Council on Organ Donation, which includes athletes, sports journalists and collegiate and professional coaches. In addition, it produces and distributes a video on organ donor awareness targeting junior high school students and their families, called *Talk, Talk, Talk.* This eight-minute video features Olympic champion Carl Lewis and liver transplant recipient Wendy Marx.
Website: http://www.transplantbook.com

World Transplant Games Federation
Fax: 011-44 -196-284-0775, E-mail: wtgf@wtgf.demon.co.uk
Highcroft, Romsey Road, Winchester, Hampshire, SO22 5DH England
   In 1978, the first Transplant Games were held in Portsmouth, England with 100 participants from only a handful of countries. In 1987, the World Transplant Games Federation was formed. Today, over 1,000 competitors from over 50 countries take part in the World Transplant Games. These Games and the World Winter Games are held every other year.
Website: http://www.wtgf.org

Fundraising and Charitable Organizations:
Children's Organ Transplant Association Inc.
Phone: 800-366-2682 or 812-336-8872, Fax: 812-336-8885,
E-mail: cota@cota.org
2501 COTA Drive, Bloomington, IN 47403
   Children's Organ Transplant Association assists transplant patients and their families in organizing fund-raising events. The association will work with adults as well as children. It has a new program that matches gifts, and patients can receive up to $10,000. All funds raised go to the individual. No administrative fees are collected.
Website: http://www.cota.org

National Foundation for Transplants (formerly Organ Transplant Fund)
Phone: 800-489-3863 or 901-684-1697 (in Memphis), Fax: 901-684-1128,
E-mail: nftpr@aol.com
1102 Brookfield, Suite 200, Memphis, TN 38119
   The National Foundation for Transplants (NFT) offers financial support services and patient advocacy for transplant candidates, recipients and their families. NFT assists in managing fund-raising campaigns for transplant candidates and recipients needing $10,000 or more for their

transplant-related care and/or medications. Also, grants for patients with smaller, nonrecurring needs for medications and other transplant-related emergencies are available. *Website:* http://www.transplants.org

National Transplant Assistance Fund
Phone: 800-642-8399 or 610-527-5056, Fax: 610-527-5210,
E-mail: NTAF@transplantfund.org
P.O. Box 258, 6 Bryn Mawr Ave., Suite 201, Bryn Mawr, PA 19010
The National Transplant Assistance Fund provides educational information, fund-raising expertise for patients raising money for transplants, and financial support to patients through medical assistance grants. *Website:* http://www.transplantfund.org

Health Insurance Information:
A.C.C.E.S.S.
(Advocating for Chronic Conditions, Entitlements and Social Services)
Phone: 888-700-7010 or 813-806-0800 (in Tampa), Fax: 813-886-1324
Gentiva Health Services, 4710 Eisenhower Blvd., Suite E3,
Tampa, FL 33634
Gentiva Health Services' A.C.C.E.S.S. program provides information on Social Security Disability, Supplemental Security Income, COBRA extensions for the disabled and the Health Insurance Portability and Accountability Act. The organization answers questions on disability issues and helps research alternative insurance sources, such as high-risk insurance pools. It also provides legal representation to individuals with pulmonary hypertension or alpha-$_1$ antitrypsin deficiency when seeking Social Security Disability and Supplemental Security Income.

Medicare Rights Center
Phone: 800-333-4114 or 212-869-3850, Fax: 212-869-3532
1460 Broadway, New York, NY 10036
The Medicare Rights Center provides assistance to people on Medicare through a national hotline counseling program, publications and public policy work. *Website:* http://www.medicarerights.org

National Organization of Social Security Claimants' Representatives
Office of Governmental Affairs
Phone: 800-431-2804 or 201-444-1415, E-mail: nosscr@worldnet.att.net
6 Prospect St., Midland Park, NJ 07432
The National Organization of Social Security Claimants' Representatives is an association of more than 3,300 attorneys and paralegals who represent Social Security and Supplemental Security Income claimants. *Website:* http://www.nosscr.org

Prescription Drug Information:
Advice for the Patient: Drug Information in Lay Language: USP DI, 1998, 18th Edition, Volume 2, written by the U.S. Pharmacopoeia Convention Inc. staff. The U.S. Pharmacopoeia is the world's oldest regularly revised national book on drug preparation and administration, and is generally accepted as being the most influential. Volume II provides information on drug use in layman's language. (United States Pharmacopeial, 1997, ISBN: 1889788015)

Fujisawa Healthcare Inc.
Customer Services: 800-888-7704
Three Parkway North, Deerfield, IL 60015-2548
Prograf Patient Assistance Program: 800-4-PROGRAF (800-477-6472)
c/o Medical Technology Hotlines, P.O. Box 7710, Washington, DC 20044
     Fujisawa Healthcare Inc. is a subsidiary of Fujisawa Pharmaceutical
Company Ltd., based in Osaka, Japan. It is the maker of the
immunosuppressive drug, Prograf. It also has produced a free "Transplant
Information Kit," which includes a video and transplant journal.
Website: http://www.Fujisawausa.com

Novartis Pharmaceutical Corp.
Patient Information: 888-NOW-NOVA (888-669-6682)
59 Route 10, East Hanover, NJ 07936
Novartis Patient Assistance Program: 800-257-3273 or 888-455-6655,
Fax: 908-277-4399
P.O. Box 52052, Phoenix, AZ 85072-0170
     Novartis, the maker of Sandimmune and Neoral, has launched The
"Transplant Learning Center (TLC)." TLC is a free, interactive education
program that provides transplant recipients with personalized feedback and
specific educational materials on such topics as adjusting to changes in your
lifestyle, relationships and personal changes that result from
transplantation. To be eligible, you need to be a recipient of a solid-organ
transplant, 18 years of age or over, and taking Neoral or Sandimmune
therapy. To enroll, call 888-TLCENTER (888-852-3683). Novartis also
offers up-to-date information in the field of transplantation on its website,
called "Transplant Square," at http://www.transplantsquare.com
Website: http://www.pharma.us.novartis.com

PDR.net
Phone: 201-358-7200, Fax: 201-573-8999,
E-mail: customer.service@medec.com
Medical Economics Co. Inc., Five Paragon Drive, Montvale, NJ 07645
     PDR.net is a medical and healthcare website created by Medical
Economics Co. Inc., publisher of healthcare magazines and directories
including the *Physicians' Desk Reference* (PDR); the most trusted source
for reliable, healthcare information used by physicians. This site includes
the PDR drug information, medical dictionary, access to MEDLINE, health
news from Reuters and more. *Website:* http://www.pdr.net

The People's Pharmacy, written by Joe Graedon and Teresa Graedon,
Ph.D., is one of the best reference books available on the subject! This book
covers side effects, interactions, home remedies and more. (St Martins,
1998, ISBN: 0312964161)

Pharmaceutical Research and Manufacturers of America
Phone: 800-762-4636
1100 15th St., N.W., Washington, DC 20005
     The Pharmaceutical Research and Manufacturers of America
membership represents approximately 100 U.S. companies that have a
primary commitment to pharmaceutical research. It publishes "The
Directory of Prescription Drug Patient Assistance Programs," which
describes more than 55 company programs that provide drugs to low-

income patients. This directory is available on its website.
Website: http://www.phrma.org

Roche Pharmaceuticals
Patient Information: 800-526-6367
Medical Needs Program: 800-285-4484
340 Kingsland St., Nutley, NJ 07110-1199
Roche Pharmaceuticals, maker of CellCept and Cytovene, has created the "Transplant Patient Partnering Program," through which transplant patients, both pre- and post-transplant, can receive current, comprehensive information about transplantation. To enroll call 800-893-1995 or visit their website at: http://www.tppp.net. After enrolling, members receive a pre-transplant or post-transplant newsletter depending on their status and can select from among more than 20 components, including books, videos and brochures. *Website:* http://www.rocheusa.com

Mail Order Pharmacies and Drug Assistance Programs:
Chronimed Inc.
Phone: 800-888-5753 or 612-979-3600, Fax: 800-395-3003,
E-mail: hsvendsen@chronimed.com
10900 Red Circle Drive, Minnetonka, Minnesota 55343
Chronimed is a specialty pharmacy that provides medication and support to transplant recipients. The Chronimed Life Management Program for Transplant was developed to increase medication awareness, understanding and adherence for patients as they face the challenges of pre- and post-transplant drug regimens. Chronimed publishes a *Transplant Support Group Directory*, updated annually and organized by state, which includes contact information for more than 350 organizations throughout the country. *Website:* http://www.chronimed.com

Continental Health Care & Lifesource Integrated Services
Phone: 800-776-4633 or 216-475-8008, Fax: 800-333-1277
or 216-475-4706
15673 NEO Parkway, Cleveland, OH 44128
Continental Health Care and Lifesource Integrated Services is a nationwide pharmacy for patients with challenging health conditions and long-term medication needs such as pre- and post-transplantation.

The Medicine Program
Phone: 573-996-7300
P.O. Box 515, Doniphan, MO 63935-0515
The Medicine Program was established as a patient advocate for those who cannot afford their prescription medication. If you do not have insurance or a government program that pays for your outpatient prescription medicines, or if the cost of your medicine causes you financial hardship, free prescription medicine is available to those who qualify.
In addition, the Medicine Program helps to simplify the application process for drug assistance programs now available from pharmaceutical manufacturers. The majority of these manufacturers provide prescription medication free-of-charge to individuals in need, regardless of age, if they meet criteria. *Website:* http://www.themedicineprogram.com

Needy Meds
E-mail: drugmaven@earthlink.net
c/o Libby Overly, P.O. Box 2372, Washington, DC 20013

Many pharmaceutical manufacturers have special programs to assist people who cannot afford the cost of their medications. One problem is that it's often hard to find these programs. Needy Meds is a website that lists more than 900 drugs that are available through these programs. Each drug listed contains a brief synopsis of the programs special requirements, forms and procedures. *Website:* http://www.needymeds.com

Stadtlanders Pharmacy
Phone: 800-238-7828, TDD: 800-336-8675, Fax: 412-824-9002,
E-mail: stadt@stadtlander.com
600 Penn Center Blvd., Pittsburgh, PA 15235-9931

Stadtlanders offers pharmacy management programs that provide medication delivery and compliance, education materials and insurance billing for transplant recipients through their "Best Care" and "On Track" programs. It also publishes *LifeTIMES*, a free magazine published twice a year, dedicated to living well after transplantation. Stadtlanders also has available a free fitness video, called *Stars for Life*, made especially for transplant recipients. It is a low-impact fitness video designed to improve circulation, increase stamina and strengthen muscles.
Website: http://www.stadtlander.com/transplant

The Transplant Pharmacy
A Division of SangStat Medical Corp./The Transplant Co.
Phone: 888-800-7264, Fax: 888-800-8322,
E-mail: customercare@transplantrx.com
945 Hamilton Ave., Menlo Park, CA 94025

SangStat, The Transplant Co., has introduced TransplantRx.com; the first online pharmacy dedicated to organ transplantation. Designed as an extension of SangStat's well-established Transplant Pharmacy, TransplantRx.com provides transplant recipients, their families and healthcare providers with a place to conveniently purchase all of their medications, and access a wealth of information and resources on transplantation online. *Website:* http://www.transplantrx.com

Support Group Information:
American Self-Help Clearinghouse
Phone: 973-625-7101, TTD: 973-625-9053, Fax: 973-625-8848,
Saint Clares Health Services, 25 Pocono Road, Denville, NJ 07834

The American Self-Help Clearinghouse maintains a database of national self-help headquarters, model one-of-a-kind groups and local self-help group clearinghouses worldwide. It also makes referrals to self-help groups nationwide, which in turn can refer people to local groups. It also offers assistance to people interested in starting new groups and publishes a directory of national support groups. *Website:* www.selfhelpgroups.org

COPD-Support Inc.

The Family of COPD Support Programs connects online individuals with chronic obstructive pulmonary disease and their caregivers through electronic mailing lists, newsletters, chatrooms, forums, a Buddy List and a "SmokeNoMore" program. *Website:* http://copd-support.com/index.html

Friends' Health Connection (formerly Long Distance Love)
Phone: 800-483-7436, Fax: 732-249-9897, E-mail: A48friend@aol.com
P.O. Box 114, New Brunswick, NJ 08903

Friends' Health Connection provides one-to-one support for people with health problems and their families. Participants are matched based on age, health problem, personal background, hobbies and interests. People of all ages participate and their health problems range from the most common to very rare disorders. Participants compare experiences, exchange questions and answers and, most importantly, share comfort and encouragement. It also publishes a newsletter twice a year, called *Health Connection. Website:* www.friendshealthconnection.org

MUMS: National Parent-to-Parent Network
Phone: 877-336-5333 (parents only) or 920-336-5333, Fax: 920-339-0995,
E-mail: mums@netnet.net
150 Custer Court, Green Bay, WI 54301-1243

MUMS is a national organization for parents or care providers of a child with any disability, disorder or health condition. MUMS' main purpose is to provide support to parents in the form of a networking system that matches them with other parents whose children have the same or similar condition. *Website:* http://www.netnet.net/mums

National Family Caregivers Association
Phone: 800-896-3650, Fax: 301-942-2302, E-mail: info@nfcacares.org
10400 Connecticut Ave., Suite 500, Kensington, MD 20895-3944

The National Family Caregivers Association provides education and information, support, public awareness and advocacy. It also publishes a quarterly newsletter, called *TAKE CARE!* and *The Resourceful Caregiver: Helping Family Caregivers Help Themselves*, which is a Yellow Pages for caregivers, including more than 500 national resources, hotlines and educational materials. (Mosby Publishing, St. Louis Mo., 1996, ISBN: 0815155565) *Website:* http://www.nfcacares.org

Organ Transplant Support Inc.
Phone: 630-527-8640, Fax: 630-527-8682, E-mail: adie2170@aol.com
P.O. Box 471, Naperville, IL 60566-0471

Organ Transplant Support provides support and comfort to transplant patients and their families by holding support and educational meetings, promoting organ donor awareness and publishing a monthly newsletter, called *The Miracle Messenger.*
Website: http://www.inil.com/users/matt/ots-1.htm

Pets Are Wonderful Support
Phone: 415-241-1460, Fax: 415-252-9471, E-mail: pawssf@dnai.com
3248 16th St., San Francisco, CA 94103

Pets Are Wonderful Support (PAWS) helps improve the quality of life for persons with HIV disease, by offering them emotional and practical support in keeping the love and companionship of their pets, and by providing information on the benefits and risk of animal companionship. It also has several brochures that may be of interest to transplant recipients, on its website including: "Safe Pet Guidelines," "Your Cat and Your Health," "Zoonoses and Your Bird," and "Pets and the Immunocompromised Patient." *Website:* http://www.pawssf.org

The Well Spouse Foundation
Phone: 800-838-0879 or 212-685-8815 (in New York), Fax: 212-685-8676,
E-mail: wellspouse@aol.com
30 E. 40th St. PH, New York, NY 10016
　　The Well Spouse Foundation provides support and information to the
well spouses of the chronically ill. It also educates human service
professionals and the public about the needs of spousal caregivers and their
families. The Foundation publishes a variety of publications, including a
bimonthly newsletter, called *Mainstay,* and has chapters throughout the
country. *Website:* http://www.wellspouse.org

Donor Family Resources:

The Compassionate Friends Inc.
Phone: 630-990-0010, Fax: 630-990-0246,
E-mail: nationaloffice@compassionatefriends.org
P.O. Box 3696, Oak Brook, IL 60522-3696
　　The Compassionate Friends is an international self-help organization
for families who have experienced the death of a child. All parents are
welcome to participate, whatever the age of their child or cause of death.
Participants include families of children who have been organ donors or
recipients. Family members contacting the national office will be sent
general information on bereavement, a national newsletter and a resource
guide. They will also be directed to the closest chapter in their community.
Website: http://www.compassionatefriends.org

Grief Recovery Institute
Phone: 323-650-1234, Fax: 323-656-9248
P.O. Box 461659, Los Angeles, CA 90046-1659
　　The Grief Recovery Institute is an internationally recognized authority
that provides educational programs and counseling services on recovering
from loss. *Website:* http://www.grief-recovery.com:80/index.htm

Growth House Inc.
E-mail: info@growthhouse.org
San Francisco, CA
　　Growth House Inc. is a resource guide to issues on death, dying, grief,
bereavement and end of life. The primary goal is to improve the quality of
compassionate care for people who are dying through public education and
global professional collaboration. *Website:* http://www.growthhouse.org

GROWW Inc.
Phone: 407-865-9249, E-mail: lfl4@att.net
931 N. State Road 434, Suite 1201-358, Altamonte Springs, FL 32714
　　Through its interactive forum on the Internet and its website, GROWW
(Grief Recovery Online founded by Widows and Widowers) exists to
inform, educate and support those who have lost loved ones. It has
numerous message boards, resource listings and chatrooms for those who
are bereaved. "Sharing Angels" is a special chatroom for organ donor
families. *Website:* http://www.groww.org

The National Donor Family Council
Phone: 800-622-9010 or 212-889-2210, Fax: 212-689-9261,
E-mail: info@kidney.org

c/o National Kidney Foundation (NKF), 30 E. 33rd St., Suite 1100, New York, NY 10016

The National Donor Family Council was started by donor families through the NKF programs based on the needs of donor families. It organizes donor family events, celebrations and support groups. It publishes a quarterly newsletter called, *For Those Who Give and Grieve*. It also has produced the following publications: *Understanding Brain Death*, *For Those Who Give and Grieve*, *National Communication Guidelines*, *Family Bill of Rights*, *The Legacy Continues* public education packet, and a library of bereavement resources.

It also maintains the "Patches of Love/National Donor Family Quilt," which travels the country to promote organ and tissue donor awareness. Donor families are encouraged to submit a square to the quilt, as long as it meets specifications. Most recently, it has created the "National Kid's Quilt" for children who have suffered the loss of a parent, sibling, grandparent or significant other. Anyone 18 years of age or younger may submit a quilt square. The National Donor Family Council holds Internet chat connecting donor families from all over the United States in a nationwide support group. Chats are held each Tuesday, from 9 to 10 p.m. EST. *Website:* http://www.kidney.org/recips/donor

Pediatric Resources:

Maxishare
Phone: 800-444-7747 or 414-266-3428, Fax: 414-266-3443
P.O. Box 2041, Milwaukee, WI 53201

Maxishare, one of the nation's leading providers of pediatric educational materials, offers a wide variety of helpful and informative brochures, videos and manuals for patients and their families, as well as training tools for health care professionals on pediatric health. Each year, Maxishare also offers conferences for those involved in the care of children. *Website:* http://maxishare.chw.org

The following resources are available from Maxishare:

Chest Physiotherapy - Infant & School Age Children: Developed as an educational and training tool for patients and their families, this 16-minute video explains chest anatomy and treatment protocols.

Metered Dose Inhaler with Holding Chamber: A Caring for Kids Video: This 10-minute video covers the use of the inhaler in a step-by-step manner, illustrated by a variety of children of different age groups. Instructions for maintaining the inhaler and monitoring the amount of medication in the inhaler are included.

Play & Your Immobilized Child: When a child requires bed rest and/or immobilization, this brochure is full of helpful hints for parents and other caregivers. It includes tips for playtime, activities to help children express and deal with feelings, and activities to help them continue to grow physically, socially and intellectually despite current physical limitations.

Smoke and How It Affects the Health Of Your Child: This brochure informs parents and caregivers about the harmful effects smoke has on the health of their child, including putting them at potentially higher risk for respiratory infections, chronic coughs and middle-ear infections. It encourages parents to eliminate any kind of smoking, including cigar and pipe smoking, around children, and make their home smoke-free.

Susan's First Surgery. This 11-minute video is ideal for teaching young patients all about surgery.

So Your Child is Going to Have Surgery. This explanation of preoperative procedures and the surgical experience makes a great "take home" piece for parents and children.

Kids and Transplant Coloring Book, written and illustrated by Ann C. Troka, a kidney recipient, is for children with organ transplants, children with family members or friends who have transplants and for other children to learn what it is like to live with a transplanted organ.

World Children's Transplant Fund
Phone: 818-905-9283, Fax: 818-905-9315
16000 Ventura Blvd., Suite 103, Encino, CA 91436
The World Children's Transplant Fund (WCTF) is dedicated to providing financial and emotional support to children and their families of the world needing organ transplants. Founded in memory of Veronica Arguello of Argentina, the WCTF has a program to build a "Veronica's House" within walking distance at all transplant centers. In addition, WCTF is dedicated to developing organ transplant centers in regions of the world where resources are scarce and transplants are most needed. WCTF helps supply the teaching, training and technology necessary to establish pediatric organ transplantation capabilities in international communities that lack these essential services. *Website:* http://www.wctf.org

Professional Organizations:
American Association of Respiratory Care
Phone: 972-243-2772, Fax: 972-484-2720, E-mail: info@aarc.org
11030 Ables Lane, Dallas, TX 75229
The American Association for Respiratory Care (AARC) is the professional organization for respiratory care practitioners. The AARC encourages professional excellence in respiratory care by advancing educational preparation and continued learning, fostering research and scientific inquiry, and exploring innovative technologies for clinical application. AARC also publishes a journal called *Respiratory Care*, featuring the foremost scientific journal in the respiratory care profession. *Website:* http://www.aarc.org

American Society of Transplantation
Phone: 856-608-1104, Fax: 856-608-1103, E-mail: ast@ahint.com
236 Route 38 W., Suite 100, Moorestown, NJ 08057
The American Society of Transplantation is a multidisciplinary group of physicians and scientists dedicated to the promotion of education and research relating to transplantation medicine and immunology. The ASTP's goal is to effect efficient transfer of information from the basic science laboratory to transplantation clinics and ultimately, to improve patient care and outcomes. It also provides current information on legislative issues and patient information on their website. It publishes the scientific journal, *Transplantation. Website:* http://www.astp.org

American Society of Transplant Surgeons
Phone: 202-416-1858, Fax: 202-416-1744
2000 L St., N.W., Suite 200, Washington, DC 20036
   The American Society of Transplant Surgeons is the professional organization for transplant surgeons and physicians designed to provide the most up-to-date information in the field of transplantation. To find out what's new in the field of transplantation, you can look up the papers presented at its annual scientific conference on their website.
Website: http://www.asts.org/index.htm

American Thoracic Society
Phone: 212-315-8700, Fax: 212-315-6498
1740 Broadway, New York, NY 10019
   The American Thoracic Society is an international professional and scientific society, which focuses on respiratory and critical care medicine. Its most notable activity is the planning and production of an international scientific conference. It publishes two highly respected journals, *The American Journal of Respiratory and Critical Care Medicine* and *The American Journal of Respiratory Cell and Molecular Biology*, both of which are available through your local medical library or you can log on at http://www.atsjournals.org to obtain articles.
Website: http://www.thoracic.org

Association of Organ Procurement Organizations
Phone: 703-573-AOPO (703-573-2676), Fax: 703-573-0578
One Cambridge Court, 8110 Gatehouse Road, Suite 101 W.,
Falls Church, VA 22042
   The Association of Organ Procurement Organizations (AOPO) is the professional organization that represents and serves organ procurement organizations through advocacy, support and development of activities that will maximize the availability of organs and tissues and enhance the quality, effectiveness and integrity of the donation process. AOPO also administers the federal accreditation process for OPOs and generates statistical reports with information on trends in donation, organ acquisition costs and personnel. *Website:* http://www.aopo.org

International Society for Heart and Lung Transplantation
Phone: 972-490-9495, Fax: 972-490-9499, E-mail: ishlt@ishlt.org
14673 Midway Road, Suite 200, Addison, TX 75001
   The International Society for Heart and Lung Transplantation is dedicated to the advancement of the science and treatment of end-stage heart and lung diseases. The society encourages basic and clinical research in the fields of heart and lung transplantation, promotes new therapeutic strategies, holds scientific meetings, sponsors a scientific journal, *The Journal of Heart and Lung Transplantation*, and maintains an international registry for heart and lung transplantation. *Website:* http://www.ishlt.org

International Transplant Nurses Society
Phone: 412-488-0240, Fax: 412-431-5911, E-mail: itns@msn.com
1739 E. Carson St., P.O. Box 351, Pittsburgh, PA 15203-1700
   Organized in 1992, the International Transplant Nurses Society was created based on a need for specifically designed training and education for nurses in the field of transplantation. *Website:* http://www.itns.org

North American Transplant Coordinators Organization
Phone: 913-492-3600, Fax: 913-541-0156
P.O. Box 15384, Lenexa, KS 66285-5384

The North American Transplant Coordinators Organization is the professional society of more than 1,750 transplant coordinators. Its mission is to provide support, develop and advance the knowledge of its members and to influence the effectiveness, quality and integrity of donation and transplantation. *Website:* http://www.natco1.org

Society of Thoracic Surgeons
Phone: 312-644-6610, Fax: 312-527-6635, E-mail: sts@sba.com
401 N. Michigan Ave., Chicago, IL 60611-4267

The Society of Thoracic Surgeons (STS) is the largest thoracic surgical organization in the world; its members include a significant majority of all board-certified thoracic surgeons in the United States and Canada. It publishes patient information on its website and its journal, *Annals of Thoracic Surgery. Website:* http://www.sts.org

Transplantation Society
Phone: 514-874-1998, Fax: 514-874-1580,
E-mail: info@transplantation-soc.org
Central Business Office, 205 Viger Ave. W., Suite 201,
Montréal (QC), Canada H2Z 1G2

The Transplantation Society serves as the principal international forum for the advancement of both basic and clinical transplantation science throughout the world. Biennial international congresses are sponsored by the society, and the official journal of the society is *Transplantation. Website:* http://www.transplantjournal.com

Government Agencies:

Centers for Disease Control and Prevention
Public Inquiries: 800-311-3435 or 404-639-3534
Phone: 404-639-3311
U.S. Department of Health and Human Services
1600 Clifton Road, Atlanta, GA 30333

The Centers for Disease Control and Prevention (CDC) is an agency of the Department of Health and Human Services. Its mission is to promote health and quality of life by preventing and controlling disease, injury and disability. The CDC includes 11 centers, institutes and offices including the Office of Health and Safety, the National Center for Chronic Disease Prevention and Health Promotion, the National Center for Environmental Health, the National Center for Health Statistics, the National Center for Infectious Diseases, among others. The CDC provides information fact sheets on disease prevention and health information from A to Z. You can also get information on the disease situation in any country you wish to travel to and the recommended shots. *Website:* http://www.cdc.gov

Division of Allergy, Immunology and Transplantation
Phone: 301-496-1886, Fax: 301-402-0175
National Institute of Allergy and Infectious Diseases
National Institutes of Health, Bethesda, MD 20892-2520

The Division of Allergy, Immunology and Transplantation supports basic and clinical research to enhance the understanding of the causes and mechanisms that lead to the development of immunologic diseases and to generate an expanded knowledge base that can be applied to the development of improved measures of diagnosis, treatment and prevention. The division supports a broad array of investigator-initiated studies as well as specific research programs including cooperative research centers in asthma, allergic and immunologic diseases; multidisciplinary program projects in autoimmunity, transplantation immunology, etc.; and cooperative multicenter clinical trials in asthma and kidney transplantation. *Website:* http://www.niaid.nih.gov/research/dait.htm

Division of Transplantation
Phone: 301-443-7577
Office of Special Programs, Health Resources and Services Administration, Department of Health and Human Services
5600 Fishers Lane, Room 7C-22, Parklawn Building, Rockville, MD 20857
      The principal responsibilities of the Division of Transplantation includes federal oversight of the Organ Procurement and Transplantation Network, the Scientific Registry of Transplant Recipients and the National Marrow Donor Program contracts; national coordination of organ donation activities, the funding of grants and special initiatives to learn more about what works to increase donation; and technical assistance to Organ Procurement Organizations and other transplant-related entities.
Website: http://www.hrsa.dhhs.gov/osp/dot

Food and Drug Administration
Phone: 888-INFO-FDA (888-463-6332), E-mail: webmail@oc.fda.gov
Public Health Service, Department of Health and Human Services
HFI-40, Rockville, MD 20857
      The Food and Drug Administration (FDA) is one of the nation's oldest consumer protection agencies. FDA is the agency charged with protecting American consumers by enforcing the Federal Food, Drug and Cosmetic Act. The FDA protects consumers by assessing the risks of prescription and over-the-counter drugs and medical devices. The FDA also checks the safety of foods, sets labeling standards and monitors the nation's blood supply. *Website:* http://www.fda.gov/fdahomepage.html

Immune Tolerance Network
Phone: 773-834-4535, Fax: 773-834-4640,
E-mail: info@immunetolerance.org
5743 S. Drexel Ave., Suite 200, Chicago, IL 60637
      The Immune Tolerance Network (ITN) is a group of scientists and clinicians whose goal is the advancement of clinical tolerance induction in a variety of diseases including: kidney and islet transplantation, autoimmune disease, and allergy and asthma. The ITN is funded by a number of cooperating government and not-for-profit organizations, including the National Institute for Allergy and Infectious Diseases and the National Institute for Diabetes and Digestive and Kidney Diseases. At present more than 70 of the world's top immune tolerance researchers from the United States, Canada, Britain, France and other countries, are united in this endeavor. The ITN will partner with both academic and industrial concerns in an effort to seek out and fund outstanding clinical research, clinical trials and the development of tolerance substances in targeted diseases.
Website: http://paramount.bsd.uchicago.edu/frameset.html

National Center for Complementary and Alternative Medicine
Phone: 888-NIH-6226 (888-644-6226) TTY/TDY, Fax: 301-495-4957
National Institutes of Health, P.O. Box 8218, Silver Springs,
MD 20907-8218

National Center for Complementary and Alternative Medicine conducts and supports basic and applied research and training, and disseminates information on complementary and alternative medicine to practitioners and the public. It also publishes a newsletter, called *Complementary & Alternative Medicine*. *Website:* http://nccam.nih.gov

National Health Information Center
Phone: 800-336-4797 or 301-565-4167 (in Maryland), Fax: 301-984-4256
Department of Health and Human Services
P.O. Box 1133, Washington, DC 20013-1133

The National Health Information Center (NHIC) is a health information referral service. NHIC puts health professionals and consumers who have health questions in touch with those organizations that are best able to provide answers. NHIC was established in 1979 by the Office of Disease Prevention and Health Promotion.
Website: http://nhic-nt.health.org

National Heart, Lung and Blood Institute
Phone: 800-575-WELL (800-575-9355) or 301-592-8573 (in Maryland),
E-mail: NHLBIinfo@rover.nhlbi.nih.gov
National Institutes of Health, 31 Center Drive, MSC 2486, Building 31,
Room 5A52, Bethesda, MD 20892-2486

The National Heart, Lung and Blood Institute plans, conducts, fosters and supports an integrated and coordinated program of basic research, clinical investigations and trials for the prevention, diagnosis and treatment of heart, blood vessel, lung, blood diseases and sleep disorders.
Website: http://www.nhlbi.nih.gov/index.htm

National Institutes of Health
Phone: 301-496-4000
Public Health Service, Department of Health and Human Services,
Bethesda, MD 20892

Consisting of 25 separate institutes, the National Institutes of Health (NIH) is one of the world's foremost biomedical research centers. The NIH conducts research in its own laboratories; supports the research of nonfederal scientists throughout the country and abroad; helps in the training of research investigators; and fosters communication of biomedical information. *Website:* http://www.nih.gov/index.html

The National Institute of Mental Health
Public Inquiries: 800-421-4211 or 301-443-4513 (in Maryland),
Fax: 301-443-4279, E-mail: nimhinfo@nih.gov
National Institutes of Health, 6001 Executive Blvd., Room 8184, MSC
9663, Bethesda, MD 20892-9663

The National Institute of Mental Health supports research nationwide on mental illness and mental health. The institute's Information Resources and Inquiries Branch responds to information requests from the public with a variety of publications and materials, such as the Depression/Awareness and Panic Disorder Education Program. *Website:* http://www.nimh.nih.gov

National Institute of Neurological Disorders and Stroke
Phone: 800-338-7657 or 301-496-6308
National Institutes of Health, Bethesda, MD 20892

The National Institute of Neurological Disorders and Stroke conducts, fosters, coordinates and guides research on the causes, prevention, diagnosis and treatment of neurological disorders and stroke. It also supports basic research in related areas. *Website:* http://www.ninds.nih.gov

National Library of Medicine
Phone: 888-FIND-NLM (888-346-3656) or 301-594-5983,
E-mail: custserv@nlm.nih.gov
National Institutes of Health, 8600 Rockville Pike, Bethesda, MD 20894

The National Library of Medicine (NLM), a part of the National Institutes of Health, is the world's largest medical library. Its collection of more than 5 million medical books, journals, pamphlets, and other items has been called the "Fort Knox of Health Information." The library also operates a computerized index, among others, known as MEDLINE, which you can access through medical libraries, universities and major hospitals in your area. Users can search by author, subject or title. If there isn't a medical library nearby, you can access MEDLINE through the NLM's website, called "PubMed," on the World Wide Web. For more information, call 800-638-8480. Reference services available.

The National Library of Medicine has also established "MEDLINEplus." Unlike MEDLINE, which is designed for scientists and health professionals, MEDLINEplus is designed for consumers. This new service provides access to extensive information about specific diseases and conditions and also has links to consumer health information from the National Institutes of Health, clearinghouses, dictionaries, lists of hospitals and physicians, health information in Spanish and other languages and clinical trials. *Website:* http://www.nlm.nih.gov

National Organ and Tissue Donation Initiative
Phone: 301-443-7577, Fax: 301-594-6095
Division of Transplantation, Health Resources and Services Administration, Department of Health and Human Services, 5600 Fishers Lane, Room 4-81, Rockville, MD 20857

The National Organ and Tissue Donation Initiative was created in 1997 to reduce the number of Americans who die each year while waiting for an organ transplant. The initiative brings together dozens of partner groups, along with the nation's OPOs and the Coalition on Donation. The campaign emphasizes the need to inform family and others about one's decision to be a donor. *Website:* http://www.organdonor.gov/initiative

Organ and Tissue Transplant Research Center
Phone: 800-441-1222 or 301-496-0670
National Institutes of Diabetes, Digestive and Kidney Disease,
National Institutes of Health, Bethesda, MD 20892

The Organ and Tissue Transplant Research Center provides a site for the development of new and promising therapies in human kidney, pancreas and pancreatic islet transplantation. The center includes a state of the art clinical transplant ward, operating facility and outpatient clinic designed for the study of new drugs or techniques that may improve the success of organ and tissue transplants. *Website:* http://www.niddk.nih.gov

Related Organizations:

Alpha 1 Association
Phone: 800-521-3025 or 952-703-9979, Fax: 952-703-9977,
E-mail: A1NA@alpha1.org
8120 Penn Ave. S., Suite 549 Minneapolis MN 55431-1326
   The Alpha 1 Association is dedicated to improving lives affected by
alpha-₁ antitrypsin deficiency through support, education, advocacy and
research. It publishes a newsletter called *Alpha 1 News*.
Website: http://www.alpha1.org

American Lung Association
Phone: 800-LUNG-USA (to connect to your local office)
National Office: 212-315-8700, E-mail: info@lungusa.org
1740 Broadway, New York, NY 10019
   The American Lung Association (ALA) offers information on lung
disease, such as asthma, emphysema and chronic bronchitis. Callers can
receive brochures on various forms of lung disease, as well as a list of
transplant centers throughout the country. The association also offers
"Better Breathers" clubs for people affected with lung disease.
   Every local ALA provides programs for asthma and smoking cessation
and offers a wide variety of information on allergies, lung cancers,
emphysema, pneumonia, tuberculosis and other types of lung disease.
Website: http://www.lungusa.org

CysticFibrosis.com
Fax: 973-237-0968, E-mail: jlb@medrise.com
190 Park Lane, Wayne NJ 07470
   CysticFibrosis.com is an online support network for adults with cystic
fibrosis. It offers education, research and the latest news on drugs and
treatment, plus online symposia, forums, support groups and chats. It
publishes a quarterly newsletter, called *CF Roundtable*.
Website: http://www.cysticfibrosis.com

Cystic Fibrosis Foundation
Phone: 800-Fight CF (800-344-4823) or 301-951-4422 (in Maryland),
Fax: 301-951-6378, E-mail: info@cff.org
6931 Arlington Road, Bethesda, MD 20814
   The Cystic Fibrosis Foundation supports a mail-order pharmacy, home
infusion services and a nationwide network of specialized care centers for
people with cystic fibrosis. Resources include fact sheets, videotapes and
HomeLines and *Commitment* newsletters. *Website:* http://www.cff.org

Cystic Fibrosis Network Inc.
E-mail: cfnetwork@juno.com
P.O. Box 1179, Broomfield, CO 80038-1179
   The Cystic Fibrosis Network is an organization operated by and for
adults with cystic fibrosis within the United States. It publishes a quarterly
newsletter called *Network* and operates a pen pal exchange.

Dailylung.com
   Dailylung.com is an online magazine covering lung disease and related
topics, such as lung transplantation. It also has an archive of journal articles
and a message board for viewers. *Website:* http://www.dailylung.com

LAM Foundation
Phone: 513-777-6889, Fax: 513-777-4109, E-mail: lam@one.net
10105 Beacon Hills Drive, Cincinnati, OH 45241

The LAM Foundation provides information, education and support; raises an awareness of lymphangioleiomyomatosis (LAM) in the medical and lay communities; sponsors conferences and a national database; provides funding of basic and clinical research. It also publishes two newsletters, *The Breath of Hope* and *Journeys*. *Website:* http://lam.uc.edu

National Emphysema Foundation
Fax: 203-854-9191, E-mail: gary@emphysemafoundation.org
Sreedhar Nair-MD, 15 Stevens St., Norwalk, CT 06856

The National Emphysema Foundation works to improve the quality of life of those with emphysema, asthma and related diseases, through education and research. It also funds and supports educational conferences and seminars. *Website:* http://emphysemafoundation.org

National Jewish Medical and Research Center
Phone: 800-222-LUNG (800-222-5864) or 303-388-4461
1400 Jackson St., Denver, CO 80206

The National Jewish Center for Immunology and Respiratory Medicine is a nonsectarian medical research center. The center provides patient care, research and medical education for chronic lung, allergic and immunologic diseases such as asthma, emphysema, chronic bronchitis, tuberculosis, among others. To listen to taped health information 24 hours a day, seven days a week, call 800-552-LUNG (800-552-5864) for Lung Facts, which is an automated information service with recorded health messages on lung, allergic and immune diseases. *Website:* www.nationaljewish.org

Primary Pulmonary Hypertension Cure Foundation
Phone: 202-518-5477, Fax: 202-518-8200,
E-mail: webmaster@pphcure.org
1826 R St., N.W., Washington, DC 20009

The Primary Pulmonary Hypertension Cure Foundation's primary goal is to find a cure for primary pulmonary hypertension by raising funds for research. The Foundation also supports a new collective group, called the International Pulmonary Hypertension Research Consortium (IPHRC). The purpose of the IPHRC is to develop an international database of diagnostic data on PPH patients, including tissue, fluid and DNA samples. *Website:* http://www.pphcure.org

Pulmonary Hypertension Central
E-mail: info@PHCentral.org
P.O. Box 1155, North Wales, PA 19454

Pulmonary Hypertension Central is an Internet resource for pulmonary hypertension information for patients, caregivers and medical professionals. This site includes a wealth of medical and financial information on pulmonary hypertension, in addition to E-mail lists, Q&A, polls and real-time chats. *Website:* http://www.PHCentral.org

Sarcoidosis Research Institute
Phone: 901-766-6951, Fax: 901-774-7294
3475 Central Ave., Memphis, TN 38111

The Sarcoidosis Research Institute provides support for individuals afflicted with the disease by disseminating information to professionals and patients, and obtaining and dispersing funds for research. *Website:* http://www.netten.net/~soskelnt/sripage.htm

Periodicals:

Breathe Well Magazine
Phone: 800-273-8985
P.O. Box 1165, West Caldwell, NJ 07006

Breathe Well Magazine, published quarterly by Boehringer Ingelheim Pharmaceuticals Inc., is a free publication that has a lot of useful information regarding pulmonary medicine.

Procure!
Phone: 312-360-9540, Fax: 312-360-9543, E-mail: wmarketing@aol.com
Witherspoon Marketing Group, Multicultural Organ Donor Programs and Publications, 601 S. LaSalle, Suite 640, Chicago, IL 60605

Procure! is a monthly newsletter that focuses on successful communication strategies for minority organ donation.

The Pulmonary Paper
Phone: 800-950-3698, Fax: 904-673-7501, E-mail: belyea@aol.com
P.O. Box 877, Ormond Beach, FL 32175

The Pulmonary Paper is a newsletter, published eight times a year, for those with respiratory problems. *Website:* http://www.pulmonarypaper.org

Transplant News
Phone: 800-689-4262 or 559-435-8098, E-mail: trannews@aol.com
Transplant Communications Inc., 1319 W. Bullard, Suite Three, Fresno, CA 93711

Transplant News, published twice monthly by Transplant Communications Inc., is an industry newsletter which offers in-depth coverage on the latest issues of interest to patients and transplant professionals. They also publish an annual *International Transplant Directory*. *Website:* http://www.trannews.com

Videos:

Advice from the Transplant Games' Athletes
Phone: 314-481-8415, E-mail: ronpete@ronpeterson.org
c/o Ron Peterson, 5353 Walsh St., Apartment 1B, St. Louis, MO 63109

Advice from the Transplant Games' Athletes is produced by Ron Peterson who traveled to the 1998 Transplant Games and videotaped advice designed to help others with lung disease. Athletes discuss topics they found to be important in maintaining their health. Joel Cooper, M.D., the father of lung transplantation, gives an introduction. Length, 33 minutes. *Website:* http://www.geocities.com/hotsprings/spa/7154

Chairobics Video Exercise Program
Phone: 800-521-7303
Chairobics, 2611 W. Fanbrook, Tucson, AZ 85741

Chairobics Video Exercise Program, created by Cheryl Spessert, a respiratory nurse, is a two-hour video of education, pulmonary rehabilitation and exercises designed for individuals with moderate to severe lung disease. It can serve as an alternative to traditional pulmonary rehabilitation for pulmonary patients who are unable to take advantage of a hospital-based program.

The Heart of a Child

Phone: 610-544-4140, E-mail: gleasonjim@aol.com
c/o TRIO Philadelphia, 407 N. Swarthmore Ave., Swarthmore, PA 19081

The Heart of a Child tells the story of the short, but inspirational, life of Amy Rose LaBarbiere, a heart-lung transplant recipient, originally broadcast by HBO. Amy undergoes a heart-lung transplant twice, and the story follows this experience with all the joys and sorrows that accompany it. There is some footage of the actual surgery that may be difficult for some viewers. Length, 60 minutes.

Maintaining Your Health with Lung Disease

Phone: 314-481-8415, E-mail: ronpete@ronpeterson.org
c/o Ron Peterson, 5353 Walsh St., Apartment 1B, St. Louis, MO 63109

Maintaining Your Health with Lung Disease, produced by Ron Peterson who was diagnosed with emphysema 11 years ago, contains advice from 18 individuals who have lung disease. Among the topics discussed are exercise, pulmonary rehabilitation, nutrition and proper breathing techniques. Thomas Petty, M.D., an internationally acclaimed expert on pulmonary rehabilitation, gives an introduction. Length, 117 minutes. *Website:* http://www.geocities.com/hotsprings/spa/7154

Patches of Love: The National Donor Family Quilt

Phone: 800-622-9010 or 212-889-2210, Fax: 212-689-9261
National Donor Family Council, c/o National Kidney Foundation, 30 E. 33rd St., New York, NY 10016

Patches of Love: The National Donor Family Quilt tells the story of the making of the quilt. Donor families share their precious memories about their loved ones and about making their squares. Three recipients, whose lives have been forever changed by the gift of donation, express their gratitude. Length, 8 minutes. *Website:* http://www.kidney.org

Receiving and Donating Organs

Phone: 800-257-5126, E-mail: custserv@films.com
c/o Films for Humanities and Sciences, Box 2053, Princeton NJ, 08543

The Doctor Is In: Receiving and Donating Organs examines how the organ transplant system works, for both donors and recipients. Viewers get to follow patients through a cornea and kidney transplant. Length, 28 minutes. *Website:* http://www.film.com

Sit and Be Fit

Phone: 800-950-3698, Fax: 904-673-7501, E-mail: belyea@aol.com
c/o The Pulmonary Paper, P.O. Box 877, Ormond Beach, FL 32175

Sit and Be Fit is a videotaped exercise program for people with COPD. Length, 23 minutes. *Website:* http://www.pulmonarypaper.org

Transplant Video Journal

Phone: 973-316-8800, Fax: 973-515-3434, E-mail: transvidjr@aol.com
c/o TransCom Media, 119 Cherry Hill Road, Parsippany, NJ, 07054

Transplant Video Journal is a video newsmagazine that reports and interprets developments and trends in the field of transplantation. It is distributed free on a quarterly basis to physicians, transplant centers, organ procurement organizations, patient support groups, managed care organizations and other interested professionals. Length, 30 minutes.

Books About Transplantation:

Defying the Gods: Inside the New Frontier of Organ Transplants, written by Scott McCartney, a Wall Street journalist, explores the world of organ transplant surgery, focusing on four Baylor University Medical Center patients, in an examination of the science and ethics of transplants. (Macmillan Publishing Co., Old Tappan, NJ, 1994, ISBN: 0025828207)

The Ethics of Organ Transplants: The Current Debate, edited by Arthur L. Caplan and Daniel H. Coelho, contains more than 30 of the most important, influential and up-to-date articles from leaders in ethics, medicine, sociology, law and politics. This book examines the numerous and tangled issues that surround organ procurement and distribution including the search for new sources of organs, new methods of procurement, new ways of managing the dying and innovative strategies for fairly distributing this scarce lifesaving resource. (Prometheus Books, 1999, ISBN: 1573922242)

Introduction to Organ Transplantation, edited by Nadey Hakim, M.D., provides an excellent overview of the tremendous progress made in recent decades in transplantation, and gives a clear description of the current status of transplant surgery for students and trainees with an interest in the field. It opens with introductory chapters on the history of transplantation and the basic science of immuno-biology, and then examines the practice of transplantation in each major system, from skin to intestine. (World Scientific Publishing, 1997, ISBN: 1860940250)

Manual of Lung Transplant Medical Care, written by the University of Minnesota Physicians Transplant Center and Fairview Health Services, is a guide for all referring and primary care physicians. It outlines optimal procedures to follow in the care of lung transplant recipients from the first referral through the rest of the recipient's life. (Fairview Press, 1999; ISBN: 1577490924)

Many Sleepless Nights, written by Lee Gutkind, is the story of transplantation as told by surgeons, candidates, recipients and others associated with the University of Pittsburgh School of Medicine. Through the use of personal accounts, this book leads the reader through the transplant process from the time of donation, through to life as an organ recipient. (University of Pittsburgh Press, 1990, ISBN: 0822959054)

Organ Transplantation: Meanings and Realities, edited by Stuart Youngner, Renee Fox and Laurence O'Connell, is a collection of essays by artists, historians and experts in other fields who were brought together by the Park Ridge Center for the Study of Health, Faith and Ethics in Chicago. These essays explore the mythology, the cultural and psychological meanings of transplantation, as well as the reasons that many people do not donate. (University of Wisconsin Press, 1996, ISBN: 0299149609)

Organ Transplants, A Patient's Guide, written by The Massachusetts General Hospital Organ Transplant Team and H.F. Pizer, is a guide to kidney, heart, heart-lung, lung, liver, pancreas and bone marrow transplants. Topics include locating organs, what happens during surgery, anti-rejection drugs and the emotional difficulties and recovery. (Harvard University Press, 1991, ISBN: 067464235X)

Organ Transplants: Making the Most of Your Gift of Life, written by Robert Finn who has interviewed patients, family members and transplant activists to give the latest facts about transplantation, as well as the stories behind them. Topics include: choosing a transplant team; anti-rejection drugs and specific situations such as living donors and transplants in children. (O'Reilly & Associates, 2000; ISBN: 156592634X)

Procuring Organs for Transplant: The Debate Over NonHeart-Beating Cadaver Protocols, edited by Robert M. Arnold, M.D. et al, explores the issues surrounding the procurement of organs for transplantation from nonheart-beating cadaver donors or from patients who have been declared dead by cardiopulmonary criteria rather than neurological criteria. (Johns Hopkins University Press, 1995; ISBN: 0801851009)

The Puzzle People: Memoirs of a Transplant Surgeon, written by Thomas E. Starzl, M.D., one of the pioneers of transplantation, documents both his life and the history of transplantation. Dr. Starzl also uses the book as a vehicle for stating his positions on many hotly debated issues, including the costs of transplant operations and the system for selecting organ recipients. (University of Pittsburgh Press, 1992, ISBN: 3714X)

Spare Parts: Organ Replacement in American Society, by Renee C. Fox and Judith B. Swazey, is a critical overview of the expansion organ transplantation has undergone since the 1970s and '80s and the ethical implications of this process. (Oxford University Press, 1992, ISBN: 0195076508)

Thoracic Transplantation, by Sara Shumway, M.D., covers the various aspects of transplantation of the heart, combined heart-lung and lung. Topics include the historical background and immunological basis of transplantation, organ preservation, donor procurement, operative techniques, postoperative care and future prospects. (Blackwell Science, 1995, ISBN: 0865422850)

Transplant: A Heart Surgeon's Account of Life-And-Death: Dilemmas of the New Medicine is written by William A. Frist, M.D., the former director of the Heart and Heart-Lung Transplant Program at Vanderbilt University Medical Center. This book provides a first-hand account of the day-to-day decisions and excitement of working on a transplant team. (Ballantine Fawcett, 1990, ISBN: 0449219054)

Trends in Organ Transplantation, written by Barbara A. H. Williams, R.N., B.S.N., and Doris M. Sandiford-Guttenbeil, R.N., B.S.N., provides information on the latest trends in the field, with an emphasis on the nursing role. Topics include the economics of transplantation; new immunosuppressive therapies; women's issues, such as pregnancy after receiving a new organ; and the experimental use of animal organs. (Springer Publishing, 1996, ISBN: 0826191509)

We Have A Donor: The Bold New World of Organ Transplantation, written by Mark Dowie, gives a behind the scenes look at the science of organ transplantation. It touches on many of the ethical issues surrounding transplantation and gives a glimpse of the human drama that is an intrinsic part of the process. (St. Martin's Press, 1994, ISBN: 0312023162)

Books About Personal Experiences:

A Change of Heart: A Memoir, written by Claire Sylvia with William Novak, is the story of one woman's life before and after her heart-lung transplant. It explores changes she experienced after having someone else's organs put inside her, including personality changes and food cravings. (Little, Brown & Co., 1997, ISBN: 0316821497)

A Gift from the Heart: A Sharing of One Man's Heart Transplant Experience, written by Jim Gleason, is about his experience with heart transplantation. It is available by contacting Jim Gleason c/o 3 Dana Drive, Collegeville, PA 19426 or call 215-986-5589 (daytime) or 610-933-7326 (evenings), or E-mail: JGLEA90698@aol.com. You can read it online at http://www.transweb.org/people/recips/experien/gleason/t_o_c.html

A Gift of Life: A Page from the Life of a Living Organ Donor, written by Lynn Cabot-Long, with Paul Jenkins as editor, is the extraordinary story of an ordinary family caught in a life-or-death struggle to save one of their own. This book has become a great resource for those families considering organ donation and those who have already donated. (JE-Lynn Publications, 1996; ISBN: 0965055558)

Dying for Life: The Journey to Transplant, written by John L. Landers, is a recipient's account of his highly personal, somewhat painful, and ultimately successful road to heart transplantation. To see a sample chapter, check out this website: http://www.transweb.org/reference/books/landers/landers5.html. To order a copy of the book, contact Distinctive Publishing Corp., P.O. Box 17868, Plantation, FL 33318-7868 or call 602-820-2806. (Distinctive Publishing Corp., 1994; ISBN: 0942963393)

Extraordinary Times, written by Sharon Torres, is a frank description of the author's experiences before and after liver transplantation. She wrote it for people who are facing transplantation and as a way to teach the general public something about transplant issues. To order a copy, contact Sharon Torres, P.O. Box 5428, San Mateo, CA 94402 or call 650-574-7740 or E-mail: bestco@pacbell.net.

Future Conditional: My Heart/Lung Transplant was written by Jo Hatton, one of the world's longest surviving heart-lung transplant recipients. In this book she describes her life and the effect her condition and her transplant had on its direction. The book is available from the publishers or from the Transplant Support Network at The Temple Row Centre, 23 Temple Row, Keighley, BD21 2AH, England or E-mail: ian.daley@geo2.poptel.org.uk. (Yorkshire Art Circus, 1996; IBSN: 1898311161)

I'm Glad You're Not Dead: A Liver Transplant Story, written by Elizabeth Parr, Ph.D., is the story about her liver transplant from her diagnosis to her transplant and recovery. (Journey Publishing, 1996, ISBN: 0965472809)

I'm Glad You're Not Dead: A Liver Transplant Story (2nd Edition), written by Elizabeth Parr, Ph.D., has an expanded glossary, an update on organ allocation and various changes throughout the text. This book is a handy way to educate worried friends and relatives about the process of transplantation. (Journey Publishing, 2000, ISBN: 0965472817)

It Gets Dark Sometimes: My Sister's Fight to Live and Save Lives, by Pulitzer Prize-winning author Jeffery Marx, is about his sister Wendy's liver transplant. This book is filled with both triumph and tragedy and is about the love of family and the power and beauty of the human spirit. For more information go to http://www.transplantbook.com or contact the Wendy Marx Foundation for Organ Donor Awareness at 202-546-7270, 322 South Carolina Ave., S.E., Suite 201, Washington, DC 20003.

I've Been Transplanted, written by Eugene Sisco, is an informative yet lighthearted look at the organ transplantation process. It is a book that the entire family can share and learn from. (PPI Publishing, 1995, ISBN: 1575150786)

The Job Club: A Guide to Job Search, Interviewing, Resumes and Cover Letters for Transplant & Dialysis Patients, written by Dennis and Kris Rager, addresses many of the different employment issues of people returning to work after a transplant. (To order a copy, contact: Rager Employment Consulting, 1104 Main St., Suite 314, Vancouver, WA 98660 or call 360-699-6165 or E-mail: RagerDK@aol.com)

Journey of the Heart: Spiritual Insights on the Road to a Transplant, written by Elizabeth Ann Bartlett, is a series of reflections on the spiritual aspects of the author's physical journey to a heart transplant. She writes about patience, hope, generosity, gratitude, humility and compassion. (Pfeifer-Hamilton Publishers, 1996, ISBN: 1570251282)

Life After Transplantation, written by Ellen Gordon Woodall, is a compilation of personal experiences by recipients and their families. This book includes a section on medications and suggestions for dealing with some of the side effects. (This publication is distributed free by the American Organ Transplant Association, 335 Cartwright Road, Missouri City, TX 77459, phone 281-261-2682.)

Lifeline: How One Night Changed Five Lives: A True Story, written by Mary Zimmeth Schomaker, follows the story of five critically ill patients whose common search for organ donors brought them together in a struggle for survival with important implications for the state of medicine today. (New Horizon Press, 1995; ISBN: 0882821350)

Life Row: A Case Study of How a Family Can Survive a Medical Crisis, written by Ed Linz, heart transplant recipient, chronicles his family's experience with the transplantation process and the triumph of a family undergoing an incredible ordeal. To order a copy, call TRIO at 800-TRIO-386. For more information, check out this website: http://www.iea.com/~adlinkex/liferow.html (Exchange Publishing; 1997, ISBN: 0965689506)

The Nicholas Effect: A Boy's Gift to the World, written by Reg Green, father of Nicholas Green, the little boy from California who was shot in Italy and whose organs were donated to seven Italians. This led to an outpouring of love by the people of Italy and a sharp increase in organ donation rates. Here is a book that will make you cry, make you glad you're a human and make you want to do something great. For more information, check out this website: http://www.nicholaseffect.com (O'Reilly & Associates, 1999, ISBN: 1565925971)

Pulse, written by Edna Buchanan, Pulitzer Prize-winning author, is a story about a man who experiences renewed health and appreciation for life after receiving a heart transplant. Against all advice, he searches for the family of the donor. Convinced the donor was murdered and not a victim of suicide, he begins a search for the truth. (Avon, 1999, ISBN: 0380728338)

Raising Lazarus, written by Robert Pensack, M.D., and Dwight Williams, is a recounting of the medical and psychological hurdles Pensack had to clear from his diagnosis through numerous operations, to his lifesaving heart transplant. His experiences led him to pursue a medical career, specializing in psychiatry. (Berkeley Publishing, 1994, ISBN: 1573225002)

Running Against Time, written by Antony C. Anjoubault, is the story of the author's 19-year struggle with hepatitis and resulting liver transplant. It has a forward by Jim Nabors, and the book is a well-written testimonial to the strength of the human spirit. (Barclay House, ISBN: 0935016295)

Second Chance, written by Diane Hebert, tells the story of her heart-lung transplant in 1985, the first in Quebec. To order a copy of the book, check out this website: http://macten.net/fdh/index-A.htm or write to The Diane Hebert Foundation, 132 Blainville est, Ste-Thérèse de Blainville QC Canada, J7E 1M2 or call 877-971-1110 or 450-971-1112, or fax 450-971-1818 or E-mail: fdh@macten.net

Surviving Transplantation: A Personal Guide for Organ Transplant Patients, their Families and Caregivers, written by John Craven, M.D., and Susan Faro, discusses coping with a serious illness and subsequent organ transplant for the layman. (University of Canada Press Inc., 1993, available online at http://www.stjosephs.london.on.ca/SJHC/programs/mental/survive/st.htm)

Sweet Reprieve, written by Frank Maier and his wife Ginny, is a journalist's story about his experiences with liver transplantation. The reader is taken from diagnosis through the pre- and post-transplant highs and lows. (Crown Publishers, 1991, ISBN: 0517581612)

Taking Heart, written by A.C. Greene, is this writer/historian's story about his heart transplant. More than just an autobiography, *Taking Heart* provides some excellent background on the history of transplantation. (Simon and Schuster, 1990, ISBN: 3621974120592)

Transplant Success Stories 1993, by Paul I. Teriyaki, Ph.D., and Jane Schoenberg, Ed., is a compilation of stories in which transplant recipients tell what transplantation has meant to them. In addition, members of three donor families give accounts of how their gift of life helped, in some measure, to reconcile them to their grief. (To order a free copy, contact the UCLA Tissue Typing Laboratory in Los Angeles at 310-825-7651.)

Books for Families with Children:

II Joshua: The Battle for Life, written by Merrily Bittler, is one baby boy's story of his birth and fight with life involving a double-lung transplant. Written by his grandmother from baby Joshua's perspective, the book chronicles Joshua's trips in and out of hospitals and shows the love, support and faith, which got Joshua and his family through the first hard years of his life. (New Horizons Publishing, 1996, ISBN: 1884687059)

An Age-Appropriate Guide to Helping your Child with a Transplant, written by Pamela Boone, R.N., M.S.N., Susan M. Kelly, R.N., B.S.N. and Katherine Oswald, R.N., B.S.N. is available on Stadtlanders Pharmacy's website at: http://www.stadtlander.com/transplant/childtx.html

A Will to Live: The Story of a Transplant Kid, written by Jessica Pace, Jane H. Talbert and Phyllis Harper (introduction), is a heartwarming story of a young girl's triumph over a double-lung and heart transplant. (Fawn Grove Press, 1998, ISBN: 0961570490)

Baby James: A Legacy of Love and Family Courage, written by Thomas and Jayne Miller, tells the story of their adopted son, Nicholas and his brief life. The parents document how the family faced their baby's four-month struggle to live and his need for a heart transplant. (Harper and Row, 1988, ISBN: 006250584X)

How to Help a Child through a Parent's Serious Illness, written by Kathleen McCue, gives practical advise on what and how you should tell your children about your illness, describes early warning signs you may see when your children aren't handling the crisis, and explains how to prepare children for visiting a sick parent in the hospital. (St. Martin Press, 1996, ISBN: 0312146191)

How Will They Get that Heart Down Your Throat? A Child's View of Transplants, written by Karen A. Walton, a kindergarten teacher and heart transplant recipient, is a book for kids about her experience. (E.M. Press Inc. 1997, ISPN: 1880664992)

Kyla's Kidney Adventure, written and illustrated by Kyla Aquino, a two-time kidney transplant recipient, is written for children with kidney disease and explains in simple terms such topics as kidney function, renal failure, dialysis and transplantation. (To order a copy, contact: The National Kidney Foundation of Northern California, 553 Pilgrim Drive, Suite C, Foster City, CA 94404.)

Lizzy Gets a New Liver, written by Lizzy Rabal and illustrated by Patricia Ritter McCracken, was written when Lizzy was just eight years old at the time of her liver transplant. (Bridge Resources, Presbyterian Distribution

Service/PDS, 100 Witherspoon St., Louisville, KY, 40202-1396, to order, call 800-524-2612)

Mira's Month, written by Deborah Weinstein-Stern, deals with the feelings of a child whose mother is hospitalized for an extended period. While the patient in this story is being treated for cancer, it can apply to any family in which a parent is being hospitalized for a serious illness. (For a free copy write to the Blood and Marrow Transplant InfoNet, 2900 Skokie Valley Road, Suite B, Highland Park, IL 60035 or call 847-433-3313, or E-mail: help@bmtnews.org).

What About Me? When Brothers and Sisters Get Sick, written by Allan Peterkin, illustrated by Frances Midendorf, is one in a series of books to help parents and their children explore the variety of feelings encountered when a brother or sister becomes seriously ill. (Magination Press, 1992, ISBN: 0945354495)

Your Child and Prednisone: Answers to Parent's Questions About Prednisone, written by Jeffery D. Punch, M.D., is an 18-page booklet. Although it was written especially for C.L.A.S.S., most of the information on side effects pertains to adults as well children. Anyone can request a free copy by writing to: C.L.A.S.S (The Children's Liver Association for Support Services), 26444 Emerald Dove Drive, Valencia, CA 91355 or call 805-255-0353 or E-mail: SupportSrv@aol.com

Miscellaneous Books:

Breathing Disorders: Your Complete Exercise Guide, written by Neil F. Gordon, M.D., is part of a series of books from the Cooper Clinic and Research Institute Fitness Series, which takes a look at the connection between breathing and exercise. (Human Kinetics, 1993; ISBN: 0873224264)

Coping with Prednisone (and Other Cortisone-Related Medicines): It May Work Miracles, But How Do You Handle the Side Effects, written by Eugenia Zukerman and Julie R. Ingelfinger, is a comprehensive, practical guide to making treatment with prednisone as effective and trouble-free as possible. (Griffin Trade Paperback, 1998; ISBN: 0312195702)

Good If Not Great Living with Lung Disease, written by Phil Petersen, is a compilation of experiences, equipment usage and easy planning for adults and children with breathing problems. (Raven Publishers Inc., 1999; ISBN: 962172642) *Website:* http://oxygenbook.com

The Merck Manual of Medical Information: Home Edition (1st Edition) is written by Robert Berkow (Preface), Mark H. Beers (Editor), Andrew J. Fletcher (Editor) and Merck & Co. staff. *The Merck Manual* is one of the most widely used sources of medical information in the world. Previously, it has been written for doctors and health-care professionals, not the general public. Now *The Merck Manual: Home Edition* contains virtually all of the information in the physician's version, but in easy-to-understand language with a reader-friendly format. (Merck & Co., 1997; ISBN: 0911910875)

The Personal Health-Care Organizer is a practical workbook and reference guide used to keep track of and manage individuals ongoing medical situations. Its workbook design allows it to be easily customized for any serious or chronic condition. To order contact: CraKel Publications, P.O. Box 51701, Irvine, CA 92619-1701 or call: 800-708-7623 or 949-249-8661, or E-mail: crakel@hydrameter.com

Prepare for Surgery, Heal Faster: A Guide of Mind-Body Techniques, written by Peggy Huddleston, takes holistic techniques such as relaxation therapy, guided imagery and meditation and uses them to overcome the anxieties before, during and after surgery. *Prepare for Surgery* allows the reader to feel calmer before surgery, have less pain, use less pain medication and recover faster. (Angel River Press, 1996, ISBN: 0964575744)

Surviving Modern Medicine: How to Get the Best from Doctors, Family and Friends, written by Peter Clarke and Susan H. Evans is an overall guide to navigating today's complicated health care system. The authors cite five critical areas for consumers to focus on to get good care: Getting your doctor to pay attention, making the best medical decisions and protecting your choices in critical-care situations. (Rutgers University Press, 1998, ISBN: 081352556X)

Organ Donor Awareness Materials:

Checks Unlimited
Phone: 800-533-3973
Check Production Division, P.O. Box 35630, Colorado Springs, CO 80935-3563

Current Inc., a mail-order check manufacturer, offers "my lines" (a space for a message above the signature line on a check). What better way to share organ and tissue donor awareness than to have it on your checks. *Website:* http://www.checksunlimited.com

Fly By Knight Designs
Phone: 401-253-5909
c/o Steve Brosnihan , P.O. Box 111, Bristol, RI 02809

Fly By Knight Designs makes an organ donor awareness T-shirt with a cartoon spelling out the slogan "Organ Donors are Heroes in the Making."

Transplant Awareness Inc.
Phone: 888-268-9232 or 703-534-8587, Fax: 703-534-7759,
E-mail: tai01@aol.com
P.O. Box 7634, Arlington, VA 22207

Transplant Awareness Inc. sells merchandise, with 100 percent of profits used to promote transplantation awareness. The group sells T-shirts, bumper stickers, pins, stickers, license plate brackets, among other items. *Website:* http://www.transplantawareness.org

Transplant Beanie Buddies
Phone: 410-451-5884, E-mail cbryon@aol.com

"Happy Henry" is 7 inches tall and comes in six colors with a nametag that states: "With a smile on my face, I will never be a loner. Give the gift of life and be an organ donor." Carol Bryon, the mother of a recipient, created "Happy Henry." All proceeds go to Johns Hopkins Pediatric Transplant Association. *Website:* http://members.aol.com/jhhptpa

Online Mailing Lists:

Alpha-1 International Support Mailing List is for people with alpha-₁ antitrypsin deficiency. To join, send an E-mail message to: LISTSERV@HOME.EASE.LSOFT.COM and type SUBSCRIBE ALPHA-1 (then insert your first and last name) in the body of the message. Once subscribed, you can send a message to the group by sending it to: ALPHA-1@HOME.EASE.LSOFT.COM You can also subscribe by visiting their website at: http://www.alphalink.org

ASSIST is an Internet mailing list devoted to the spouses and family members of those who have chronic lung disorders including lung transplantation. To subscribe send an E-mail message to: ASSIST-REQUEST@HOME.EASE.LSOFT.COM and type: SUBSCRIBE ASSIST (then insert your first and last name) in the body of the message. Once subscribed, you can send a message to the group by sending it to: ASSIST@HOME.EASE.LSOFT.COM

Cystic Fibrosis Discussion Group is an mailing list for patients and family members affected by cystic fibrosis. To join, send an E-mail message to: LISTSERV@HOME.EASE.LSOFT.COM and type: SUBSCRIBE CYSTIC-L (then insert your first and last name) in the body of the message. Once subscribed, you can send a message to the group by sending it to: CYSTIC-L@HOME.EASE.LSOFT.COM

The Idiopathic Pulmonary Fibrosis (IPFer) **Mailing List** is a discussion group for anyone who suffers from idiopathic pulmonary fibrosis and/or their caregiver. To join, send an E-mail message to: LISTSERV@HOME.EASE.LSOFT.COM and type: SUBSCRIBE IPFER (then insert your first and last name) in the body of the message. Once subscribed, you can send a message to the group by sending it to: IPFER@HOME.EASE.LSOFT.COM

Medical Meanderings is an online newsletter that provides medical information and transplant news articles. To subscribe, check out their website at: http://organtx.org/sub.htm. Subscribers can also receive topic-specific newsletters, such as Transplant, Heart/Circulation, Lung and Cancer. For more information, E-mail: Info@organtx.org

Second Wind Lung Transplant Association Inc. Mailing List is a discussion group for those who are interested in lung transplantation and its related problems. To subscribe, fill out the application found on their website at: http://www.2ndwind.org. Once subscribed, you can send a message to the group via E-mail at: secondwind@home.ease.lsoft.com. For more information, see their website at: http://www.2ndwind.org

TransplantBuddies.com is a group of bulletin boards lists for transplant recipients and people awaiting or considering a future transplant. To post a message or to review past messages, go to their website at: http://www.transplantbuddies.com

TRNSPLNT is a mailing list for organ transplant recipients and anyone interested in the issues. To subscribe, send the following message via E-mail to: LISTSERV@WUVMD.WUSTL.EDU or LISTSERV@WUVMD.BITNET, and type: SUB TRNSPLNT (insert your first and last name). Once online, you can send a message to the group via E-mail by sending a message to: trnsplnt@wuvmd.wustl.edu

TRXSUPPORT is a mailing list for pre- and post-transplant support. To subscribe, send an E-mail message to: majordomo@listserv.prodigy.com and type: SUBSCRIBE TRXSUPPORT (then insert your first and last name) in the body of the message.

TXLONGTERM is a mailing list meant for long-term transplant recipients. To subscribe, use the online form at http://www.onelist.com/ subscribe.cgi/txlongterm

Weekly Transplant Chats Online:

Sunday, 9 p.m. EST, Organ Transplant Chat
Talk City http://www.geocities.com/~rolo1/community.html
Contact: gmreilly@snet.net

Sunday, 8 to 9 p.m. EST, Lung Transplant Chat
Second Wind Lung Transplant Association: http://www.2ndwind.org/ main.htm. Contact: luckylungsforjo@aol.com

Monday, 8 to 9 p.m. EST, Lung Transplant Chat
Second Wind Lung Transplant Association: http://www.2ndwind.org/ main.htm. Contact: luckylungsforjo@aol.com

Monday, 8 p.m. EST, Donor Awareness
AOL: allHealth, aol://2719:3-1453-Helping%20Hand%20Cafe
Contact: BHostMich@aol.com or HOST AHTH Blu@aol.com

Tuesday, 8 to 9 p.m. EST, Lung Transplant Chat
Second Wind Lung Transplant Association: http://www.2ndwind.org/ main.htm. Contact: luckylungsforjo@aol.com

Tuesday, 9 p.m. EST, Carol's LungTx Room AOL: private room, go to any chat room, click on private chat, type in Carols LungTx Room. Contact: Michele Trunnell: BHostMich@aol.com or MTrunn5402@aol.com

Wednesday, 1 to 2 p.m. EST, Lung Transplant Chat
Second Wind Lung Transplant Association: http://www.2ndwind.org/ main.htm. Contact: luckylungsforjo@aol.com

Wednesday, 7 p.m. EST, All Organs & Tissues Transplant
DrKoop: Communities: Health Central: https://www.drkoop.com/ _mem_bin/formslogin.asp?http://drkoop.com/community/chat/ chat.asp?room=healthcentral

Wednesday, 7 p.m. EST, The Lung Transplant Page: Psychological Issues and Concerns. *Website:* http://homestead.deja.com/user.lungtxpsych/ index.html

Wednesday, Midnight to 1 a.m. EST, Lung Transplant Chat
Second Wind Lung Transplant Association: http://www.2ndwind.org/
main.htm. Contact: luckylungsforjo@aol.com

Thursday, 9 to 10 p.m. EST, Lung Transplant Chat
Second Wind Lung Transplant Association: http://www.2ndwind.org/
main.htm. Contact: luckylungsforjo@aol.com

Thursday, 11 p.m. to Midnight EST, Lung Transplant Chat
Second Wind Lung Transplant Association: http://www.2ndwind.org/
main.htm. Contact: luckylungsforjo@aol.com

Friday, 9 p.m. EST, All Organs & Tissues Transplant
AOL: allHealth, aol://2719:3-49-Positive%20Reflections
Contact: HOST AHTH Kandy@aol.com or HOST AHTH Liv@aol.com

Saturday 9 p.m. EST, Transplant Pre-n-Post Support Community
Talk City: www.tpnp.org/community.html, #Transplant channel
Contact: gmreilly@snet.net

APPENDIX A:

LUNG AND HEART-LUNG TRANSPLANT CENTERS:

- *The following list of lung and heart-lung transplant centers includes only those centers actively accepting new patients as of Sept. 15, 2000.*

- *The number of single and bilateral-lung and heart-lung transplants performed includes adults and pediatrics, cadaveric and living-related transplants.*

- *Waiting times reported are purely speculative for individual patients since they are a function of many different variables (e.g., number of patients currently listed, blood type, body size, waiting time accrued, the success of your local Organ Procurement Agency, etc.) Therefore, the time you will wait for your transplant cannot be predicted.*

- *Survival rates can also be misleading. A low survival rate might indicate that a particular center does more high-risk transplants, while a higher survival rate might indicate that another center does not.*

- *To provide the most complete and accurate information, all centers have been contacted numerous times. If an asterisk appears next to the name, it indicates a center that did not respond to our requests for information. In addition, these listing may not reflect current conditions. Although centers supplied this information, we cannot guarantee accuracy or assume responsibility for errors. ALWAYS REFER TO THE TRANSPLANT CENTER IN QUESTION FOR MORE UP-TO-DATE INFORMATION.*

- *n. a. denotes not available.*

ALABAMA   UNOS Region: 3

University of Alabama Hospital
618 S. 20th St., Birmingham, AL 35233
Main Phone: 205-934-3411
Website: http://www.health.uab.edu

Cardiothoracic Transplant Program: 800-822-8816 or
    205-975-8615, Fax: 205-975-9792
Program Established: 1988
1-Year Patient Survival Rate: 83%
    (based on 187 patients transplanted from 1988 to 1999)

Median Waiting Time (days): 352 (range 30 to 817)
Medicare Designated Center: Yes
Pediatric Transplantation: Yes (2 performed)
Living-Lobar Lung Donor Transplantation: No
Lung Retransplantation: Yes (7 performed)

OPO: Alabama Organ Center
301 S. 20th St., Suite 1001, Birmingham, AL 35233-2033
Main Phone: 205-731-9200/9250, Fax: 205-731-9250
Website: http://www.uab.edu/aoc

Transplants Performed:	1988	1989	1990	1991	1992	1993	1994	1995	1996	1997	1998	1999	2000	Total
Single or Bilateral-Lung	0	1	2	6	9	11	23	27	25	27	30	31	39	231
Heart-Lung	1	2	2	0	1	1	2	4	1	1	2	2	5	24

ARIZONA   UNOS Region: 5

**University Medical Center
at the University of Arizona**
1501 N. Campbell Ave., Tucson, AZ 85724
Main Phone: 520-694-6000

Cardiothoracic Transplantation Program: 800-524-5927 or
    520-694-6299, Fax: 520-694-2692
Program Established: 1979
1-Year Patient Survival Rate: 61% (based on 50 patients
    transplanted from 5/19/90 to 9/12/00)
Median Waiting Time (days): 212 (range 1 to 726)

Medicare Designated Center: No
Pediatric Transplantation: Yes (1 performed)
Living-Lobar Lung Donor Transplantation: No
Retransplantation: No (but, have performed 2 heart-lung retransplants)
Website: http://www.azumc.com/specialtycare/types/heartlung.htm

OPO: Donor Network of Arizona
3877 N. 7th St., Suite 200, Phoenix, AZ 85014-5084
Main Phone: 602-222-2200, Fax: 602-222-2202,
E-mail: dna1@dnaz.org
Website: http://www.dnaz.org

Transplants Performed:	1988	1989	1990	1991	1992	1993	1994	1995	1996	1997	1998	1999	2000	Total
Single or Bilateral-Lung	0	0	4	4	4	5	6	7	6	7	4	2	4	53
Heart-Lung	3	8	1	4	1	2	7	5	2	3	3	1	4	44

CALIFORNIA

UNOS Region: 5

Cedars-Sinai Medical Center
8700 W. Beverly Blvd., Suite 6215, Los Angeles, CA 90048-1869
Main Phone: 310-423-5000

Lung Transplantation Program: 310-423-3851, Fax: 310-423-0852
Program Established: 1988
1-Year Patient Survival Rate: 88.9%
  (based on 18 patients transplanted from 1997 to 2000)
Median Waiting Time (days): 181 (range 3 to 1,270)
Medicare Designated Center: No

Pediatric Transplantation: No
Living-Lobar Lung Donor Transplantation: No
Retransplantation: Yes (3 performed)
Website: http://www.csmc.edu/mktg/professionals/services/
  lungtransplant.html

OPO: Southern California Organ Procurement Center
2200 W. 3rd St., Suite 200, Los Angeles, CA 90057
Main Phone: 213-413-6219, Fax: 213-413-5373

Transplants Performed:	1988	1989	1990	1991	1992	1993	1994	1995	1996	1997	1998	1999	2000	Total
Single or Bilateral-Lung	1	9	12	8	9	5	7	11	7	5	1	3	4	79
Heart-Lung	0	0	0	0	0	0	0	0	0	1	0	0	0	1

Children's Hospital Los Angeles
4650 Sunset Blvd., Los Angeles, CA 90027
Main Phone: 323-660-2450

Cardiothoracic Transplant: 323-669-5965, Fax: 323-668-7979
Program Established: 1993
1-Year Patient Survival Rate: 100%
  (based on 16 patients transplanted from 1999 to 2000)
Median Waiting Time (days): 300 (range 4 to 1,424)
Medicare Designated Center: No

Pediatric Transplantation: Yes (91 performed)
Living-Lobar Lung Donor Transplantation: Yes (34 performed)
Lung Retransplantation: Yes (2 performed, but only on a case-by-
  case basis)
Website: http://www.chla.org/cardiothoracic.cfm

OPO: Southern California Organ Procurement Center
2200 W. 3rd St., Suite 200, Los Angeles, CA 90057
Main Phone: 213-413-6219, Fax: 213-413-5373

Transplants Performed:	1988	1989	1990	1991	1992	1993	1994	1995	1996	1997	1998	1999	2000	Total
Single or Bilateral-Lung	0	0	0	0	0	2	3	9	5	8	8	8	5	48
Heart-Lung	0	0	0	0	0	1	4	2	2	1	0	1	1	12

Stanford University Hospital
300 Pasteur Drive, Stanford, CA 94305
Main Phone: 650-723-4000

Lung and Heart-Lung Transplant Program: 650-723-5771,
  Fax: 650-725-3846
Program Established: 1981
1-Year Patient Survival Rate: 87.5%
  (based on 43 patients transplanted from 1/1/97 to 12/31/98)
Median Waiting Time (days): 243 (range 1 to 999)

Medicare Designated Center: Yes
Pediatric Transplantation: Yes (30 performed)
Living-Lobar Lung Donor Transplantation: No
Lung Retransplantation: Yes (3 performed)
Website: http://www-med.stanford.edu/shs/txp

OPO: California Transplant Donor Network
55 Francisco St., Suite 510, San Francisco, CA 94133-2115
Main Phone: 415-837-5888, Fax: 415-837-5880
Website: http://www.ctdn.org

Transplants Performed:	1988	1989	1990	1991	1992	1993	1994	1995	1996	1997	1998	1999	2000	Total
Single or Bilateral-Lung	0	8	9	9	6	9	8	14	14	24	21	9	21	152
Heart-Lung	16	14	14	11	4	7	13	16	6	10	6	7	11	135

University of California/Davis Medical Center
2315 Stockton Blvd., Sacramento, CA 95817
Main Phone: 916-734-2111

Lung Transplant Program: 800-821-9912 or 916-734-5360,
  Fax: 916-734-5582, E-mail: transplant@ucdavis.edu
Program Established: 1994
1-Year Patient Survival Rate: 69.2%
  (based on 55 patients transplanted since program inception)
Median Waiting Time (days): 79.5 (range 1 to 290)

Medicare Designated Center: Yes
Pediatric Transplantation: No
Living-Lobar Lung Donor Transplantation: No
Lung Retransplantation: Yes (2 performed)
Website: http://transplant.ucdmc.ucdavis.edu/lung/index.html

OPO: Golden State Donor Services
1760 Creekside Oaks Drive, Suite 160, Sacramento, CA 95833-3632
Main Phone: 916-567-1600, Fax: 916-567-8300,
Website: http://www.gsds.org

Transplants Performed:	1988	1989	1990	1991	1992	1993	1994	1995	1996	1997	1998	1999	2000	Total
Single or Bilateral-Lung	0	0	0	0	0	0	1	6	17	10	8	13	1	56
Heart-Lung	0	0	0	0	0	0	0	0	0	0	0	0	0	0

University of California at Los Angeles Medical Center

10833 Le Conte Ave., Los Angeles, CA 90095
Main Phone: 310-825-6301

Heart-Lung and Lung Transplant Programs: 310-825-6068,
 Fax: 310-206-6301
Program Established: 1988
1-Year Patient Survival Rate: 69.9%
 (based on 28 patients transplanted from 1995 to 1997)
Median Waiting Time (days): 442 (range not available)

Medicare Designated Center: Yes
Pediatric Transplantation: No
Living-Lobar Lung Donor Transplantation: No
Lung Retransplantation: Yes (1 performed; but only on their own
 patients, and only on a case-by-case basis)
Website: http://healthcare.ucla.edu/transplant/lung.html

OPO: Southern California Organ Procurement Center
2200 W. 3rd St., Suite 200, Los Angeles, CA 90057
Main Phone: 213-413-6219, Fax: 213-413-5373

Transplants Performed:	1988	1989	1990	1991	1992	1993	1994	1995	1996	1997	1998	1999	2000	Total
Single or Bilateral-Lung	0	0	3	0	3	11	21	25	13	12	17	10	8	123
Heart-Lung	1	1	0	0	0	0	0	1	0	0	0	1	0	4

University of California at San Diego Medical Center

200 W. Arbor Drive, San Diego, CA 92103-8401
Main Phone: 619-543-6222

Lung Transplantation Program: 619-543-7300, Fax: 619-543-7334
Program Established: 1990
1-Year Patient Survival Rate: 75.6%
 (based on 45 patients transplanted from 1/1/97 to 12/31/98)
Average Waiting Time (days): 2 years

Medicare Designated Center: Yes
Pediatric Transplantation: Yes (5 performed)
Living-Lobar Lung Donor Transplantation: Yes (3 performed)
Lung Retransplantation: Yes (1 performed, but only on a case-by-
 case basis)
Website: http://www-surgery.ucsd.edu/heart/transplantation.htm

OPO: Organ and Tissue Acquisition Center of Southern California
3665 Ruffin Road, Suite 120, San Diego, CA 92123
Main Phone: 619-292-8750, Fax: 619-560-5945

Transplants Performed:	1988	1989	1990	1991	1992	1993	1994	1995	1996	1997	1998	1999	2000	Total
Single or Bilateral-Lung	0	0	3	15	12	18	17	15	17	27	19	17	18	178
Heart-Lung	0	0	1	1	1	2	2	0	2	2	0	2	0	13

University of California at San Francisco Medical Center

505 Parnassus Ave., Moffit 884, Box 0116, San Francisco,
CA 94143-0116
Main Phone: 415-476-1000

Heart and Lung Transplant Program: 415-476-3503,
 Fax: 415-502-5316

Website: http://www.surgery.ucsf.edu/clinical/index.html

OPO: California Transplant Donor Network
55 Francisco St., Suite 510, San Francisco, CA 94133-2115
Main Phone: 415-837-5888, Fax: 415-837-5880
Website: http://www.ctdn.org

Transplants Performed:	1988	1989	1990	1991	1992	1993	1994	1995	1996	1997	1998	1999	2000	Total
Single or Bilateral-Lung	0	0	0	1	4	11	6	10	10	12	10	6	6	76
Heart-Lung	0	0	0	0	0	0	1	0	0	0	0	0	0	1

University of Southern California-University Hospital

1510 San Pablo St., Los Angeles, CA 90033
Main Phone: 800-USA-CARE (800-872-2273) or 323-442-8500
Website: http://www.uscuh.com

Lung and Heart-Lung Transplant Program: 323-442-5849,
 Fax: 323-442-6201
Program Established: 1991

1-Year Patient Survival Rate: 100%
 (based on 14 patients transplanted from 1/1/97 to 12/31/98)
Pediatric Transplantation: No
Living-Lobar Lung Donor Transplantation: Yes
Lung Retransplantation: Yes

OPO: Southern California Organ Procurement Center
2200 W. 3rd St., Suite 200, Los Angeles, CA 90057
Main Phone: 213-413-6219, Fax: 213-413-5373

Transplants Performed:	1988	1989	1990	1991	1992	1993	1994	1995	1996	1997	1998	1999	2000	Total
Single or Bilateral-Lung	0	0	0	0	1	10	17	13	15	11	14	12	23	116
Heart-Lung	0	0	0	0	0	0	0	0	0	0	0	0	0	0

COLORADO

Children's Hospital
1056 E. 19th Ave., Denver, CO 80218-1088
Main Phone: 800-624-6553 or 303-861-8888
Website: http://www.tchden.org/clinicalindex.html

Lung Transplant Program: 303-837-2921, Fax: 303-837-2924
Program Established: 1995
1-Year Patient Survival Rate: 100%
   (based on 2 patients transplanted from 1995 to 1998)

UNOS Region: 8

Medicare Designated Center: No
Pediatric Transplantation: Yes (2 performed)
Living-Lobar Lung Donor Transplantation: Yes
Lung Retransplantation: (will consider on a case-by-case basis)

OPO: Donor Alliance Inc.
3773 Cherry Creek N. Drive, Suite 601, Denver, CO 80209-3826
Main Phone: 303-329-4747, Fax: 303-321-1183
Website: http://www.donoralliance.org

Transplants Performed:	1988	1989	1990	1991	1992	1993	1994	1995	1996	1997	1998	1999	2000	Total
Single or Bilateral-Lung	0	0	0	0	0	0	0	1	0	0	1	0	0	2
Heart-Lung	0	0	0	0	0	0	0	0	0	0	0	0	0	0

University Hospital at the
University of Colorado Health Science Center
4200 E. 9th Ave., Denver, CO 80262
Main Phone: 800-638-3503 or 303-372-0000
Website: http://uch.uchsc.edu/sotx

Lung and Heart-Lung Transplant Programs: 303-372-8748,
   Fax: 303-372-6516
Program Established: 1992
1-Year Patient Survival Rate: 85%
   (based on 144 patients transplanted since program inception)

Median Waiting Time (days): 206 (range 2 to 1,000)
Medicare Designated Center: Yes
Pediatric Transplantation Center: No
Living Donor Lobar Transplantation Center: Yes
Lung Retransplantation: Yes
Website: http://www.uchsc.edu/sm/surgery/translung.html

OPO: Donor Alliance Inc.
3773 Cherry Creek N. Drive, Suite 601, Denver, CO 80209-3826
Main Phone: 303-329-4747, Fax: 303-321-1183
Website: http://www.donoralliance.org

Transplants Performed:	1988	1989	1990	1991	1992	1993	1994	1995	1996	1997	1998	1999	2000	Total
Single or Bilateral-Lung	0	0	0	0	9	14	20	20	19	21	20	21	29	173
Heart-Lung	0	0	0	0	0	0	1	0	0	0	0	2	0	3

FLORIDA

Jackson Memorial Hospital at the
University of Miami School of Medicine
1611 N.W. 12th Ave., Miami, FL 33136-1094
Main Phone: 305-585-1281

Cardiopulmonary Transplant Program: 305-355-5120,
   Fax: 305-355-5207
Program Established: 1996
1-Year Patient Survival Rate: 71%
   (based on 14 patients transplanted from 1/1/99 to 9/29/00)

UNOS Region: 3

Median Waiting Time (days): 90 (range 7 to 356)
Medicare Designated Center: No
Pediatric Transplantation: Yes
Living-Lobar Lung Donor Transplantation: No
Lung Retransplantation: Yes (but only on a case-by-case basis)
Website: http://www.um-jmh.org/Departments/Transplant_Services.html

OPO: University of Miami Organ Procurement Organization
1150 N.W. 14th St., Suite 208, Miami, FL 33136
Main Phone: 305-243-7622, Fax: 305-243-7628
Website: http://www.med.miami.edu/OPO

Transplants Performed:	1988	1989	1990	1991	1992	1993	1994	1995	1996	1997	1998	1999	2000	Total
Single or Bilateral-Lung	0	0	0	0	0	0	0	0	6	2	1	5	8	22
Heart-Lung	0	0	0	0	0	0	0	0	0	0	0	0	1	1

Shands Hospital at the University of Florida
1600 S.W. Archer Road, Gainesville, FL 32611
Main Phone: 352-395-8000

Lung Transplant Program: 800-749-7424 or 352-265-8940,
Fax: 352-265-8970
Program Established: 1994
1-Year Patient Survival Rate: 82%
   (based on 97 patients transplanted from 1/1/94 to 9/27/00)
Median Waiting Time (days): 356 (range 60 to 712)
Medicare Designated Center: Yes

Pediatric Transplantation: Yes (19 performed)
Living-Lobar Lung Donor Transplantation: No
Lung Retransplantation: Yes (6 performed, but only on a case-by-
   case basis and only on their own patients)
Website: http://www.shandstransplant.org/lung

OPO: Organ Procurement Organization at University of Florida
Ayers Medical Plaza, 720 S.W. 2nd Ave., Suite 570,
Gainesville, FL 32601
Main Phone: 352-395-0632, Fax: 352-338-9886
Website: http://www.surgery.ufl.edu/divisions/OPO/Opo.html

Transplants Performed:	1988	1989	1990	1991	1992	1993	1994	1995	1996	1997	1998	1999	2000	Total
Single or Bilateral-Lung	0	0	0	0	0	0	17	24	14	28	27	19	19	148
Heart-Lung	0	0	0	0	0	0	0	0	0	1	2	0	0	3

GEORGIA

UNOS Region: 3

Emory University Hospital
1364 Clifton Road, N.E., Atlanta, GA 30322
Main Phone: 404-712-7021

Lung and Heart-Lung Transplant Program: 404-727-9650,
Fax: 404-727-1516, E-mail: transplant_info@emory.org
Program Established: 1993
1-Year Patient Survival Rate: 75.96%
(based on 61 patients transplanted since program inception)
Median Waiting Time (days): not available

Medicare Designated Center: Yes
Pediatric Transplantation: Yes (3 performed)
Living-Lobar Lung Donor Transplantation: No
Lung Retransplantation: Yes (1 performed)
Website: http://www.emory.org/transplant/homepage/cgi

OPO: LifeLink of Georgia
3715 Northside Parkway, Suite 300, 100 N. Creek, Atlanta, GA 30327
Main Phone: 404-266-8884, Fax: 404-266-0592
Website: http://www.lifelinkfound.org/pro.html

Transplants Performed:	1988	1989	1990	1991	1992	1993	1994	1995	1996	1997	1998	1999	2000	Total
Single or Bilateral-Lung	0	0	0	0	0	3	7	7	9	11	11	9	9	66
Heart-Lung	1	2	0	1	0	0	0	0	0	0	0	0	0	4

ILLINOIS

UNOS Region: 7

Children's Memorial Hospital
2300 Children's Plaza, Chicago, IL 60614
Main Phone: 773-880-4000

Pulmonary Division: 773-880-8150, Fax: 773-880-4057
Program Established: 1997
1-Year Patient Survival Rate: not available
Median Waiting Time (days): 435 (range 30 to 820)
Medicare Designated Center: No
Pediatric Transplantation: Yes

Living-Lobar Lung Donor Transplantation: No
Lung Retransplantation: not applicable
Website: http://www.childmmc.edu/cmhweb/cmhdepts/CVSurgeryWeb/
TX.HTM

OPO: Regional Organ Bank of Illinois
800 S. Wells, Suite 190, Chicago, IL 60607-4529
Main Phone: 312-431-3600, Fax: 312-803-7643
Website: http://www.robi.org

Transplants Performed:	1988	1989	1990	1991	1992	1993	1994	1995	1996	1997	1998	1999	2000	Total
Single or Bilateral-Lung	0	0	0	0	0	0	0	0	0	0	0	1	0	1
Heart-Lung	0	0	0	0	0	0	0	0	0	0	0	0	0	0

Loyola University Medical Center
2160 S. First Ave., Maywood, IL 60153
Main Phone: 708-216-9000

Lung and Heart-Lung Transplantation: 800-424-6313 or 708-327-5864,
Fax: 708-327-2424
Program Established: 1990
1-Year Patient Survival Rate: 73%
(based on 20 patients transplanted in 1998)
Median Waiting Time (days): 610 (range 245 to 1,003)

Medicare Designated Center: Yes
Pediatric Transplantation: Yes (18 performed)
Living-Lobar Lung Donor Transplantation: No
Lung Retransplantation: Yes (but only on a case-by-case basis)
Website: http://www.luhs.org/svcline/transplant/specialty/d100hl.htm

OPO: Regional Organ Bank of Illinois
800 S. Wells, Suite 190, Chicago, IL 60607-4529
Main Phone: 312-431-3600, Fax: 312-803-7643
Website: http://www.robi.org

Transplants Performed:	1988	1989	1990	1991	1992	1993	1994	1995	1996	1997	1998	1999	2000	Total
Single or Bilateral-Lung	1	1	4	9	28	50	33	32	37	22	20	33	35	305
Heart-Lung	0	1	0	3	1	4	3	2	0	2	0	0	0	16

University of Illinois Hospital & Clinics

1740 W. Taylor St., Chicago, IL 60612
Main Phone: 312-996-7000
Website: http://www.hospital.uic.edu

Lung Transplant Program: 312-413-1831, Fax: 312-413-7839
Program Established: 1994
1-Year Patient Survival Rate: 81.8%
  (based on 11 patients transplanted from 1/1/97 to 12/31/98)
Waiting Time (days): 712

Medicare Designated Center: No
Pediatric Transplantation Center: No
Living-Lobar Lung Donor Transplantation: No
Lung Retransplantation: Yes

OPO: Regional Organ Bank of Illinois
800 S. Wells, Suite 190, Chicago, IL 60607-4529
Main Phone: 312-431-3600, Fax: 312-803-7643
Website: http://www.robi.org

Transplants Performed:	1988	1989	1990	1991	1992	1993	1994	1995	1996	1997	1998	1999	2000	Total
Single or Bilateral-Lung	0	0	0	0	0	0	3	10	6	8	3	2	4	36
Heart-Lung	1	0	0	0	0	0	0	2	1	0	0	0	0	4

INDIANA

Clarian Health-Methodist Hospital of Indiana

I-65 at 21 St., P.O. Box 1367, Indianapolis, IN 46206-1367
Main Phone: 317-929-2000

Transplant Center: 800-510-2725 or 317-929-8677, Fax: 317-929-5768
Program Established: 1989
1-Year Patient Survival Rate: 75%
  (based on 44 patients transplanted from 1/13/97 to 7/7/99)
Median Waiting Time (days): 623 (range 211 to 937)

UNOS Region: 10

Medicare Designated Center: Yes
Pediatric Transplantation: No
Living-Lobar Lung Donor Transplantation: No
Lung Retransplantation: Yes (1 performed)

OPO: Indiana Organ Procurement Organization
429 N. Pennsylvania St., Suite 201, Indianapolis, IN 46204-1816
Main Phone: 317-685-0389, Fax: 317-685-1687

Transplants Performed:	1988	1989	1990	1991	1992	1993	1994	1995	1996	1997	1998	1999	2000	Total
Single or Bilateral-Lung	0	1	4	16	10	15	11	10	14	15	21	16	32	165
Heart-Lung	0	1	1	0	1	1	0	2	0	1	0	0	0	7

KENTUCKY

Jewish Hospital

217 E. Chestnut St., Louisville, KY 40202
Main Phone: 502-587-4011

Lung Transplant Program: 800-866-7539 or 502-587-4939,
  Fax: 502-587-4184, E-mail: transplant@jewishhospital.org
Program Established: 1991
1-Year Patient Survival Rate: 72%
  (based on 25 patients transplanted from 1/1/97 to 12/31/98)
Median Waiting Time (days): 243 (range 133 to 300)

UNOS Region: 11

Medicare Designated Center: Yes
Pediatric Transplantation Center: Yes
Living-Lobar Lung Donor Transplantation: No
Lung Retransplantation: Yes (2 performed)
Website: http://www.jhhs.org/orgalung.html

OPO: Kentucky Organ Donor Affiliates
106 E. Broadway, Louisville, KY 40202
Main Phone: 502-581-9511, Fax: 502-589-5157

Transplants Performed:	1988	1989	1990	1991	1992	1993	1994	1995	1996	1997	1998	1999	2000	Total
Single or Bilateral-Lung	0	0	0	1	0	1	7	15	12	15	10	14	9	84
Heart-Lung	1	0	0	0	0	1	0	1	0	1	0	0	0	4

University of Kentucky Medical Center

800 Rose St., Lexington, KY 40536-0084
Main Phone: 859-323-5000

Heart and Lung Transplant Center: 800-456-5287 or 859-257-5188,
  Fax: 859-323-1700
Program Established: 1991
1-Year Patient Survival Rate: 41.5%
  (based on 7 patients transplanted from 1/1/97 to 12/31/98)
Median Waiting Time (days): not available

Medicare Designated Center: No
Pediatric Transplantation Center: Yes
Living-Lobar Lung Donor Transplantation: No
Lung Retransplantation: Yes (2 performed)
Website: http://www.mc.uky.edu/transplant/lung.htm

OPO: Kentucky Organ Donor Affiliates
106 E. Broadway, Louisville, KY 40202
Main Phone: 502-581-9511, Fax: 502-589-5157

Transplants Performed:	1988	1989	1990	1991	1992	1993	1994	1995	1996	1997	1998	1999	2000	Total
Single or Bilateral-Lung	0	0	0	1	5	12	19	23	8	1	6	16	13	104
Heart-Lung	0	0	0	0	0	2	2	1	1	0	0	0	0	6

LOUISIANA

Ochsner Foundation Hospital
Ochsner Clinic, 1514 Jefferson Highway, New Orleans, LA 70121
Main Phone: 504-842-3925

Lung Transplant Program: 800-643-1635 or 504-842-3925,
   Fax: 504-842-6228
Program Established: 1990
1-Year Patient Survival Rate: 84.5%
   (based on 96 patients from 5/1/95 to 4/30/00)
Median Waiting Time (days): 42 (range 2 to 202)

UNOS Region: 3

Medicare Designated Center: Yes
Pediatric Transplantation: Yes (9 performed)
Living-Lobar Lung Donor Transplantation: No
Lung Retransplantation: Yes (5 performed)
Website: http://www.ochsner.org/transplant/lungprogram.html

OPO: Louisiana Organ Procurement Agency
3501 N. Causeway Blvd., Suite 940, Metairie, LA 70002-3626
Main Phone: 504-837-3355, Fax: 504-837-3587
Website: http://www.lopa.org

Transplants Performed:	1988	1989	1990	1991	1992	1993	1994	1995	1996	1997	1998	1999	2000	Total
Single or Bilateral-Lung	0	0	0	2	5	5	9	12	18	23	18	19	23	134
Heart-Lung	0	0	1	0	0	0	0	0	0	0	0	0	0	1

MARYLAND

Johns Hopkins Hospital
600 N. Wolfe St., Baltimore, MD 21205
Main Phone: 410-955-5000

Adult Lung and Heart-Lung Transplant Program: 888-304-5069 or
   410-614-4898, Fax: 410-614-7008
Pediatric Lung Transplant Program: 888-304-5069 or 410-955-2035
Program Established: 1993
1-Year Patient Survival Rate: 72%
   (based on 86 patients transplanted from 2/1/93 to 6/15/00)
Median Waiting Time (days): 361 (range 2 to 1,653)

UNOS Region: 2

Medicare Designated Center: Yes
Pediatric Transplantation Center: Yes (4 performed)
Living-Lobar Lung Donor Transplantation: Yes (2 performed)
Lung Retransplantation: Yes (but only on a case-by-case basis)
Website: http://www.med.jhu.edu/transplant/lung_intro.html

OPO: Transplant Resource Center of Maryland
1540 Caton Center Drive, Suite R, Baltimore, MD 21227
Main Phone: 410-242-7000, Fax: 410-242-1871
Website: http://www.mdtransplant.org

Transplants Performed:	1988	1989	1990	1991	1992	1993	1994	1995	1996	1997	1998	1999	2000	Total
Single or Bilateral-Lung	0	0	0	0	0	1	3	7	9	6	18	29	19	92
Heart-Lung	4	2	3	0	0	0	0	0	0	0	0	1	2	12

University of Maryland Medical System
22 S. Greene St., Baltimore, MD 21201
Main Phone: 800-492-5538 or 410-328-8667

Thoracic Transplant Program: 410-328-2736, Fax: 410-328-1311
Program Established: 1992
1-Year Patient Survival Rate: 75%
   (based on 64 patients transplanted from 1/92 to 9/2000)
Median Waiting Time (days): not available
Medicare Designated Center: Yes

Pediatric Transplantation: No
Living-Lobar Lung Donor Transplantation: No
Lung Retransplantation: No
Website: http://www.umm.edu/transplant/lung/index.html

OPO: Transplant Resource Center of Maryland
1540 Caton Center Drive, Suite R, Baltimore, MD 21227
Main Phone: 410-242-7000, Fax: 410-242-1871
Website: http://www.mdtransplant.org

Transplants Performed:	1988	1989	1990	1991	1992	1993	1994	1995	1996	1997	1998	1999	2000	Total
Single or Bilateral-Lung	0	0	0	0	2	3	2	10	20	8	11	4	6	66
Heart-Lung	0	0	0	0	0	0	0	0	1	0	0	0	0	1

MASSACHUSETTS

Brigham and Women's Hospital
75 Francis St., Boston, MA 02115
Main Phone: 888-294-5864 or 617-732-5500

Lung Transplantation Program: 617-732-7269, Fax: 617-582-6102
Program Established: 1990
1-Year Patient Survival Rate: 76%
   (based on 144 patients transplanted from 1990 to 2000)
Median Waiting Time (days): 383 (range 38 to 1,856)
Medicare Designated Center: Yes

UNOS Region: 1

Pediatric Transplantation: No
Living-Lobar Lung Donor Transplantation: Yes
Lung Retransplantation: Yes (3 performed; but only on a case-by-
   case basis)
Website: http://www.chestsurg.org

OPO: New England Organ Bank
Washington St. at Newton Corner, One Gateway Center,
Newton, MA 02158-2803
Main Phone: 617-244-8000, Fax: 617-244-8755
Website: http://www.neob.org

Transplants Performed:	1988	1989	1990	1991	1992	1993	1994	1995	1996	1997	1998	1999	2000	Total
Single or Bilateral-Lung	0	0	6	8	12	12	9	23	17	15	12	18	18	132
Heart-Lung	0	0	0	0	1	1	1	0	0	0	0	0	0	3

Children's Hospital

300 Longwood Ave., Boston, MA 02115
Main Phone: 617-355-6000

Lung Transplant Program: 617-355-6681, Fax: 617-566-7810
Program Established: 1990
1-Year Patient Survival Rate: 75%
  (based on 4 patients transplanted from 1/1/97 to 12/31/98)
Median Waiting Time (days): 240 (range 60 to 640)
Medicare Designated Center: No

Pediatric Transplantation: Yes (16 performed)
Living-Lobar Lung Donor Transplantation: Yes (1 performed)
Lung Retransplantation: No
Website: http://www.childrenshospital.org/surgery/lungtx.html

OPO: New England Organ Bank
Washington St. at Newton Corner, One Gateway Center,
Newton, MA 02158-2803
Main Phone: 617-244-8000, Fax: 617-244-8755
Website: http://www.neob.org

Transplants Performed:	1988	1989	1990	1991	1992	1993	1994	1995	1996	1997	1998	1999	2000	Total
Single or Bilateral-Lung	0	0	1	1	4	4	2	0	3	3	2	3	4	27
Heart-Lung	0	0	0	0	1	1	1	0	0	0	1	0	0	4

Massachusetts General Hospital

55 Fruit St., Boston, MA 02114-2696
Main Phone: 617-726-2000
Website: http://www.mgh.harvard.edu

Lung Transplantation Program: 617-726-6162, Fax: 617-726-2581
Program Established: 1990
1-Year Patient Survival Rate: 81%
  (based on 100 patients transplanted since program inception)
Average Waiting Time (days): 725

Medicare Designated Center: Yes
Pediatric Transplantation: No
Living-Lobar Lung Donor Transplantation: Yes (12 performed)
Lung Retransplantation: Yes (1 performed)

OPO: New England Organ Bank
Washington St. at Newton Corner, One Gateway Center,
Newton, MA 02158-2803
Main Phone: 617-244-8000, Fax: 617-244-8755
Website: http://www.neob.org

Transplants Performed:	1988	1989	1990	1991	1992	1993	1994	1995	1996	1997	1998	1999	2000	Total
Single or Bilateral-Lung	0	0	3	11	7	6	7	12	10	11	8	9	16	100
Heart-Lung	0	0	0	0	0	0	0	0	0	0	0	0	0	0

MICHIGAN

Henry Ford Hospital

2799 W. Grand Blvd., Detroit, MI 48202
Main Phone: 800-999-4340 or 313-916-2600
Website: http://www.henryfordhealth.org

Lung Transplant Program: 313-916-1258 or 313-916-1471,
  Fax: 313-916-9102
Program Established: 1994
1-Year Patient Survival Rate: 78.7%
  (based on 17 patients transplanted from 1/1/97 to 12/31/98)

UNOS Region: 10

Average Waiting Time (days): 534 (range 10 to 1,068)
Medicare Designated Center: Yes
Pediatric Transplantation: No
Living-Lobar Lung Donor Transplantation: No
Lung Retransplantation: Yes (1 performed, but only on a case-by-case
  basis and on their own patients)

OPO: Transplantation Society of Michigan
2203 Platt Road, Ann Arbor, MI 48104
Main Phone: 734-973-1577, Fax: 734-973-3133

Transplants Performed:	1988	1989	1990	1991	1992	1993	1994	1995	1996	1997	1998	1999	2000	Total
Single or Bilateral-Lung	0	0	0	0	0	0	1	6	14	12	5	9	9	56
Heart-Lung	0	0	0	0	0	0	0	0	0	0	0	0	0	0

University of Michigan Medical Center *

1500 E. Medical Center Drive, Ann Arbor, MI 48109
Main Phone: 734-936-4000

Lung Transplant Program: 734-936-8535, Fax: 734-936-5048
1-Year Patient Survival Rate: 78.3%

  (based on 46 patients transplanted from 1/1/97 to 12/31/98)
Website: http://www.med.umich.edu/trans/public

OPO: Transplantation Society of Michigan
2203 Platt Road, Ann Arbor, MI 48104
Main Phone: 734-973-1577, Fax: 734-973-3133

Transplants Performed:	1988	1989	1990	1991	1992	1993	1994	1995	1996	1997	1998	1999	2000	Total
Single or Bilateral-Lung	0	0	3	19	17	10	16	20	18	19	27	25	40	214
Heart-Lung	1	0	0	2	2	1	2	1	1	1	1	1	0	13

MINNESOTA

Fairview University Medical Center *

Harvard St. at E. River Road, Minneapolis, MN 55455
Main Phone: 800-688-5252 or 612-273-3000

Lung Transplant Program: 800-888-8942 or 612-625-9922,
    Fax: 612-626-6968
Program Established: 1986
1-Year Patient Survival Rate: 78.7%

UNOS Region: 7

(based on 61 patients transplanted from 1/1/97 to 12/31/98)
Medicare Designated Center: Yes
Website: http://www.fairviewtransplant.org/lungtx.htm

OPO: LifeSource/Upper Midwest Organ Procurement Organization
2550 University Ave. W., Suite 315 S., St Paul, MN 55114-1904
Main Phone: 612-603-7800, Fax: 612-603-7801
Website: http://www.life-source.org

Transplants Performed:	1988	1989	1990	1991	1992	1993	1994	1995	1996	1997	1998	1999	2000	Total
Single or Bilateral-Lung	2	6	11	16	25	29	31	31	24	35	29	39	30	308
Heart-Lung	2	9	6	3	1	3	5	1	1	5	3	0	1	40

St. Mary's Hospital *

1216 2nd St. S.W., Rochester, MN 55902
Main Phone: 507-284-2511

Heart & Lung Transplant Program: 800-422-6296 or
    507-266-4034, Fax: 507-266-0731
1-Year Patient Survival Rate: 33.3%

(based on 3 patients transplanted from 1/1/97 to 12/31/98)
Medicare Designated Center: No

OPO: LifeSource/Upper Midwest Organ Procurement Organization
2550 University Ave. W., Suite 315 S., St Paul, MN 55114-1904
Main Phone: 612-603-7800, Fax: 612-603-7801
Website: http://www.life-source.org

Transplants Performed:	1988	1989	1990	1991	1992	1993	1994	1995	1996	1997	1998	1999	2000	Total
Single or Bilateral-Lung	0	0	3	3	12	6	2	3	2	0	3	1	n. a.	35
Heart-Lung	0	0	0	0	0	0	1	0	1	1	0	1	n. a.	4

MISSOURI

Barnes-Jewish Hospital

One Barnes Hospital Plaza, St. Louis, MO 63110
Main Phone: 314-362-5000

Lung Transplant Program: 800-321-4054 or 314-362-5378,
    Fax: 314-362-9272
Program Established: 1988
1-Year Patient Survival Rate: 84%
    (based on 491 patients transplanted from 1988 to 1999)
Average Waiting Time (days): 18 to 24 months

UNOS Region: 8

Medicare Designated Center: Yes
Pediatric Transplantation: No
Living-Lobar Lung Donor Transplantation: No
Lung Retransplantation: Yes (8 performed, but only on a case-by-
    case basis)
Website: http://www.bjc.org/bjh.html

OPO: Mid-American Transplant Services
1139 Olivette Executive Parkway, St Louis, MO 63132-3205
Main Phone: 314-991-1661, Fax: 314-991-2805

Transplants Performed:	1988	1989	1990	1991	1992	1993	1994	1995	1996	1997	1998	1999	2000	Total
Single or Bilateral-Lung	5	23	37	42	46	48	48	45	43	57	55	47	52	548
Heart-Lung	1	0	0	0	0	0	0	1	0	1	0	1	1	5

St. Louis Children's Hospital
at the Washington University Medical Center

One Children's Place, St. Louis, MO 63110-1077
Main Phone: 314-454-6000

Lung Transplant Program: 314-454-4131, Fax: 314-454-4280
Program Established: 1990
1-Year Patient Survival Rate: 80% to 85%
    (based on 187 patients transplanted from 1990 to 1998)
Median Waiting Time (days): <1 year old, 81; 1 to 5 years old, 99;

6 to 10 years old, 270; 11 to 17 years old, 429; 18 years + up 1,254
Medicare Designated Center: No
Pediatric Transplantation: Yes (226 performed)
Living-Lobar Lung Donor Transplantation: Yes (38 performed)
Lung Retransplantation: Yes (25 performed)
Website: http://ssweet.carenet.org/lungtxp

OPO: Mid-American Transplant Services
1139 Olivette Executive Parkway, St Louis, MO 63132-3205
Main Phone: 314-991-1661, Fax: 314-991-2805

Transplants Performed:	1988	1989	1990	1991	1992	1993	1994	1995	1996	1997	1998	1999	2000	Total
Single or Bilateral-Lung	0	0	3	12	16	15	22	27	22	27	33	19	14	210
Heart-Lung	0	0	0	0	0	4	1	3	2	0	0	0	2	12

NEBRASKA

BryanLGH Medical Center East

1600 S. 48th St., Lincoln, NE 68506-1299
Main Phone: 402-489-0200
Website: http://www.bryan.org

Lung Transplant Program: 402-481-3933, Fax: 402-481-3918
Program Established: 1992
1-Year Patient Survival Rate: 100%
   (based on 4 patients transplanted from 7/1/95 to 12/30/99)

UNOS Region: 8

Median Waiting Time (days): range 100 to 855
Medicare Designated Center: No
Pediatric Transplantation: No
Living-Lobar Lung Donor Transplantation: No
Lung Retransplantation: No

OPO: Nebraska Organ Retrieval System Inc.
4060 Vinton St., Suite 200, Omaha, NE 68105
Main Phone: 402-553-7952, Fax: 402-553-0933

Transplants Performed:	1988	1989	1990	1991	1992	1993	1994	1995	1996	1997	1998	1999	2000	Total
Single or Bilateral-Lung	0	0	0	0	3	4	3	1	1	1	0	1	3	17
Heart-Lung	0	0	0	0	0	0	0	0	0	0	0	0	0	0

NEW YORK

Mount Sinai Medical Center

One Gustave Levy Place, New York, NY 10029
Main Phone: 212-241-6500
Website: http://www.mssm.edu/rmti

Lung Transplant Program: 212-241-3079, Fax: 212-534-3186
Program Established: 1992
1-Year Patient Survival Rate: 100%
   (based on 3 patients transplanted in 1999)

UNOS Region: 9

Median Waiting Time (days): 534 (range not available)
Medicare Designated Center: No
Pediatric Transplantation: No
Living-Lobar Lung Donor Transplantation: No
Lung Retransplantation: No (but only on a case-by-case basis)

OPO: New York Organ Donor Network
475 Riverside Drive, Suite 1244, New York, NY 10115-1244
Main Phone: 212-870-2240, Fax: 212-870-3299

Transplants Performed:	1988	1989	1990	1991	1992	1993	1994	1995	1996	1997	1998	1999	2000	Total
Single or Bilateral-Lung	0	0	0	0	2	3	4	0	0	0	0	3	3	15
Heart-Lung	0	0	0	0	3	2	2	0	0	0	0	0	0	7

New York University Medical Center

530 1st Ave., New York, NY 10016
Main Phone: 212-263-7300

Lung Transplant Program: 212-263-7461, Fax: 212-263-2042
Program Established: 1996
1-Year Patient Survival Rate: 66%
   (based on 5 patients transplanted since program inception)
Median Waiting Time (days): 765 (range 730 to 820)

Medicare Designated Center: N
Pediatric Transplantation: No
Living-Lobar Lung Donor Transplantation: No
Lung Retransplantation: No
Website: http://mcrcr4.med.nyu.edu/Transplant/TX.html

OPO: New York Organ Donor Network
475 Riverside Drive, Suite 1244, New York, NY 10115-1244
Main Phone: 212-870-2240, Fax: 212-870-3299

Transplants Performed:	1988	1989	1990	1991	1992	1993	1994	1995	1996	1997	1998	1999	2000	Total
Single or Bilateral-Lung	0	0	0	0	0	0	0	0	1	0	1	3	0	5
Heart-Lung	0	0	0	0	0	0	0	0	0	0	0	0	0	0

Presbyterian Hospital in New York City

Columbia Presbyterian Medical Center
622 W. 168th St., New York, NY 10032-3784
Main Phone: 212-305-2323

Lung and Heart-Lung Transplant Program: 212-305-LUNG
   (212-305-7771), Fax: 212-342-5382
Program Established: 1989
1-Year Patient Survival Rate: 78.2%
   (based on 22 patients transplanted in 1999)

Median Waiting Time (days): 623 (range 14 to 1,068)
Medicare Designated Center: No
Pediatric Transplantation: No
Living-Lobar Lung Donor Transplantation: No
Lung Retransplantation: not available
Website: http://www.nyp.org/transplant/mainbody.html

OPO: New York Organ Donor Network
475 Riverside Drive, Suite 1244, New York, NY 10115-1244
Main Phone: 212-870-2240, Fax: 212-870-3299

Transplants Performed:	1988	1989	1990	1991	1992	1993	1994	1995	1996	1997	1998	1999	2000	Total
Single or Bilateral-Lung	0	3	15	19	18	32	20	21	26	25	14	21	18	232
Heart-Lung	2	3	3	3	1	2	2	2	1	7	7	2	0	35

NORTH CAROLINA

Duke University Medical Center and Durham VA Medical Center

Erwin Road, Durham, NC 27710
Main Phone: 919-684-8111

Lung Transplant Program: 800-249-5864 or 919-684-2240,
Fax: 919-681-9571
Heart-Lung Transplant Program: 800-249-5864 or 919-684-2651
Program Established: 1992
1-Year Patient Survival Rate: 81%
(based on all patients transplanted from 1992 to 1999)
Average Waiting Time (days): 270

UNOS Region: 11

Medicare Designated Center: Yes
Pediatric Transplantation: Yes
Living-Lobar Lung Donor Transplantation: Yes (3 performed)
Lung Retransplantation: Yes (12 performed; will accept patients from other centers, but only on a case-by-case basis)
Website: http://organtransplant.mc.duke.edu/transplant.nsf

OPO: Carolina Donor Services
702 Johns Hopkins Drive, Greenville, NC 27834
Main Phone: 919-757-0090, Fax: 919-757-0708
E-mail: copanc@mindspring.com
Website: http://www.copanc.org

Transplants Performed:	1988	1989	1990	1991	1992	1993	1994	1995	1996	1997	1998	1999	2000	Total
Single or Bilateral-Lung	0	0	0	0	5	15	25	37	33	53	35	52	53	308
Heart-Lung	0	0	0	0	1	0	2	3	0	3	4	2	2	17

University of North Carolina Hospitals

101 Manning Drive, Chapel Hill, NC 27514
Main Phone: 919-966-4131

Lung Transplant Program: 888-263-5293 or 919-966-6457,
Fax: 919-843-0564, E-mail: transplant@unch.unc.edu
Program Established: 1990
1-Year Patient Survival Rate: 72.6%
(based on 33 patients transplanted from 1/1/97 to 12/31/98)
Median Waiting Time (days): 568 (range 163 to 1,401)
Medicare Designated Center: Yes

Pediatric Transplantation: Yes (23 performed)
Living-Lobar Lung Donor Transplantation: Yes (8 performed)
Lung Retransplantation: Yes (2 performed)
Website: http://www.med.unc.edu/transplant

OPO: Carolina Donor Services
702 Johns Hopkins Drive, Greenville, NC 27834
Main Phone: 800-220-2672, Fax: 252-757-0708,
E-mail: copanc@mindspring.com
Website: http://www.carolinadonorservices.org

Transplants Performed:	1988	1989	1990	1991	1992	1993	1994	1995	1996	1997	1998	1999	2000	Total
Single or Bilateral-Lung	0	0	11	26	22	20	19	18	18	23	12	17	13	186
Heart-Lung	0	0	0	2	0	1	1	2	0	0	1	0	2	7

OHIO

Cleveland Clinic Foundation

Desk A1109, 9500 Euclid Ave., Cleveland, OH 44195
Main Phone: 800-223-2273 or 216-444-2200

Lung Transplant Program: 216-445-1115, Fax: 216-445-3127
Program Established: 1990
1-Year Patient Survival Rate: 82.9%
(based on 21 patients transplanted from 1990 to 1999)
Median Waiting Time (days): 328 (range 1 to 1251)
Medicare Designated Center: Yes

UNOS Region: 10

Pediatric Transplantation: Yes (5 performed)
Living-Lobar Lung Donor Transplantation: No
Lung Retransplantation: Yes
Website: http://www.clevelandclinic.org/transplant/services/lung.htm

OPO: LifeBanc of Ohio
20600 Chagrin Blvd., Suite 350, Cleveland, OH 44122-5343
Main Phone: 888-306-4273 or 216-752-5433, Fax: 216-751-4204,
E-mail: lifebanc@clevelandnet.com

Transplants Performed:	1988	1989	1990	1991	1992	1993	1994	1995	1996	1997	1998	1999	2000	Total
Single or Bilateral-Lung	0	0	5	18	19	21	16	18	11	14	29	32	45	228
Heart-Lung	0	0	0	0	1	2	1	0	1	0	0	0	1	6

Ohio State University Hospital

410 W. 10th Ave., Columbus, OH 43210
Main Phone: 614-293-8000

Lung Transplant Program: 800-293-5123 or 614-293-7153,
Fax: 614-293-9820
Program Established: 1998
1-Year Patient Survival Rate: 77%
(based on 13 patients transplanted from 1998 to 1999)
Median Waiting Time (days): 120 (range 90 to 180)

Medicare Designated Center: No
Pediatric Transplantation: No
Living-Lobar Lung Donor Transplantation: No
Lung Retransplantation: Yes (but only on a case-by-case basis)
Website: http://www.osumedcenter.edu/health_services/services.asp?servicearea=12

OPO: Lifeline of Ohio
770 Kinnear Road, Suite 200, Columbus, OH 43212
Main Phone: 614-291-5667, Fax: 614-291-0660

Transplants Performed:	1988	1989	1990	1991	1992	1993	1994	1995	1996	1997	1998	1999	2000	Total
Single or Bilateral-Lung	0	0	0	0	0	0	0	0	0	0	1	12	9	22
Heart-Lung	0	0	0	0	0	0	0	0	0	0	0	0	1	1

University Hospitals of Cleveland
11100 Euclid Ave., Cleveland, OH
Main Phone: 216-844-1000

Lung Transplant Program: 216-844-3947, Fax: 216-844-8479
Program Established: 1998
1-Year Patient Survival Rate: 100%
  (based on 3 patients transplanted from 2/6/99 to 5/10/00)
Median Waiting Time (days): 42 (range 13 to 497)

Medicare Designated Center: No
Pediatric Transplantation: Yes
Living-Lobar Lung Donor Transplantation: No
Lung Retransplantation: No (but will evaluate on a case-by-case basis)

OPO: LifeBanc of Ohio
20600 Chagrin Blvd., Suite 350, Cleveland, OH 44122-5343
Main Phone: 888-306-4273 or 216-752-5433, Fax: 216-751-4204,
E-mail: lifebanc@clevelandnet.com

Transplants Performed:	1988	1989	1990	1991	1992	1993	1994	1995	1996	1997	1998	1999	2000	Total
Single or Bilateral-Lung	0	0	0	0	0	0	0	0	0	0	0	1	10	11
Heart-Lung	0	0	0	0	0	0	0	0	0	0	0	0	0	0

OKLAHOMA

UNOS Region: 4

Baptist Medical Center
3300 N.W. Expressway, Oklahoma City, OK 73112
Main Phone: 405-949-3349

Lung Transplant Program: 800-991-3349 or 405-949-3349,
  Fax: 405-945-5467
Program Established: 1990
1-Year Patient Survival Rate: 80%
  (based on 46 patients transplanted from 6/23/90 to 6/30/2000)
Median Waiting Time (days): 537 (range 147 to 1,182)
Medicare Designated Center: No

Pediatric Transplantation: No
Living-Lobar Lung Donor Transplantation: No
Lung Retransplantation: No
Website: http://www.integris-health.com/servicearea.asp?ID=20

OPO: Oklahoma Organ Sharing Network
5801 N. Broadway, Suite 100, Oklahoma City, OK 73118-7489
Main Phone: 888-580-5680, Fax: 405-840-9748,
E-mail: oosn@oosn.com

Transplants Performed:	1988	1989	1990	1991	1992	1993	1994	1995	1996	1997	1998	1999	2000	Total
Single or Bilateral-Lung	0	0	1	5	2	7	5	2	4	4	4	6	9	49
Heart-Lung	2	1	0	0	0	0	0	0	0	0	0	0	0	3

OREGON

UNOS Region: 6

Oregon Health Sciences University Hospital and Portland VA Medical Center
3181 S.W. Sam Jackson Park Road, Portland, OR 97201-3098
Main Phone: 503-494-8311

Lung and Heart-Lung Transplant Program: 503-494-7820,
  Fax: 503-494-5049
Program Established: 1992
1-Year Patient Survival Rate: 68.9%
  (based on 4 patients transplanted from 1/1/97 to 12/31/98)

Average Waiting Time (days): 181 (range 3 to 819)
Medicare Designated Center: No
Pediatric Transplantation: No
Living-Lobar Lung Donor Transplantation: No
Lung Retransplantation: No
Website: http://www.ohsu.edu/transplant

OPO: Pacific N.W. Transplant Bank
2611 S.W. 3rd Ave, Suite 320, Portland, OR 97201-4952
Main Phone: 503-494-5560

Transplants Performed:	1988	1989	1990	1991	1992	1993	1994	1995	1996	1997	1998	1999	2000	Total
Single or Bilateral-Lung	0	0	0	0	2	3	3	3	1	2	2	1	2	19
Heart-Lung	0	0	0	0	0	2	0	0	1	0	0	0	1	4

PENNSYLVANIA

UNOS Region: 2

Children's Hospital of Philadelphia
324 S. 34th St., Philadelphia, PA 19104
Main Phone: 215-590-1000

Thoracic Organ Transplant Program: 215-590-6051,
  Fax: 215-590-1340
Program Established: 1994
1-Year Patient Survival Rate: 63%
  (based on 43 patients transplanted from 1994 to 1999)

Median Waiting Time (days): varies depending on age
Medicare Designated Center: No
Pediatric Transplantation: Yes
Website: http://heart.chop.edu/chrtlng.shtml
Lung Retransplantation: Yes (1 performed)

OPO: Delaware Valley Transplant Program
Rodin Place, 2000 Hamilton St., Suite 201,
Philadelphia, PA 19130-3813
Main Phone: 800-543-6391 or 215-557-8090, Fax: 215-557-9359

Transplants Performed:	1988	1989	1990	1991	1992	1993	1994	1995	1996	1997	1998	1999	2000	Total
Single or Bilateral-Lung	0	0	0	0	1	0	1	9	5	8	8	3	6	41
Heart-Lung	0	0	0	0	0	0	0	1	3	3	6	7	1	21

Children's Hospital of Pittsburgh
3705 5th Ave., One Children's Place, Pittsburgh, PA 15213-3584
Main Phone: 412-648-3200

Lung Transplant Program: 412-692-5325, Fax: 412-692-6991,
  E-mail: info@chplink.chp.edu
Program Established: 1985
1-Year Patient Survival Rate: 70%; 74% for those with non-infective
  lung disease (based on 70 patients transplanted from 1985 to 1999)
Median Waiting Time (days): 534 (range 356 to 890)

Medicare Designated Center: Yes
Pediatric Transplantation: Yes (76 performed)
Living-Lobar Lung Donor Transplantation: Yes (2 performed)
Lung Retransplantation: Yes (9 performed)
Website: http://www.chp.edu/03clinserv/03heart/
  03heart_serv_pedheartlung.htm

OPO: Center for Organ Recovery and Education
204 Sigma Drive, RIDC Park, Pittsburgh, PA 15238-2825
Main Phone: 412-963-3550, Fax: 412-963-3563

Transplants Performed:	1988	1989	1990	1991	1992	1993	1994	1995	1996	1997	1998	1999	2000	Total
Single or Bilateral-Lung	0	1	1	4	8	4	4	5	0	6	6	0	6	45
Heart-Lung	0	1	0	4	6	5	1	3	2	0	2	5	1	30

Hospital of the University of Pennsylvania
3400 Spruce St., Philadelphia, PA 19104
Main Phone: 215-662-4000

Lung Transplant Program: 215-662-2365, Fax: 215-349-8235
Program Established: 1991
1-Year Patient Survival Rate: 71%
  (based on 227 patients transplanted from 1993 to 2000)
Average Waiting Time (days): 540 -712 (range 3 to 1,068)
Medicare Designated Center: Yes

Pediatric Transplantation: No
Living-Lobar Lung Donor Transplantation: No
Lung Retransplantation: Yes (7 performed)
Website: http://www.med.upenn.edu/health/hi_files/transplant/tp_lung/
  lu_stats.html

OPO: Gift of Life Donor Program
2000 Hamiliton Rodan Place, Philadelphia, PA 19131
Main Phone: 215-557-8091, Fax: 215-963-0498

Transplants Performed:	1988	1989	1990	1991	1992	1993	1994	1995	1996	1997	1998	1999	2000	Total
Single or Bilateral-Lung	0	0	0	3	12	30	32	39	30	29	33	24	31	263
Heart-Lung	0	0	0	0	0	0	0	0	1	0	0	0	0	1

Temple University Hospital *
320 Parkinson Pavilion, Broad and Tioga St.,
Philadelphia, PA 19140
Main Phone: 215-707-2000

Lung Transplant Program: 215-707-1722, Fax: 215-707-4327
1-Year Patient Survival Rate: 61.1%
  (based on 31 patients transplanted from 1/1/97 to 12/31/98)

Medicare Designated Center: No
Website: http://www.temple.edu/pulmonary/profess/lungtrans.html

OPO: Delaware Valley Transplant Program
Rodin Place, 2000 Hamiliton St., Suite 201,
Philadelphia, PA 19130-3813
Main Phone: 800-543-6391 or 215-557-8090, Fax: 215-557-9359

Transplants Performed:	1988	1989	1990	1991	1992	1993	1994	1995	1996	1997	1998	1999	2000	Total
Single or Bilateral-Lung	0	0	0	0	0	0	13	17	8	19	13	9	n. a.	79
Heart-Lung	3	0	0	0	0	0	0	1	2	3	3	1	n. a.	13

**University of Pittsburgh Medical Center
and Oakland VA Medical Center**
200 Lothrop St., Pittsburgh, PA 15213-2582
Main Phone: 412-647-2345

Lung and Heart-Lung Transplant Program: 800-533-8762 or
412-648-9136, Fax: 412-648-1029
Program Established: 1982 (701 lung-related transplants to date)
1-Year Patient Survival Rate: 72%
 (based on 80 patients transplanted from 1/1/97 to 12/31/98)

Mean Waiting Time (days): 534 single-lung; 712 bilateral-lung
Medicare Designated Center: Yes
Pediatric Transplantation: Yes (279 performed)
Living-Lobar Lung Donor Transplantation: Yes (4 performed)
Lung Retransplantation: Yes (26 performed)
Website: http://www.upmc.edu/clc/lungtransplantation.htm

OPO: Center for Organ Recovery and Education
204 Sigma Drive, RIDC Park, Pittsburgh, PA 15238-2825
Main Phone: 412-963-3550, Fax: 412-963-3563

Transplants Performed:	1988	1989	1990	1991	1992	1993	1994	1995	1996	1997	1998	1999	2000	Total
Single or Bilateral-Lung	5	5	13	54	55	63	38	47	34	48	33	34	39	468
Heart-Lung	11	3	4	3	8	5	3	3	3	2	2	2	1	50

TENNESSEE

Baptist Memorial Hospital
6019 Walnut Grove Road, Memphis, TN 38120
Main Phone: 901-227-2727
Website: http://www.bmhcc.org/baptistonline/home

Thoracic Transplant Services: 901-226-2000, Fax: 901-226-2010,
E-mail: transplantservices@bmhcc.org
Program Established: 1991
1-Year Patient Survival Rate: 75%
 (based on 17 patients transplanted from 1/1/93 to 12/31/99)

UNOS Region: 11

Average Waiting Time: 18 to 24 months
Medicare Designated Center: No
Pediatric Transplantation: No
Living-Lobar Lung Donor Transplantation: No
Lung Retransplantation: No

OPO: Mid-South Transplant Foundation
910 Madison Ave., Suite 1002, Memphis, TN 38103
Main Phone: 901-328-4438, Fax: 901-328-4462
Website: http://www.jericho.org/_transpl.html

Transplants Performed:	1988	1989	1990	1991	1992	1993	1994	1995	1996	1997	1998	1999	2000	Total
Single or Bilateral-Lung	0	0	0	2	5	2	2	2	2	5	3	1	0	24
Heart-Lung	0	0	0	1	0	2	2	1	0	3	0	0	0	9

Vanderbilt University Medical Center
and Nashville VA Medical Center
1211 22nd Ave. S., Nashville, TN 37232-4734
Main Phone: 615-322-5000

Lung Transplant Program: 615-936-0393, Fax: 615-936-0396
Program Established: 1988
1-Year Patient Survival Rate: 74%
 (based on 140 patients transplanted since program inception)
Median Waiting Time (days): 110 (range 1 to 924)

Medicare Designated Center: Yes
Pediatric Transplantation: Yes (4 performed)
Living-Lobar Lung Donor Transplantation: Yes
Lung Retransplantation: Yes (3 performed)
Website: http://www.mc.vanderbilt.edu/transplant/hrtlung.htm

OPO: Tennessee Donor Services
1714 Hayes St., Nashville, TN 37203
Main Phone: 615-327-2247, Fax: 615-320-1655

Transplants Performed:	1988	1989	1990	1991	1992	1993	1994	1995	1996	1997	1998	1999	2000	Total
Single or Bilateral-Lung	0	0	5	9	9	8	14	13	16	16	20	19	17	146
Heart-Lung	3	0	0	0	0	0	0	4	1	0	0	2	1	11

TEXAS

Baylor University Medical Center
3500 Gaston Ave., Dallas, TX 75246
Main Phone: 214-820-0111
Website: http://www.bhcs.com

Cardio-Thoracic Transplantation: 214-820-6856, Fax: 214-820-4527
Program Established: 1990
1-Year Patient Survival Rate: 67%
 (based on 93 patients transplanted since program inception)
Median Waiting Time (days): 419 (range 118 to 705)

UNOS Region: 4

Medicare Designated Center: Yes
Pediatric Transplantation: No
Living-Lobar Lung Donor Transplantation: No
Lung Retransplantation: No (1 performed)

OPO: Southwest Transplant Alliance
3710 Rawlins, Suite 1100, Dallas, TX 75219
Main Phone: 800-788-8058 or 214-821-1910, Fax: 214-827-8352,
E-mail: sta@organ.org
Website: http://www.organ.org/donors.html

Transplants Performed:	1988	1989	1990	1991	1992	1993	1994	1995	1996	1997	1998	1999	2000	Total
Single or Bilateral-Lung	0	0	2	2	5	4	16	16	9	22	14	11	8	109
Heart-Lung	0	2	0	0	0	1	1	0	0	0	0	0	1	5

Christus Santa Rosa Medical Center

2827 Babcock Road, San Antonio, TX 78229
Main Phone: 210-705-6300

Christus Transplant Institute: 210-705-6700
Heart-Lung Transplant Program: 888-481-4800 or 210-705-6700,
 Fax: 210-705-6748
Program Established: 1999 (heart-lung only center)
1-Year Patient Survival Rate: 100%
 (based on 3 patients transplanted from 1995 to 1999)

Average Waiting Time for Heart-Lung: 2 years
Medicare Designated Center: No, application in progress
Pediatric Transplantation: No
Living-Lobar Lung Donor Transplantation: No
Lung Retransplantation: Yes
Website: http://www.santarosahealth.org/TransplantInstitute.html

OPO: Texas Organ Sharing Alliance
8121 Datapoint Drive, Suite 1150, San Antonio, TX 78229
Phone: 210-614-7030, Fax: 210-614-2129

Transplants Performed:	1988	1989	1990	1991	1992	1993	1994	1995	1996	1997	1998	1999	2000	Total
Single or Bilateral-Lung	0	0	0	0	0	0	0	0	0	0	0	0	0	0
Heart-Lung	0	0	0	0	0	0	0	2	0	0	0	1	0	3

Columbia Hospital at Medical City Dallas

7777 Forest Lane, Dallas, TX 75230
Main Phone: 972-566-7000

Lung Transplant Program: 972-566-7199, Fax: 972-566-4872
Program Established: 1995
1-Year Patient Survival Rate: 75%
 (based on 37 patients transplanted since program inception)
Median Waiting Time (days): 150 (range 2 to 471)
Medicare Designated Center: application in progress

Pediatric Transplantation: No
Living-Lobar Lung Donor Transplantation: No
Lung Retransplantation: Yes (but only on a case-by-case basis)
Website: http://www.medicalcitytransplants.com

OPO: Southwest Transplant Alliance
3710 Rawlins, Suite 1100, Dallas, TX 75219
Main Phone: 800-788-8058 or 214-821-1910, Fax: 214-827-8352,
E-mail: sta@organ.org
Website: http://www.organ.org/donors.html

Transplants Performed:	1988	1989	1990	1991	1992	1993	1994	1995	1996	1997	1998	1999	2000	Total
Single or Bilateral-Lung	0	0	0	0	0	0	0	0	6	13	12	4	2	37
Heart-Lung	0	0	0	0	0	0	0	0	0	1	1	0	0	2

Methodist Hospital at Baylor College of Medicine

6565 Fannin, Houston, TX 77030
Main Phone: 713-790-3333

Lung Transplant Program: 713-790-2501, Fax: 713-793-1335
Program Established: 1986
1-Year Patient Survival Rate: 76%
 (based on 47 patients transplanted from Sept. 1996 to 2000)
Median Waiting Time (days): 65 (range 210 to 712)
Medicare Designated Center: No, application in progress
Pediatric Transplantation: No

Living-Lobar Lung Donor Transplantation: No
Lung Retransplantation: Yes (3 performed, but only on a case-by-
 case basis)
Website: http://www.methodisthealth.com/motc/lung.htm

OPO: LifeGift Organ Donation Center
5615 Kirby Drive, Suite 900, Houston, TX 77005-2405
Main Phone: 800-633-6562, 713-523-4438, Fax: 713-737-8100,
E-mail: webmastr@mail.lifegift.org
Website: http://www.lifegift.org

Transplants Performed:	1988	1989	1990	1991	1992	1993	1994	1995	1996	1997	1998	1999	2000	Total
Single or Bilateral-Lung	3	6	5	10	16	15	14	14	8	19	12	8	16	146
Heart-Lung	4	4	1	0	0	0	0	0	0	0	0	0	0	9

St. Luke's Episcopal Hospital

6720 Bertner St., Houston, TX 77030
Main Phone: 713-791-2011
Website: http://www.sleh.com

Lung Transplant Program: 713-791-3952, Fax: 713-794-6696
Program Established: 1994
1-Year Patient Survival Rate: 75%
 (based on 12 patients transplanted from 1/1/97 to 12/31/98)
Waiting Time (days): single 180 to 356; double 356 to 712
 (range 9 to 1,068)

Medicare Designated Center: No, application in progress
Pediatric Transplantation: No
Living-Lobar Lung Donor Transplantation: No
Lung Retransplantation: Yes (4 performed, but only on a case-by-
 case basis)

OPO: LifeGift Organ Donation Center
5615 Kirby Drive, Suite 900, Houston, TX 77005-2405
Main Phone: 800-633-6562, 713-523-4438, Fax: 713-737-8100,
E-mail: webmastr@mail.lifegift.org
Website: http://www.lifegift.org

Transplants Performed:	1988	1989	1990	1991	1992	1993	1994	1995	1996	1997	1998	1999	2000	Total
Single or Bilateral-Lung	0	0	0	0	0	0	3	3	3	4	8	8	8	37
Heart-Lung	0	0	0	0	0	0	0	1	0	0	0	1	1	3

St. Paul Medical Center at the University of Texas Southwestern

5909 Harry Hines Blvd., Dallas, TX 75235
Main Phone: 214-879-1000

Heart and Lung Transplant Program: 800-458-3278 or
   214-879-6210, Fax: 214-879-6209
Program Established: 1990
1-Year Patient Survival Rate: 82%
   (based on 53 patients transplanted from 9/24/90 to 1/1/00)
Median Waiting Time (days): 436 (range 328 to 589)

Medicare Designated Center: Yes
Pediatric Transplantation: Yes (2 performed)
Living-Lobar Lung Donor Transplantation: Yes
Lung Retransplantation: Yes (but only on a case-by-case basis)
Website: http://www.stpauldallas.com/area3/a3b.html

OPO: Southwest Transplant Alliance
3710 Rawlins, Suite 1100, Dallas, TX 75219
Main Phone: 800-788-8058 or 214-821-1910, Fax: 214-827-8352,
E-mail: sta@organ.org
Website: http://www.organ.org/donors.html

Transplants Performed:	1988	1989	1990	1991	1992	1993	1994	1995	1996	1997	1998	1999	2000	Total
Single or Bilateral-Lung	0	0	1	1	1	2	4	4	6	14	11	9	8	61
Heart-Lung	0	0	0	0	0	0	0	0	0	0	0	0	0	0

University Hospital of the University of Texas Health Science Center

4502 Medical Drive, San Antonio, TX 78229
Main Phone: 210-567-5777

Lung Transplant Program: 210-567-5777, Fax: 210-567-5122
Program Established: 1987
1-Year Patient Survival Rate: 83%
   (based on 19 patients transplanted from 71/1/97 to 12/31/98)
Median Waiting Time (days): Single, 330 (range 20 to 666);

Bilateral, 330 (range 206 to 410)
Medicare Designated Center: No
Pediatric Transplantation: Yes (2 performed)
Living-Lobar Lung Donor Transplantation: No
Lung Retransplantation: No
Website: http://www.uthscsa.edu/general_info.htm

OPO: Texas Organ Sharing Alliance
8121 Datapoint Drive, Suite 1150, San Antonio, TX 78229
Phone: 210-614-7030, Fax: 210-614-2129

Transplants Performed:	1988	1989	1990	1991	1992	1993	1994	1995	1996	1997	1998	1999	2000	Total
Single or Bilateral-Lung	2	13	22	18	15	14	12	11	7	7	12	12	7	152
Heart-Lung	3	1	0	0	0	0	0	0	0	0	0	0	0	4

University of Texas Medical Branch at Galveston

301 University Blvd., Galveston, TX 77555-0536
Main Phone: 409-772-1011

Heart and Lung Transplant Program: 800-323-4109 (in Texas only)
   or 409-772-6839, Fax: 409-772-5054
Program Established: 1994
1-Year Patient Survival Rate: 50%
   (based on 17 patients transplanted from 1996 to 1999)
Waiting Time (days): varies
Medicare Designated Center: No

Pediatric Transplantation: Yes
Living-Lobar Lung Donor Transplantation: No
Lung Retransplantation: not available
Website: http://surgery.uth.tmc.edu/organ_transplant

OPO: Southwest Transplant Alliance
3710 Rawlins, Suite 1100, Dallas, TX 75219
Main Phone: 800-788-8058 or 214-821-1910, Fax: 214-827-8352,
E-mail: sta@organ.org
Website: http://www.organ.org/donors.html

Transplants Performed:	1988	1989	1990	1991	1992	1993	1994	1995	1996	1997	1998	1999	2000	Total
Single or Bilateral-Lung	0	0	0	0	0	0	0	0	1	6	5	5	n. a.	17
Heart-Lung	0	0	0	0	0	0	1	0	0	1	0	0	n. a.	2

UTAH

University of Utah Medical Center

50 N. Medical Drive, Salt Lake City, UT 84132
Main Phone: 801-581-2121

Lung Transplant Program: 800-456-8341 or 801-585-3697,
   Fax: 801-585-5685
Program Established: 1992
1-Year Patient Survival Rate: 84%
   (based on 35 patients transplanted from 1992 to 1999)
Median Waiting Time (days): 129 (range 0 to 540)

UNOS Region: 5

Medicare Designated Center: Yes
Pediatric Transplantation: No
Living-Lobar Lung Donor Transplantation: No
Lung Retransplantation: Yes (4 performed)
Website: http://www.med.utah.edu/transplant/lngtrnsplnt.htm

OPO: Intermountain Organ Recovery System
230 S. 500 E., Suite 290, Salt Lake City, UT 84102
Main Phone: 800-83-DONOR (800-833-6667) or 801-521-1755,
Fax: 801-364-8815
Website: http://www.iors.com

Transplants Performed:	1988	1989	1990	1991	1992	1993	1994	1995	1996	1997	1998	1999	2000	Total
Single or Bilateral-Lung	0	0	0	0	1	3	0	8	5	9	9	13	9	57
Heart-Lung	1	0	0	0	0	0	0	0	0	0	1	0	0	2

VIRGINIA

Hunter Holmes McGuire Veterans Administration Medical Center

1201 Broad Rock Blvd., Richmond, VA 23249
Main Phone: 804-675-5000

Lung Transplant Program: 804-675-5442, Fax: 804-675-5400
1-Year Patient Survival Rate: 75%
  (based on 8 patients transplanted from 7/1/95 to 6/30/97)

UNOS Region: 11

Average Waiting Time (days): 534 to 712 (range 90 to 890)
Medicare Designated Center: not applicable
Pediatric Transplantation: No
Living-Lobar Lung Donor Transplantation: No
Lung Retransplantation: (does not have an established policy)

OPO: LifeNet
5809 Ward Court, Virginia Beach, VA 23455
Main Phone: 757-464-4761, Fax: 757-464-5721

Transplants Performed:	1988	1989	1990	1991	1992	1993	1994	1995	1996	1997	1998	1999	2000	Total
Single or Bilateral-Lung	0	0	0	1	1	1	1	3	4	2	4	2	n. a.	19
Heart-Lung	1	0	1	0	1	0	1	0	0	0	0	0	n. a.	4

Inova Fairfax Hospital

3300 Gallows Road, Falls Church, VA 22046
Main Phone: 703-698-1110

Inova Transplant Center
Lung Transplant Program: 703-698-3388 or 703-698-2213,
  Fax: 703-698-2797, E-mail: steven.nathan@inova.com,
  E-mail: transplant.center@inova.com
Program Established: 1991
1-Year Patient Survival Rate: 84%
  (based on 38 patients transplanted from 1991 to July 1999)

Median Waiting Time (days): 131 (range 32 to 566)
Medicare Designated Center: Yes
Pediatric Transplantation: Yes (1 performed)
Living-Lobar Lung Donor Transplantation: No
Lung Retransplantation: No
Website: http://www.inova.com/fh/transplant/lung/index.html

OPO: Washington Regional Transplant Consortium
8110 Gatehouse Road, Suite 101, W. Falls Church, VA 22042
Main Phone: 703-641-0100, Fax: 703-641-0211
Website: http://www.wrtc.org

Transplants Performed:	1988	1989	1990	1991	1992	1993	1994	1995	1996	1997	1998	1999	2000	Total
Single or Bilateral-Lung	0	0	0	1	1	2	6	2	4	3	10	13	19	61
Heart-Lung	0	0	0	0	0	0	0	0	0	1	0	0	0	1

Medical College of Virginia Hospitals

401 N. 12th St., P.O. Box 980204, Richmond, VA 23298-0510
Main Phone: 804-828-9000

Heart & Lung Transplant Program: 800-628-4141 or
  804-828-4571, Fax: 804-828-5192
Program Established: 1991
1-Year Patient Survival Rate: 75%
  (based on 4 patients transplanted from 1/1/97 to 12/31/98)

Average Waiting Time (days): 712 days
Medicare Designated Center: No
Pediatric Transplantation: No
Living-Lobar Lung Donor Transplantation: No
Lung Retransplantation: No
Website: http://views.vcu.edu/hltransplant

OPO: LifeNet
5809 Ward Court, Virginia Beach, VA 23455
Main Phone: 757-464-4761, Fax: 757-464-5721

Transplants Performed:	1988	1989	1990	1991	1992	1993	1994	1995	1996	1997	1998	1999	2000	Total
Single or Bilateral-Lung	0	0	0	3	4	5	0	4	4	4	0	0	n. a.	24
Heart-Lung	1	0	1	2	1	1	0	0	0	0	0	0	n. a.	6

Sentara Norfolk General Hospital

600 Gresham Drive, Norfolk, VA 23507
Main Phone: 757-668-3000

Lung Transplant Program: 757-668-2831, Fax: 757-668-2814
Program Established: 1992
1-Year Patient Survival Rate: 100%
  (based on 3 patients transplanted from 1/1/97 to 12/31/98)
Median Waiting Time (days): not available

Medicare Designated Center: No
Pediatric Transplantation: No
Living-Lobar Lung Donor Transplantation: No
Lung Retransplantation: not available
Website: http://www.sentara.com/transplant/pulmonary.htm

OPO: LifeNet
5809 Ward Court, Virginia Beach, VA 23455
Main Phone: 757-464-4761, Fax: 757-464-5721

Transplants Performed:	1988	1989	1990	1991	1992	1993	1994	1995	1996	1997	1998	1999	2000	Total
Single or Bilateral-Lung	0	0	0	0	3	3	2	4	6	1	2	0	3	24
Heart-Lung	0	0	0	0	0	1	1	1	1	0	0	0	0	4

University of Virginia Health Sciences Center

Lee St., Charlottesville, VA 22908
Main Phone: 804-924-0211

Cardiopulmonary Transplant Program: 800-257-0757 or
804-982-4456, Fax: 804-924-2359
Program Established: 1990
1-Year Patient Survival Rate: 83.3%
(based on 12 patients transplanted during 1998)
Median Waiting Time (days): 315 (range 60 to 990)

Medicare Designated Center: Yes
Pediatric Transplantation: Yes (6 performed)
Living-Lobar Lung Donor Transplantation: Yes (2 performed)
Lung Retransplantation: No
Website: http://www.med.virginia.edu/heart/patients/lungtrans.html

OPO: LifeNet
5809 Ward Court, Virginia Beach, VA 23455
Main Phone: 757-464-4761, Fax: 757-464-5721

Transplants Performed:	1988	1989	1990	1991	1992	1993	1994	1995	1996	1997	1998	1999	2000	Total
Single or Bilateral-Lung	0	0	3	8	17	18	13	16	15	13	12	16	22	153
Heart-Lung	0	0	0	2	0	0	0	0	0	1	0	0	0	3

WASHINGTON

UNOS Region: 6

University of Washington Medical Center

1959 N.E. Pacific St., P.O. Box 356310, Seattle, WA 98195
Main Phone: 206-543-3093

Lung Transplant Program: 206-543-3093, Fax: 206-543-0325
Program Established: 1991
1-Year Patient Survival Rate: 77%
(based on 113 patients transplanted from 1992 to 1997)
Median Waiting Time (days): 272 (range 10 to 694)

Medicare Designated Center: Yes
Pediatric Transplantation: Yes
Living-Lobar Lung Donor Transplantation: No
Lung Retransplantation: No (1 performed)
Website: http://www.washington.edu/medical/uwmc

OPO: LifeCenter Northwest
2553 S.E. 76th Ave., Mercer Island, WA 98040
Main Phone: 888-543-3287, Fax: 206-230-5806

Transplants Performed:	1988	1989	1990	1991	1992	1993	1994	1995	1996	1997	1998	1999	2000	Total
Single or Bilateral-Lung	0	0	0	0	12	13	13	13	14	12	12	26	26	141
Heart-Lung	0	0	0	0	0	0	0	0	0	0	0	0	0	0

WISCONSIN

UNOS Region: 7

Children's Hospital of Wisconsin

9000 W. Wisconsin Ave., P.O. Box 1997, Milwaukee, WI 53201
Main Phone: 414-266-2000

Lung Transplant Program: 414-266-6458, Fax: 414-266-6742
Program Established: 1994
1-Year Patient Survival Rate: under 10 years 100% ; 11 to 17 years
66.7% (based on 1 and 3 patients respectively, transplanted from
1/1/97 to 12/31/98)

Median Waiting Time (days): not available
Medicare Designated Center: No
Pediatric Transplantation: Yes (17 performed)
Living-Lobar Lung Donor Transplantation: No
Lung Retransplantation: Yes (2 performed)
Website: http://www.chw.org/Specialty/program.htm

OPO: Wisconsin Donor Network
9200 W. Wisconsin Ave., Milwaukee, WI 53226
Phone: 414-259-2024, Fax: 414-259-8059, E-mail: pvolelk@fmlh.edu

Transplants Performed:	1988	1989	1990	1991	1992	1993	1994	1995	1996	1997	1998	1999	2000	Total
Single or Bilateral-Lung	0	0	0	0	0	0	0	2	4	3	2	1	2	14
Heart-Lung	0	0	0	0	0	0	1	0	0	0	0	1	1	3

Froedtert Memorial Lutheran Hospital
at the Medical College of Wisconsin *

9200 W. Wisconsin Ave., Milwaukee, WI 53226
Main Phone: 414-259-3000

Lung Transplant Program: 414-456-6756, Fax: 414-456-6203
1-Year Patient Survival Rate: 80%
(based on 15 patients transplanted from 1/1/97 to 12/31/98)

Medicare Designated Center: No
Pediatric Transplantation: No
Website: http://www.froedtert.com/healthcare/centers/transplant

OPO: Froedtert Memorial Hospital OPO
9200 W. Wisconsin Ave., Milwaukee, WI 53226
Phone: 414-259-2024, Fax: 414-259-8059,
E-mail: pvolelk@fmlh.edu

Transplants Performed:	1988	1989	1990	1991	1992	1993	1994	1995	1996	1997	1998	1999	2000	Total
Single or Bilateral-Lung	0	0	0	0	0	0	0	0	4	7	8	3	7	29
Heart-Lung	0	1	0	0	0	0	0	0	0	0	0	0	0	1

St. Luke's Medical Center

2900 W. Oklahoma Ave., Milwaukee, WI 53215
Main Phone: 414-649-6000

Lung and Heart-Lung Transplant Program: 414-649-5410,
   Fax: 414-649-5452
Program Established: 1992
1-Year Patient Survival Rate: 70%
   (based on 10 patients transplanted from 1/95 to 7/99)

Median Waiting Time (days): 176 (range 7 to 812)
Medicare Designated Center: No
Pediatric Transplantation: No
Living-Lobar Lung Donor Transplantation: No
Lung Retransplantation: Yes (but only on a case-by-case basis)

OPO: Froedtert Memorial Hospital OPO
9200 W. Wisconsin Ave., Milwaukee, WI 53226
Phone: 414-259-2024, Fax: 414-259-8059, E-mail: pvolelk@fmlh.edu

Transplants Performed:	1988	1989	1990	1991	1992	1993	1994	1995	1996	1997	1998	1999	2000	Total
Single or Bilateral-Lung	0	0	0	0	5	1	1	5	2	1	1	2	3	21
Heart-Lung	0	0	0	0	0	0	0	0	0	0	0	0	0	0

University of Wisconsin Hospital and Clinics

600 Highland Ave., Madison, WI 53792-3236
Main Phone: 608-263-6400

Heart and Lung Transplant Program: 608-263-7832,
   Fax: 608-263-0597
Program Established: 1988
1-Year Patient Survival Rate: 84%
   (based on 151 patients transplanted from 10/1/88 to 12/31/99)
Median Waiting Time (days): 271 (range 1 to 776)
Medicare Designated Center: Yes

Pediatric Transplantation: Yes
Living-Lobar Lung Donor Transplantation: No
Lung Retransplantation: Yes (8 performed, but only on their own
   patients)
Website: http://www.surgery.wisc.edu/patient/txcar
   diac01_overview.html

OPO: Organ Procurement Organization at University of Wisconsin
600 Highland Ave., F4/316, Madison, WI 53792
Main Phone: 608-263-1341, Fax: 608-262-9099
Website: http://www.surgery.wisc.edu/patient/patient_txindex.html

Transplants Performed:	1988	1989	1990	1991	1992	1993	1994	1995	1996	1997	1998	1999	2000	Total
Single or Bilateral-Lung	1	0	0	1	2	8	16	26	22	25	23	35	20	179
Heart-Lung	0	1	0	0	2	0	1	0	1	1	0	2	0	8

Transplant Center	City/State	Medicare-Designated Center	Pediatric Transplant-ation	Living-Lobar Lung Donor	Lung Retransplant-ation	No. of Transplants 1988 - 2000
Baptist Medical Center	Oklahoma City, OK					52
Baptist Memorial Hospital	Memphis, TN					33
Barnes-Jewish Hospital	St. Louis, MO	X			8	553
Baylor University Medical Center	Dallas, TX	X			1	114
Brigham and Women's Hospital	Boston, MA	X		X	3	153
BryanLGH Medical Center East	Lincoln, NE					17
Cedars-Sinai Medical Center	Los Angeles, CA				3	80
Children's Hospital	Boston, MA		16	1		31
Children's Hospital	Denver, CO		2	X	X	2
Children's Hospital	Los Angeles, CA		91	34	2	60
Children's Hospital of Philadelphia	Philadelphia, PA		X		1	62
Children's Hospital of Pittsburgh	Pittsburgh, PA	X	76	2	9	75
Children's Hospital of Wisconsin	Milwaukee, WI		17		2	17
Children's Memorial Hospital	Chicago, IL		X			1
Christus Santa Rosa Medical Center	San Antonio, TX	in progress			X	3
Clarian Health-Methodist Hospital	Indianapolis, IN	X			1	172
Cleveland Clinic Foundation	Cleveland, OH	X	5		X	234
Columbia Hospital/Medical City Dallas	Dallas, TX	in progress			X	39
Duke University Medical Center	Durham, NC	X	X	3	12	325
Emory University Hospital	Atlanta, GA	X	3		1	70
Fairview University Medical Center	Minneapolis, MN	X				348
Froedtert Memorial Lutheran Hospital	Milwaukee, WI					30
Henry Ford Hospital	Detroit, MI	X			1	56
Hospital of the U. of Pennsylvania	Philadelphia, PA	X			7	264
Hunter Holmes McGuire Veterans Ad.	Richmond, VA					23
Inova Fairfax Hospital	Falls Church, VA	X	1			62
Jackson Memorial Hospital	Miami, FL		X		X	23
Jewish Hospital	Louisville, KY	X	X		2	88
Johns Hopkins Hospital	Baltimore, MD	X	4	2	X	104
Loyola University Medical Center	Maywood, IL	X	18		X	321
Massachusetts General Hospital	Boston, MA	X		12	1	100
Medical College of Virginia Hospitals	Richmond, VA					30
Methodist Hospital/Baylor College	Houston, TX	in progress			3	155
Mount Sinai Medical Center	New York, NY					22
New York University Medical Center	New York, NY					5

Transplant Center	City/State	Medicare-Designated Center	Pediatric Transplant-ation	Living-Lobar Lung Donor	Lung Retransplant-ation	No. of Transplants 1988 - 2000
Ochsner Foundation Hospital	New Orleans, LA	X	9		5	135
Ohio State University Hospital	Columbus, OH				X	23
Oregon Health Sciences U. Hospital	Portland, OR					23
Presbyterian Hospital in NY City	New York, NY					267
Sentara Norfolk General Hospital	Norfolk, VA					28
Shands Hospital at the U. of Florida	Gainesville, FL	X	19		6	151
Stanford University Hospital	Stanford, CA	X	30		3	287
St. Louis Children's Hospital	St. Louis, MO		226	38	25	226
St. Luke's Episcopal Hospital	Houston, TX	in progress			4	40
St. Luke's Medical Center	Milwaukee, WI				X	21
St. Mary's Hospital	Rochester, MN					39
St. Paul Medical Center	Dallas, TX	X	2	X	X	61
Temple University Hospital	Philadelphia, PA					92
University of Alabama Hospital	Birmingham, AL	X	2		7	255
U. of California/Davis Medical Center	Sacramento, CA	X			2	56
U. of Ca. at Los Angeles Medical Ct.	Los Angeles, CA	X			1	127
U. of Ca. at San Diego Medical Center	San Diego, CA	X	5	3	1	191
U. of Ca. at San Francisco Medical Ct.	San Francisco, CA					77
University Hospital of U. of Texas	San Antonio, TX		2			156
University Hospital at U. of Co.	Denver, CO	X		X	X	176
University Hospitals of Cleveland	Cleveland, OH		X			11
U. of Illinois Hospital and Clinics	Chicago, IL				X	40
U. of Kentucky Medical Center	Lexington, KY		X		2	110
U. of Maryland Medical System	Baltimore, MD	X				67
University Medical Center/U. Arizona	Tucson, AZ		1			97
U. of Michigan Medical Center	Ann Arbor, MI					227
U. of North Carolina Hospitals	Chapel Hill, NC	X	23	8	2	208
U. of Pittsburgh Medical Center	Pittsburgh, PA	X	279	4	26	518
University of Southern California	Los Angeles, CA			X	X	116
U. of Texas Medical Branch	Galveston, TX		X			19
U. of Utah Medical Center	Salt Lake City, UT	X			4	59
U. of Virginia Health Sciences Center	Charlottesville, VA	X	6	2		156
U. of Washington Medical Center	Seattle, WA	X	X		1	141
U. of Wisconsin Hospital & Clinics	Madison, WI	X	X		8	187
Vanderbilt University Medical Center	Nashville, TN	X	4	X	3	157

APPENDIX B:

MEDIAN WAITING TIME TO LUNG TRANSPLANT:

Based on the 1997 Report of the OPTN: Waiting List Activity and Donor Procurement, UNOS, Richmond, Va. and the Division of Transplantation, Office of Special Programs, Health Resources and Services Administration, U.S. Department of Health and Human Services, Rockville, Md.

- *Includes the median waiting time for transplants performed between Jan. 1, 1994 and Dec. 31, 1996.*

- *No. of Regs indicates the number of all registrations added between 1994 and 1996.*

- *MWT (Median Waiting Time) indicates the estimated number of days by which 50% of the study population had received a transplant.*

- *95% C.I. (Confidence Interval) represents a 95% confidence that the range of days in which the true median is expected to fall is within the lower and upper limits.*

- *+ Indicates not calculated or not estimable. Because of the great variability in waiting times for small groups, median waiting times were not calculated for categories with fewer than 10 registrations.*

UNOS Region: 1

Connecticut, Maine, Massachusetts, New Hampshire, Rhode Island, Vermont

		No. of Regs	MWT	95% C.I.
Blood Type:	A	80	+	(+, +)
	AB	9	+	(+, +)
	B	24	+	(+, +)
	O	87	+	(+, +)
Age Group:	0 - 5	2	+	(+, +)
	6 - 10	2	+	(+, +)
	11 - 17	15	757	(663, +)
	18 +	181	+	(+, +)
Race:	White	183	+	(+, +)
	Black	5	+	(+, +)
	Hispanic	10	+	(+, +)
	Asian	0	+	(+, +)
	Other	2	+	(+, +)

UNOS Region: 2

Delaware, District of Columbia, Maryland, New Jersey, Pennsylvania, West Virginia

		No. of Regs	MWT	95% C.I.
Blood Type:	A	320	686	(601, 1,006)
	AB	39	1,027	(232, +)
	B	105	611	(523, 1,160)
	O	476	1,038	(887, 1,166)
Age Group:	0 - 5	35	+	(+, +)
	6 - 10	10	+	(+, +)
	11 - 17	35	1,166	(767, +)
	18 +	860	910	(707, 1,038)
Race:	White	797	920	(767, 1,088)
	Black	96	672	(553, +)
	Hispanic	43	661	(339, +)
	Asian	2	+	(+, +)
	Other	2	+	(+, +)

UNOS Region: 3

Alabama, Arkansas, Florida,
Georgia, Louisiana, Mississippi,
Puerto Rico

		No. of Regs	MWT	95% C.I.
Blood Type:	A	121	77	(60, 98)
	AB	16	110	(35, 166)
	B	23	123	(54, 202)
	O	136	153	(127, 204)
Age Group:	0 - 5	0	+	(+, +)
	6 - 10	1	+	(+, +)
	11 - 17	9	+	(+, +)
	18 +	286	113	(86, 127)
Race:	White	258	110	(82, 125)
	Black	24	133	(98, 251)
	Hispanic	11	148.5	(102, +)
	Asian	1	+	(+, +)
	Other	2	+	(+, +)

UNOS Region: 4

Oklahoma, Texas

		No. of Regs	MWT	95% C.I.
Blood Type:	A	99	147	(108, 198)
	AB	5	+	(+, +)
	B	26	247	(135, 353)
	O	136	302	(239, 422)
Age Group:	0 - 5	0	+	(+, +)
	6 - 10	1	+	(+, +)
	11 - 17	12	247	(179, 278)
	18 +	253	218	(174, 295)
Race:	White	219	232	(174, 280)
	Black	17	203	(87, 378)
	Hispanic	27	312	(187, 492)
	Asian	3	+	(+, +)
	Other	0	+	(+, +)

UNOS Region: 5

Arizona, California, Hawaii,
Nevada, New Mexico, Utah

		No. of Regs	MWT	95% C.I.
Blood Type:	A	203	416	(311, 494)
	AB	25	173	(71, 365)
	B	57	1,036	(429, +)
	O	253	446	(385, 512)
Age Group:	0 - 5	7	+	(+, +)
	6 - 10	2	+	(+, +)
	11 - 17	26	331	(169, 687)
	18 +	503	428	(386, 487)
Race:	White	422	416	(368, 454)
	Black	29	512	(462, +)
	Hispanic	70	524	(314, 795)
	Asian	13	328	(211, +)
	Other	4	+	(+, +)

UNOS Region: 6

Alaska, Idaho, Montana, Oregon, Washington

		No. of Regs	MWT	95% C.I.
Blood Type:	A	34	178	(129, 320)
	AB	1	+	(+, +)
	B	4	+	(+, +)
	O	36	295	(202, 649)
Age Group:	0 - 5	0	+	(+, +)
	6 - 10	0	+	(+, +)
	11 - 17	2	+	(+, +)
	18 +	73	244	(178, 322)
Race:	White	67	246	(160, 336)
	Black	2	+	(+, +)
	Hispanic	3	+	(+, +)
	Asian	2	+	(+, +)
	Other	1	+	(+, +)

UNOS Region: 7

Illinois, Minnesota, North Dakota, South Dakota, Wisconsin

		No. of Regs	MWT	95% C.I.
Blood Type:	A	233	326	(260, 373)
	AB	20	106	(41, 168)
	B	45	241	(227, 293)
	O	208	280	(260, 307)
Age Group:	0 - 5	2	+	(+, +)
	6 - 10	3	+	(+, +)
	11 - 17	19	257	(139, 467)
	18 +	482	281	(260, 301)
Race:	White	454	281	(257, 307)
	Black	32	275	(222, 370)
	Hispanic	15	274	(217, 336)
	Asian	3	+	(+, +)
	Other	2	+	(+, +)

UNOS Region: 8

Colorado, Iowa, Kansas, Missouri, Nebraska, Wyoming

		No. of Regs	MWT	95% C.I.
Blood Type:	A	294	697	(639, 782)
	AB	19	545	(406, 640)
	B	60	573	(454, +)
	O	326	770	(690, 1,083)
Age Group:	0 - 5	24	23	(11, 44)
	6 - 10	23	543	165, 722
	11 - 17	56	469	(286, 605)
	18 +	596	760	(698, 904)
Race:	White	640	722	(658, 770)
	Black	29	1,083	(526, +)
	Hispanic	21	701	(404, +)
	Asian	6	+	(+, +)
	Other	3	+	(+, +)

UNOS Region: 9

New York

		No. of Regs	MWT	95% C.I.
Blood Type:	A	108	+	(+, +)
	AB	13	+	(+, +)
	B	23	+	(+, +)
	O	116	914	(676, +)
Age Group:	0 - 5	2	+	(+, +)
	6 - 10	5	+	(+, +)
	11 - 17	11	+	(+, +)
	18 +	242	1,191	(741, +)
Race:	White	216	993	(737, +)
	Black	31	+	(+, +)
	Hispanic	10	+	(+, +)
	Asian	1	+	(+, +)
	Other	2	+	(+, +)

UNOS Region: 10

Indiana, Michigan, Ohio

		No. of Regs	MWT	95% C.I.
Blood Type:	A	164	825	(755, 958)
	AB	17	876	(291, +)
	B	46	857	(698 +)
	O	162	610	(547, 716)
Age Group:	0 - 5	0	+	(+, +)
	6 - 10	0	+	(+, +)
	11 - 17	4	+	(+, +)
	18 +	385	755	(698, 828)
Race:	White	345	755	(669, 828)
	Black	33	+	(+, +)
	Hispanic	9	+	(+, +)
	Asian	1	+	(+, +)
	Other	1	+	(+, +)

UNOS Region: 11

Kentucky, North Carolina, South
Carolina, Tennessee, Virginia

		No. of Regs	MWT	95% C.I.
Blood Type:	A	242	307	(240, 373)
	AB	25	152	(97, 202)
	B	80	446	(283, 587)
	O	344	618	(528, 828)
Age Group:	0 - 5	4	+	(+, +)
	6 - 10	1	+	(+, +)
	11 - 17	26	543	(295, 777)
	18 +	660	453	(397, 513)
Race:	White	600	450	(373, 500)
	Black	71	798	(473, +)
	Hispanic	17	129	(46, 332)
	Asian	2	+	(+, +)
	Other	1	+	(+, +)

TRANSPLANT CENTER WORKSHEET:

TRANSPLANT CENTER:		
City/State:		
Phone:		
Fax:		
Coordinator Contact:		
Medical Director:		
How Many Surgeons Available?		
Program Established:		
Total No. of Lung Transplants Performed:		
No. of Single, Bilateral and Heart-Lung:		
Recommended Transplant Type:		
Total No. of Transplants on My Disease:		
How Many Transplants Do You Do Per Year?		
What is Your Patient Survival Rate at 1 Year?		
3 Years? 5 Years?		
How Long Do You Think I Will Have to Wait?		
No. of Patients on the Local Waiting List?		
No. of Patients with My Blood Type?		
No. of Your Patients Who Died While Waiting?		
Do I Need to Move Closer to the Transplant Center?		
Pre-Transplant Housing Available/Cost?		
How Will I Get to the Hospital When Called?		
How Much Will My Transplant Cost?		
How Much Will I Have to Pay?		
How Long is the Average Hospital Stay?		
Post-Transplant Housing Available/Cost?		
Do You Have A Support Group?		

EXERCISE LOG:

The Borg Scale of Perceived Rate of Exertion:

0 - Nothing at all	2 - Weak	5 - Strong	8 - Very Strong	* Maximal
0.5 - Very, Very Weak	3 - Moderate	6 - Strong	9 - Very Strong	
1- Very Weak	4 - Somewhat Strong	7 - Very Strong	10 - Very, Very Strong	

DATE:	Exercise Type:	Resting Heart Rate:	Exercise Heart Rate:	Rate of Exertion:	Distance:	Time:	Comments:

HEALTH INSURANCE WORKSHEET:

INSURANCE COMPANY:		
Phone:		
Monthly Premium Cost:		
Annual Deductible:		
Out-of-Pocket Maximum:		
Lifetime Maximum:		
Out-of-Network:		
When Will I Be Eligible?		
Pre-existing Condition Clause:		
Inpatient Hospital Care:		
Deductible?		
Lung/Heart-Lung Transplantation?		
Prescription Drug Coverage:		
Annual Maximum:		
Lifetime Maximum:		
Co-Payments:		
Mail Order Available?		
Office Visits:		
Specialists:		
Lab Work:		
X-rays:		
Diagnostic Tests:		
Preventative Screening:		
Other:		

PERSONAL HEALTH INFORMATION:

DATE: _____

PATIENT NAME: _____ PHONE: _____

ADDRESS: _____ FAX: _____

CITY: _____ STATE: _____ ZIP: _____

PRIMARY CARE PHYSICIAN: _____ PHONE: _____

ADDRESS: _____ FAX: _____

CITY: _____ STATE: _____ ZIP: _____

TRANSPLANT PHYSICIAN: _____ PHONE: _____

TRANSPLANT COORDINATOR: _____ PHONE: _____

ADDRESS: _____ FAX: _____

CITY: _____ STATE: _____ ZIP: _____

PRIMARY HEALTH INSURANCE: _____ PHONE: _____

ADDRESS: _____ FAX: _____

CITY: _____ STATE: _____ ZIP: _____

POLICY NO: _____

PATIENT SOCIAL SECURITY NO: _____ DATE OF BIRTH: _____

IN CASE OF EMERGENCY CONTACT: _____ PHONE: _____

ALLERGIES: _____

PRIOR SURGERIES AND DATES: _____

_____

PRIMARY DIAGNOSIS: _____ DATE: _____

SECONDARY DIAGNOSIS: _____ DATE: _____

MEDICATIONS:	DOSE:	MEDICATIONS:	DOSE:

DAILY LOG:

DATE:	Weight:	Body Temperature:	Blood Pressure:	Heart Rate:	FVC:	FEV$_1$
	lbs.					
	lbs.					
	lbs.					
	lbs.					
	lbs.					
	lbs.					
	lbs.					
	lbs.					
	lbs.					
	lbs.					
	lbs.					
	lbs.					
	lbs.					
	lbs.					
	lbs.					
	lbs.					
	lbs.					
	lbs.					
	lbs.					
	lbs.					
	lbs.					
	lbs.					
	lbs.					
	lbs.					
	lbs.					

WEIGHT LIFTING LOG:

	SEAT:	DATE:	DATE:	DATE:	DATE:	DATE:	DATE:	DATE:	DATE:	DATE:	DATE:	DATE:
UPPER BODY:												
Chest Press:		lbs.	lbs.	lbs.	lbs.	lbs.	lbs.	lbs.	lbs.	lbs.	lbs.	lbs.
Lat. Pulldown		lbs.	lbs.	lbs.	lbs.	lbs.	lbs.	lbs.	lbs.	lbs.	lbs.	lbs.
Back Extensions:		lbs.	lbs.	lbs.	lbs.	lbs.	lbs.	lbs.	lbs.	lbs.	lbs.	lbs.
Shoulder Press:		lbs.	lbs.	lbs.	lbs.	lbs.	lbs.	lbs.	lbs.	lbs.	lbs.	lbs.
Biceps Curls:		lbs.	lbs.	lbs.	lbs.	lbs.	lbs.	lbs.	lbs.	lbs.	lbs.	lbs.
Tricep Extension:		lbs.	lbs.	lbs.	lbs.	lbs.	lbs.	lbs.	lbs.	lbs.	lbs.	lbs.
Seated Row:		lbs.	lbs.	lbs.	lbs.	lbs.	lbs.	lbs.	lbs.	lbs.	lbs.	lbs.
LEGS:												
Leg Press:		lbs.	lbs.	lbs.	lbs.	lbs.	lbs.	lbs.	lbs.	lbs.	lbs.	lbs.
Leg Extension:		lbs.	lbs.	lbs.	lbs.	lbs.	lbs.	lbs.	lbs.	lbs.	lbs.	lbs.
Leg Curl:		lbs.	lbs.	lbs.	lbs.	lbs.	lbs.	lbs.	lbs.	lbs.	lbs.	lbs.
Calf Raise:		lbs.	lbs.	lbs.	lbs.	lbs.	lbs.	lbs.	lbs.	lbs.	lbs.	lbs.
Hip Abductor:		lbs.	lbs.	lbs.	lbs.	lbs.	lbs.	lbs.	lbs.	lbs.	lbs.	lbs.
Hip Adductor:		lbs.	lbs.	lbs.	lbs.	lbs.	lbs.	lbs.	lbs.	lbs.	lbs.	lbs.
Squats:		lbs.	lbs.	lbs.	lbs.	lbs.	lbs.	lbs.	lbs.	lbs.	lbs.	lbs.
ABDOMINALS:												
Stomach Crunches:		lbs.	lbs.	lbs.	lbs.	lbs.	lbs.	lbs.	lbs.	lbs.	lbs.	lbs.
OTHER:												
		lbs.	lbs.	lbs.	lbs.	lbs.	lbs.	lbs.	lbs.	lbs.	lbs.	lbs.
		lbs.	lbs.	lbs.	lbs.	lbs.	lbs.	lbs.	lbs.	lbs.	lbs.	lbs.
		lbs.	lbs.	lbs.	lbs.	lbs.	lbs.	lbs.	lbs.	lbs.	lbs.	lbs.
		lbs.	lbs.	lbs.	lbs.	lbs.	lbs.	lbs.	lbs.	lbs.	lbs.	lbs.

To Contact the Publisher:

Trafford Publishing
1663 Liberty Drive
Bloomington, IN 47403

Toll-free: 888-232-4444
E-mail: CustomerSupport@trafford.com
Website: https://www.trafford.com

To Contact the Author:

Karen A. Couture
8315 SW 108th Loop
Ocala, FL 34481 USA
cosimotto8@gmail.com

Ordering Information:

For additional copies of this book,
The Lung Transplantation Handbook
contact Trafford Publishing by phone or mail
    or
visit Trafford's online bookstore at
https://www.trafford.com
    or
visit the online bookstores Amazon.com or
BarnesandNoble.com
    or
inquire at your local bookstore.

Volume discounts are available.

Printed in the United States
By Bookmasters